ADVANCES IN CANCER RESEARCH

VOLUME 14

Contributors to This Volume

G. I. Abelev

Georges Mathé

Donald Metcalf

Georges Meyer

Roland Motta

Kusuya Nishioka

Alice Stewart

Ernest Winocour

ADVANCES IN CANCER RESEARCH

GEORGE KLEIN

Department of Tumor Biology
Karolinska Institutet
Stockholm, Sweden

SIDNEY WEINHOUSE

Fels Research Institute
Temple University Medical School
Philadelphia, Pennsylvania

Consulting Editor

ALEXANDER HADDOW

Chester Beatty Research Institute
Institute of Cancer Research
Royal Cancer Hospital
London, England

Volume 14

 ACADEMIC PRESS New York and London 1971

CONTENTS

Active Immunotherapy

GEORGES MATHÉ

The Investigation of Oncogenic Viral Genomes in Transformed Cells by Nucleic Acid Hybridization

ERNEST WINOCOUR

Viral Genome and Oncogenic Transformation: Nuclear and Plasma Membrane Events

GEORGES MEYER

Passive Immunotherapy of Leukemia and Other Cancer

ROLAND MOTTA

Humoral Regulators in the Development and Progression of Leukemia

Donald Metcalf

Complement and Tumor Immunology

Kusuya Nishioka

Alpha-Fetoprotein in Ontogenesis and Its Association with Malignant Tumors

G. I. Abelev

Low Dose Radiation Cancers in Man

ALICE STEWART

CONTRIBUTORS TO VOLUME 14

Numbers in parentheses refer to the pages on which the authors' contributions begin.

G. I. ABELEV, *Laboratory of Tumor Immunochemistry, N. F. Gamaleya Institute for Epidemiology and Microbiology, Moscow, USSR* (295)

GEORGES MATHÉ, *Institut de Cancérologie et d'Immunogénétique, Hôpital Paul-Brousse, 94-Villejuif, France* (1)

DONALD METCALF, *Cancer Research Unit, Walter and Eliza Hall Institute, Melbourne, Australia* (181)

GEORGES MEYER, *Research Department of the Regional Cancer Center of Marseilles, 13, Marseilles, France* (71)

ROLAND MOTTA, *Institut de Cancérologie et d'Immunogénétique, Hôpital Paul-Brousse, 94-Villejuif, France and Unite de Génétique, Université Paris VI, Paris, France* (161)

KUSUYA NISHIOKA, *Virology Division, National Cancer Center Research Institute, Tokyo, Japan* (231)

ALICE STEWART, *Department of Social Medicine, Oxford University, Oxford, England* (359)

ERNEST WINOCOUR, *Department of Genetics, Weizmann Institute of Science, Rehovot, Israel* (37)

CONTENTS OF PREVIOUS VOLUMES

ACTIVE IMMUNOTHERAPY

Georges Mathé

Institut de Cancérologie et d'Immunogénétique,
Hôpital Paul-Brousse, 94-Villejuif, France

I. Introduction

Specific active immunotherapy is defined as the stimulation of immune reactions directed against tumor-associated antigens; nonspecific active immunotherapy is the general stimulation of the host's immune reactions by "adjuvants" of immunity.

There is an extensive literature on experimental immunological prevention, describing experiments in which the antitumor effects of immunization (Glynn et al., 1963; Mathé et al., 1969b) or stimulation of immune reactions (Old et al., 1959; Biozzi et al., 1960; Amiel, 1967; Mathé et al., 1969b) have been tested by carrying out these procedures prior to grafting or inducing a tumor. On the other hand, far less attention has been paid to immunotherapy, the objective of which is to devise immunological procedures to inhibit established tumors. Immunotherapy is applicable to man at present, while our knowledge of tumor associated antigens in man is far too small to warrant any attempts at tumor prevention.

1

One of the main reasons for the paucity of experiments on specific immunization after grafting or inducing a tumor can be found by analogy between cancers and infections, against which immunotherapy is no longer used in a curative role. However, it now seems that when immunotherapy is used to cure cancer, it can sometimes be efficacious, though this varies according to different circumstances; but occasionally remarkable effects have been observed in several experimental systems and have already shown to act in man.

This review will be limited as far as possible to a consideration of isogenic tumors grafted into hosts with identical histocompatibility antigens, or autologous tumors, either induced by carcinogens or which occur spontaneously. Only passing reference will be made to studies on tumor grafted into incompatible hosts.

Clinical trials have often preceded studies in experimental animals or have been made at the same time. We made our first clinical trial of immunotherapy in acute lymphoblastic leukemia in 1964. Provided these trials are carried out in a scientific fashion, their results can be just as valuable as experiments in animals. However, the results of clinical and experimental studies will not be mixed in this article, but will be described consecutively.

II. Experimental Basis

A. Specific Immunotherapy

Various antigenic stimulants can be used for specific immunotherapy, namely tumor cells, purified antigens, or oncogenic viruses.

1. *Tumor Cells*

In mice, grafted subcutaneously with 10^4 L 1210 leukemia cells, a significant increase of survival time has been obtained by injecting them 24 hours or even 4 days after grafting, with 10^7 isogenic leukemic cells irradiated with 15,000 rads *in vitro* (Mathé 1968; Mathé *et al.*, 1969b) (Fig. 1). In these experiments tumor cells had been injected subcutaneously, and the leukemia had been transmitted over so many generations that it might have produced a certain withdrawal of histocompatibility with the mice to which it had been grafted (the latter were Fl(DBA/2 $\times$ C57Bl/6) mice).

Two other experiments were made in which we treated mice, inoculated intravenously with 10^4 living cells of very recently induced leukemias. The RC19 leukemia, induced by Rauscher virus, and the E ♀ Kl leukemia, induced by Gross virus in C57Bl/6 mice were used. Specific active immunotherapy applied 24 hours after an isogenic graft of E ♀ Kl leukemia had a noticeable effect (Mathé *et al.*, 1971). Iris

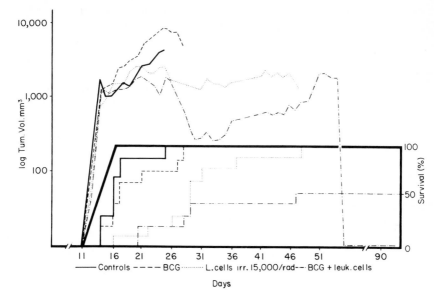

FIG. 1. Tumor volume and cumulative survival of mice grafted with L 1210 leukemia and not treated or treated by BCG (first injection 24 hours after the graft and injections repeated each 4 days), or irradiated leukemic cells (one injection 24 hours after the graft), or association of both.

Parr (1971) obtained similar results on 5178Y tumor grafted intraperitoneally with 10^3 live tumor cells.

Kronman *et al.* (1970) obtained remarkable results in pure strain guinea pigs in which they had grafted hepatomas intramuscularly. Intradermal injections of living hepatoma cells (three injections per week on alternate weeks) induced an immunological reaction against the hepatomas.

2. *Purified Antigens*

Though several groups of chemists are now working on the extraction and characterization of "tumor-associated antigens," up until now they have only been testing their value in preventing the take of tumors. In our laboratory, Martyré and Halle-Pannenko (1968) have been working along these lines studying the antigens of the virus-induced Charlotte Friend leukemia.

3. *Vaccination by Oncogenic Viruses*

Even when the vaccination is commenced after the inoculation of the animal with the virus to induce a tumor, an antitumor effect can be achieved during the latent period. It has been shown that the administration of homologous virus during the course of the latent period to hamsters inoculated neonatally with SV4O or adenovirus reduced the incidence of tumors as compared to controls receiving only a single inoculation of virus (Eddy et al., 1964; Deichman and Kluchareva, 1964; Allison, 1964). Repeated doses of adenovirus 7 in the latent period had an inhibitory effect on adenovirus 12 tumor induction (Periés et al., 1966; Eddy, 1965).

4. Tumors Carrying Embryonic Antigens

As it is known that tumors of the digestive system, especially hepatomas, carry embryonic antigens (Abelev et al., 1963), it would be very interesting to test embryonic extracts as antigens for active immunotherapy (Sedallian and Triau, 1968).

B. NONSPECIFIC IMMUNOTHERAPY

A number of "adjuvants" have been used for nonspecific immunotherapy.

1. Freund's Adjuvant

Freund's adjuvant is the classical example of a stimulant of immunity (Freund, 1953). It has only rarely been used to try to cure tumors; that is, given after the establishment of the tumor. Hirano and his colleagues (1967) described how this adjuvant given 1 week after animals had been grafted with a lymphoma inhibited the tumor growth.

Allison (1964) observed that giving Freund's complete adjuvant to hamsters during the latent period following neonatal inoculation with adenovirus type 12 affected tumor production and the production of complement-fixing antibodies to adenovirus virions and T-antigens.

2. Zymosan

Zymosan, first used as an immunosuppressive agent (Mathé and Bernard, 1956), was later shown by Bradner et al. (1958) to be able to stimulate antitumor immunity and has been used to attempt to cure various nonspecific grafted tumors (Sokoloff et al., 1961) as well as spontaneous tumors (Martin et al., 1964). Under certain conditions, which are described later, it can have a beneficial effect.

3. BCG

BCG has been shown in our laboratory to prolong slightly the survival of mice carrying L 1210 leukemia, when it is injected 24 hours after a graft of 10^4 leukemic cells (Mathé, 1968; Mathé et al., 1969b). Better results have been obtained on RC19 leukemia transplanted intravenously; this leukemia is particularly sensitive to the immune reactions promoted by BCG (Mathé *et al.*, 1971).

Iris Parr (1971) obtained comparable results on 5178Y grafted tumor. Lemonde and Clode-Hyde (1966) gave BCG to mice that had been inoculated with polyoma virus at birth, and obtained a moderate but noteworthy prolongation of survival time.

4. *Corynebacterium parvum*

Corynebacterium parvum has been shown by Smith and Woodruff (1968) to inhibit the growth of mammary carcinoma in A line mice. This effect has been confirmed by Currie and Bagshawe (1970) using fibrosarcomas. On the other hand, *Corynebacterium parvum* has no effect on L 1210 leukemia (Mathé *et al.*, 1969b).

5. *Bordetella pertussis*

Bordetella pertussis has been reported by Wissler *et al.* (1968) as being able to enhance the rejection of transplanted tumors. In our study of the action of adjuvants on L 1210 leukemia it was found to be ineffective (Mathé *et al.*, 1969b).

6. *Polynucleotides*

Polynucleotides are a group of compounds whose immunoadjuvant properties have only been recognized recently. It was first shown that oligonucleotides derived from natural sources delayed the appearance of spontanous mammary cancer in C3H mice (Braun *et al.*, 1963).

Then interest focused on synthetic double-stranded polynucleotides, in particular, polyinosinic-cytidylic acid (poly-IC) and poly-adenylic-uracylic acid (poly-AU). The ability of these substances to induce the production of interferon led to their effects on virus-induced tumor growth being studied. First the capacity of poly-IC to act prophylactically as well as therapeutically in a variety of virus-induced tumors (Baron and Levy, quoted by Braun, 1970; Jung Koo Youn *et al.*, 1968).

However, search for a mode of action other than interferon production was begun once it was established that poly-IC acted equally well against the growth of transplanted tumors (Baron and Levy, quoted by Braun, 1970; Braun, 1970; Hayat and Mathé, 1971). Furthermore, the timing and nature of the antitumor effect makes it clear that it is related to factors other than stimulation of interferon production. Poly-AU is known to be a relatively poor inducer of interferon, but has been demonstrated by Braun and his collaborators, Webb, Plescia, and Raskova (quoted by Braun, 1970) to have a pronounced antitumor effect.

C. Parameters of Action of Active Immunotherapy
   and Possible Side Effects

Such are the main experiments, most of them are very recent, that show that specific or nonspecific immune stimulation applied after the establishment of a malignant neoplasm can have an antitumor action. The results appear to be very variable from one experiment to another. Factors influencing the results will be analyzed as far as possible.

1. Factors Related to the Immunostimulating Agent

a. *The Specificity of the Stimulation.* Specific active immunotherapy in L 1210 leukemia appears to be definitely more effective than BCG, which is the best of the adjuvants, although in preventive treatment, BCG given 14 days before a graft of living L 1210 cells is clearly more effective than immunization with irradiated tumor cells (Mathé *et al.,* 1969b) (Fig. 2).

b. *Combination.* The combination of two adjuvants for the treatment of L 1210 leukemia has never given us a better but never a poorer result than the most efficient agent used alone (unpublished).

The combination of active specific and nonspecific immunotherapy

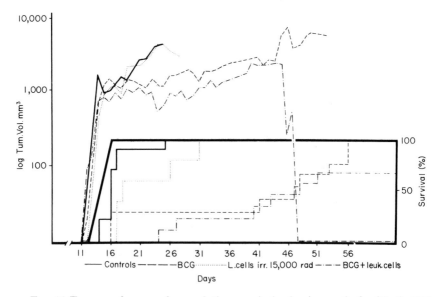

Fig. 2. Tumor volume and cumulative survival of mice grafted with L 1210 leukemia and not treated or treated by BCG (first injection 14 days before the graft and injections repeated each 4 days), or irradiated leukemic cells (one injection 14 days before the graft), or association of both.

(leukemic cells and BCG injected separately) has given better results in L 1210 leukemia than immunization with leukemia cells alone, which is the more effective of these two agents (Fig. 1) (Mathé, 1968; Mathé et al., 1969b).

There are several examples in the literature of experiments designed to cure various tumors with a combination of an adjuvant and immunization by tumor cells, in which favorable results have been achieved. Unfortunately, there were only a few attempts to compare the effects of the combination with each procedure given alone. Iris Parr (1971) obtained a beneficial effect by giving simultaneously irradiated tumor cells and Bordetella pertussis vaccine or BCG, 24 hours after a graft of L 5178 lymphoma. Emerson and Emerson (1965) observed regression of spontaneous mammary cancers in certain strains of mice following the injection of a mixture of tumor homogenates and Freund's adjuvant. Berman et al. (1967) treated hamsters with virus and Freund's adjuvant during the latent period following their neonatal inoculation with adenovirus 12, and obtained a reduction in the frequency of tumors.

c. *Adjuvantlike Effects.* Some adjuvant effect may be achieved if noncompatible cells are used as the tumor cells to immunize an animal. We have observed that when tumor cells that are allogenic with respect to the host are used to immunize against a tumor carrying the same antigens as these cells, a better result is obtained than with tumor cells that are isogenic with the host (not published). Lin and Murphy (1969) attributed adjuvant effect of this magnitude to a lipoprotein present in the cells.

One special use of an adjuvant is the xenogenization of tumor elements given to initiate the immunization or its intensification. Czajkowski et al. (1966) proposed a method for enhancing the antigenicity of neoplastic cells. A highly antigenic foreign protein carrier was chemically coupled with bis-diazobenzidine to cancer cells obtained from animals. When incorporated in Freund's complete adjuvant and reinjected into the animals, this tumor foreign protein complex elicited active immunity to autologous tumor tissue in C3H mice bearing spontaneous mammary adenocarcinomas and methylcholanthrene-induced squamous cell carcinomas.

Plescia and Braun (quoted by Braun, 1970) have tried to enhance immunogenicity of tumor cells by complexing these cells with foreign basic proteins, either methylated bovine serum albumin or methylated bovine γ-globulin. The protective immunity elicited by small complexes in prophylactic experiments was good, but was less favorable when used for tumor therapy.

Isogenic hosts can reject a small skin graft of virus-infected skin

(Mathé, 1967) and a virus infection can even alter tumor antigenicity (Stück *et al.*, 1964; Svet-Moldavsky and Hamburg, 1964; Sjögren and Hellström, 1965). These observations led Kobayashi *et al.* (1970) to successfully vaccinate rats against a tumor by injecting them prophylactically with tumor cells infected with Friend virus. An experiment to test the therapeutic antitumor effects of this method needs to be made. It is possible that increased immunogenicity of host cells is the main mechanism of viral oncolysis (Lindenmann and Klein, 1967).

d. *Increase of Specific Immunogenicity.* It is possible that cells used as a specific vaccine may have little effect or none at all, either because they are poor in tumor-associated antigens or perhaps the cell surface sialomucins act as a barrier between them and the immunological machinery. Treatment of the cells with neuraminidase could possibly increase their immunogenicity (Bagshawe and Currie, 1968).

e. *Methods of Administration.* The way in which specific or nonspecific stimulants of immunity are used needs to be examined. We have shown in L 1210 leukemia that a single injection of irradiated leukemia cells given 24 hours after the graft of living leukemia cells had the same antitumor effect as a series of injections given every 4 days. The reverse occurs with BCG, where repeated injections are more active than a single injection (Mathé *et al.*, 1969b).

f. *Dose.* The amount of antigen or adjuvant appears to be important. Our experiments made with Hayat have shown that small doses of poly-IC are more effective as adjuvants than large doses (Hayat and Mathé, 1971). This idea could not be extrapolated to all adjuvants.

g. *Microorganisms.* When microorganisms are used as adjuvants, other factors have to be considered. Living BCG is more active than killed BCG; we have found certain preparations of BCG are more active than others. There is a marked difference in the adjuvant activity of various strains of *Corynebacterium parvum* (Smith and Woodruff, 1968).

2. Factors Related to the Tumor and the Host

a. *Tumor Volume.* This seems to be the most important factor influencing the outcome of active immunotherapy. In our experience using L 1210 leukemia (Mathé, 1968; Mathé *et al.*, 1969b), immunotherapy is only effective when the number of leukemic cells is 10^5 or less (Fig. 3). This figure shows how this fundamental concept applies equally to the action of adjuvants and active specific immunotherapy, as well as the combination of these methods. Later in this article I explain how this consideration has influenced the selection of patients for the first trials of active immunotherapy.

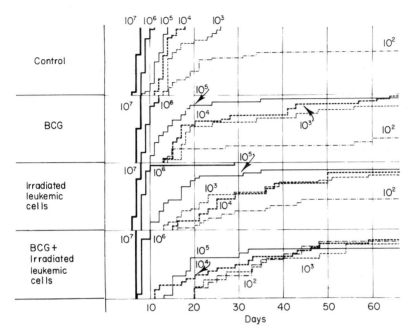

Fig. 3. Cumulative survival of mice grafted with 10^2 to 10^7 L 1210 leukemia cells, not treated or treated in the 24 hours following the graft by BCG (repeated injections) or irradiated leukemic cells (one injection), or association of both.

b. *Localization.* Needless to say, the localization of the tumor could be a major factor. Certain sites, in particular the nervous system, are probably less accessible to immunological effects.

c. *Genetic Factors.* Variations in the host's response to active immunotherapy are further influenced by genetic factors. Emerson and Emerson (1965) have shown that susceptibility to active immunotherapy of spontaneous adenocarcinoma varies from one substrain of mice to another.

d. *Age.* The animal's age might influence the result, since it is known that immune responses become depressed in old age, at least in some strains of mice. Mice bearing tumors can develop an overall or dissociated immunological insufficiency (Doré *et al.*, 1969). It can be questioned in such a case whether active immunotherapy is able to restore specific or overall immunity; for if it does not, it could potentiate the growth of the tumor.

e. *Tolerance.* Under certain conditions, the failure to obtain an effect with active immunotherapy could be explained by the fact that some animals carrying tumors will be tolerant to the tumor antigens. This tolerance could result from oncogenic viruses infecting the animals at birth, or by vertical transmission during fetal life. This type of tolerance has been suspected in AkR mice in relation to leukemia induced by Gross virus. Meanwhile, it has been observed that immune stimulation by *Corynebacterium parvum* (Lamensans *et al.*, 1968) or BCG (Doré *et al.*, 1970) given to 2-month-old AkR mice, before an isogenic graft of K36 leukemia, an AkR leukemia, delayed and reduced the mortality. With Doré *et al.* (1970), we found that a preventive action against the leukemia could be obtained by injecting allogenic E ♂ G2 leukemia cells (a leukemia induced in C57Bl/6 mice by Gross virus). Mice vaccinated in this way, and overcoming a graft of K36 leukemia, formed cytotoxic antibodies against a leukemia induced in C3H mice by Passage A (Gross) virus and against cells from a spontaneous AkR leukemia.

Tolerance has also been suspected in murine spontaneous mammary tumors, but evidence has already been cited that immunotherapy has given positive results against this tumor, which is against the idea of tolerance in this situation (Emerson and Emerson, 1965).

The studies of Berman *et al.* (1967) provided more evidence against the tolerance theory. They inoculated adenovirus type 12 into newborn hamsters, then during the latent period injected them with more virus, or Freund's adjuvant, or both agents; these animals then produced antibodies against the virion and against T antigen. Hence tolerance by neonatal or perinatal exposure to oncogenic virus, supposing that it exists, is not a constant or absolute phenomenon.

It has been shown that immunological tolerance against various antigens can also be induced in adults. But if tolerance exists at any time in a disease, it is not unthinkable that it could be broken. Orbach-Arbouys (1968a,b,c) has broken tolerance in rats to sheep red cells by total body irradiation, with drugs used in cancer chemotherapy (6-mercaptopurine, methotrexate, cyclophosphamide) and with antilymphocyte serum (ALS).

f. *Immunoresistance.* It is not impossible that the failures could one day be explained by the development of immunoresistance related to the selection of cells with decreased concentration of tumor-specific surface antigens; Fenÿo *et al.* (1968) have demonstrated that this phenomenon is a real possibility.

3. *Side Effects*

The beneficial effects obtained with active immunotherapy vary under different conditions, to such an extent that it is not always possible to reproduce in a second experiment the results of a preceding one. Sometimes a small difference that passes unnoticed can reduce or annul the effect. Occasionally it is possible to observe facilitation of the tumor growth which is opposed to the therapeutic effect that is sought.

Cruse (1967) reported tumor growth facilitation following the administration of a mixture of ground tumor tissue and Freund's adjuvant after a graft of an isogenic tumor. Hirano *et al.* (1967) injected *Bordetella pertussis* vaccine intravenously on the seventh day after the transplantation of a lymphoma and obtained an enhancement of tumor growth. A similar result was obtained by Floersheim (1967). Giving *Corynebacterium parvum* abolished the hosts' resistance against certain types of transplanted tumors (Cudkowicz, 1968). Donner *et al.* (1970) facilitated solid tumor growth by injecting polysaccharides from proteus.

Goldner *et al.* (1965) reported that in hamsters inoculated neonatally with SV40, administration of adjuvant during the latent period appeared to cause some increase in tumor development. In hamsters inoculated with the Bryan strain of Rous sarcoma virus, the injection of Freund's complete adjuvant seems to increase the incidence of tumors (Allison and Berman, quoted by Berman *et al.*, 1967).

The factors that direct the effect of adjuvants in the direction of enhancement of tumor growth are not precise and require further investigation. The dose of adjuvant may be important; Schoenberg and Moore (1960) showed that Freund's adjuvant induced a more rapid death and larger tumor formation in mice if given in large doses. This makes us ask whether this untoward action operates through "tumor enhancement" as described by Kaliss (1966) which essentially involves blocking antibodies. G. Möller (1964) demonstrated that tumor associated antigens in the same way as H-2 antigens, can raise blocking antibodies. When this type of result is observed, it would be valuable to confirm the truth of this hypothesis by the passive transfer of the antibody. The phenomenon of immunological enhancement is more to be feared in solid tumors than in the leukemias. The spleen is suspected to play a major role in the production of enhancement antibodies, as demonstrated in mice by Ferrer (1966). The therapeutic importance of splenectomy has been suggested and shown to be valuable in inhibiting the growth of sarcoma 180 (Ferrer and Mihich, 1968).

D. Modalities and Mechanisms of Action of Active Immunotherapy

In contrast to chemotherapy, active immunotherapy does not appear to conform to rules of a first-order kinetic reaction, since it does not destroy a given percentage of tumor cells independent of the total number of cells (Mathé *et al.*, 1969b). Though this gives the therapy a disadvantage, it is advantageous, for it enables all the tumor cells to be destroyed when their number is small. In all cases when experimental tumors have been cured by chemotherapy, it seems that the final cure can be attributed to immunization of the animal that occurs spontaneously (Glynn *et al.*, 1963; Schabel *et al.*, 1966). Furthermore, this appears to be the same for certain other types of cancer therapy; Apffel *et al.* (1966) have shown in mice bearing transplantable ascitic tumors and treated daily by aspiration of the ascites, recovered completely; these animals were immune to the original tumor or subsequent challenge.

In experimental tumors grafted subcutaneously, the growth curve can be measured; this follows a Gompertz function. Active immunotherapy only acts during the saturation phase and is without effect in the exponential phase (Fig. 4) (Mathé *et al.*, 1969b); there is reason to think that this is because active immunotherapy requires a certain number of days for the immunization to be established.

In Fig. 6 it can be seen that immunotherapy is not an all-or-none phenomenon. In some animals it can induce a complete regression of tumors and they are cured, in others the tumor growth will enter a plateau. We have wondered if in the latter case whether the action of immunotherapy is to hold the tumor cells in the G0 phase; recently,

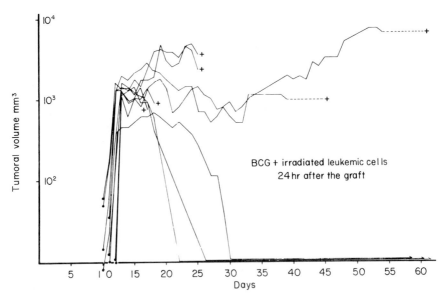

FIG. 4. Tumoral volume of each mouse in a group of mice carrying L 1210 leukemia and treated by the association of BCG and irradiated leukemic cells 24 hours after the graft.

Lhéritier *et al.* (1971) have shown that active immunotherapy does not prolong the cell cycle and does not increase the percentage of cells in G0.

The mechanism of action of active immunotherapy still remains a matter for speculation. I have regrouped under the wide and imprecise term "adjuvants" methods such as the use of living BCG, killed *Corynebacterium parvum*, synthetic polynucleotides, given intravenously or intraperitoneally, which can be very different from the classical method for adjuvance produced by giving the antigen mixed with Freund's adjuvant.

I propose to call "systemic adjuvants" those procedures which are not administered with the antigen but can stimulate general immune reactions, and "local adjuvants" those which are administered mixed with antigen. The action of the local adjuvants is generally thought to be brought about by macrophages and lymphocytes at the site of the injection of the antigen. This leads to a stimulation of immunoglobulin production (Freund, 1953), through the proliferation of antibody-synthesizing cells (Talmage and Pearlman, 1963), and an increase of cell-mediated immunity in a variety of systems (White, 1967).

Though Freund's adjuvant is generally administered, mixed with the antigen, as a local adjuvant, it is not less active if it is given separately from the antigen, as a systemic adjuvant, as has been shown in some of the experiments of Berman *et al.* (1967).

The mechanism of action of systemic adjuvants seems to be complex. It has been shown that the majority of them, BCG (Biozzi *et al.*, 1960), *Corynebacterium parvum* (Halpern *et al.*, 1964) and polynucleotides (Braun and Nakano, 1967; Braun, 1970) increase phagocytosis by the reticuloendothelial system. However, Smith and Woodruff (1968) did not observe a correlation between the effect of *Corynebacterium parvum* on phagocytic activity and its antitumor action.

Another effect of systemic adjuvants is the augmentation of the numbers of immunocompetent cells in the peripheral lymphoid tissue. This can be shown by the "rosettes" test or by the Jerne test (Jerne *et al.*, 1963) which allows the number of cells capable of forming "rosettes" or lytic plaques in the spleen of a mouse immunized with sheep red cells to be counted. This increase has been demonstrated for BCG and *Corynebacterium parvum* (Biozzi *et al.*, 1968), poly-IC and poly-AU (Braun, 1970; Hayat and Mathé, 1971).

It has also been shown that these adjuvants increase the production of a variety of serum antibodies and delayed hypersensitivity reactions against several antigens. The important studies on this topic have been made by Dubost and Schaedler (1957) on BCG, Neveu *et al.* (1964) on

Corynebacterium parvum, Finger *et al.* (1967) on *Bordetella pertussis vaccine,* Braun *et al.* (quoted by Braun, 1970) and Johnson *et al.* (1970) on polynucleotides.

It is known that the phagocytic and immunostimulant actions of polynucleotides are not the only ways they can exert their antitumor effects. At the same time polynucleotides have cytotoxic effects and are interferon inducers; interferon itself can have a degree of cytotoxicity (Macieira-Coelhol *et al.,* 1971). But it seems that these three effects do not occur at the same dose; the immunoadjuvant effect of poly-IC occurs when it is given in small doses (Hayat and Mathé, 1971; Braun, 1970).

Bordetella pertussis vaccine exerts a very special effect on lymphoid tissue: a marked blood lymphocytosis, ranging from 50,000 to 120,000 per cm³ is usually induced in 1-month-old mice by injecting them with 0.3 ml. of vaccine; small lymphocytes in lymphoid follicles are depleted, there is little activity in the germinal centers and the number of nucleated cells in the red pulp is generally considerably reduced (Hirano *et al.,* 1967).

Several workers have attempted to isolate the active substances from mycobacteria that are responsible for their adjuvant activity, waxes (Jollès *et al.,* 1962; Hiu *et al.,* 1969), methanol-extracted residue (MER) (Weiss *et al.,* 1961, 1966). A substance called reticulostimulin has been isolated from *Corynebacteria* by Prevot (1965); it appears to be the active factor but it has not been fully identified.

The list of adjuvants in the wide sense is certainly not complete, and it is to be hoped that there will be a systematic testing on various tumors of bacterial endotoxins (see Braun and Kessel, 1964) and various polyanions (Regelson, 1967; Regelson and Munson, 1971; Braun *et al.,* 1968) which have been shown to stimulate the hosts' defense system, but have not been used practically due to their toxic side effects. The bacterial lipopolysaccharides (Shilo, 1960), statolon (Probst, quoted by Regelson *et al.,* 1971), protodyne (Berger *et al.,* 1968) merit further investigation. Phytohemaglutinin has the special property of transforming a large proportion of small lymphocytes into immunoblasts *in vitro;* but *in vivo* its paramount action is immunosuppressive (Stevens and Willoughby, 1967).

The mechanism of action of active specific immunotherapy is probably affected by a combination of two immune cytotoxic processes: cytotoxic antibodies, which fix complement, and the "killing" action of lymphocytes. Denham *et al.* (1970) raised the hypothesis that the cells responsible for the cytotoxicity are "immunoblasts" (or lymphocytes transformed by the antigen); these cells are rich in RNA, their cytoplasms contain many ribosomes but are deprived of endoplasmic reticulum. An injection of tumor cells on animal will induce between the sixth and twelfth days a great number of immunoblasts that are cytotoxic to the tumor cells; these are then replaced by lymphocytes which are morphologically normal but potentially cytotoxic against the same tumor cells; their cytotoxicity will not appear until after their transformation into immunoblasts under the influence of a further injection of antigen. The respective roles of cytotoxic antibodies and cells are not very clear. It is probable that final immunotherapeutic action is the algebraic sum of these two beneficial effects, and the harmful effects of enhancement antibodies which protect the tumor cells against the other two cytotoxic effects. The detailed mechanism of the mode of potentiation of specific and nonspecific immunotherapy merits further study.

Are other effects produced by immunotherapy that are not directly immunological, for example, inhibition of tumor growth by lymphocytes acting by virtue of the allogenic inhibition phenomenon described by the Möllers (E. Möller, 1965; G. Möller and Möller, 1966)? Lamensans et al. (1968) suspected that this effect might explain the action of Corynebacterium parvum, for this microorganism protects F1 hybrid mice against homologous disease induced by injecting them with parental spleen cells (Biozzi et al., 1965). They have also noticed that the effect of Corynebacterium parvum against grafted AkR leukemia is more pronounced in hybrid mice than in AkR mice.

Without doubt immunotherapy cannot only strengthen immunity against tumor associated antigens, but immunity against oncogenic viruses. Rauscher and his colleagues (1963) observed that Freund's adjuvant, injected after an inoculation of Rous sarcoma virus, increased the production of antibody against this virus.

E. THE SPECIAL CASE OF ANTITUMOR IMMUNOTHERAPY INDUCED BY LOCAL HYPERSENSITIVITY REACTIONS

Zbar et al. (1970) have shown that the growth of strain-2 hepatoma could be suppressed at the site of delayed hypersensitivity skin reaction to another antigenically different, transplantable hepatoma, and at the site of delayed hypersensitivity skin reactions to bacterial antigens.

F. STRATEGY OF USING ACTIVE IMMUNOTHERAPY IN CANCER

The preceding arguments have indicated that active immunotherapy in treatment of cancer is best suited for situations where the total number of cells is small. In view of the possible clinical application, it is interesting to try immunotherapy as a second treatment on tumors whose mass has been first reduced by surgery, radiotherapy, or chemotherapy.

Another justification for the use of active immunotherapy in this sequence comes from the studies of Gershon et al. (1968). They found that hamsters grafted with an allotransplantable lymphoma that does not metastasize, develop a state of concomitant immunity; removal of the tumor 7 days after transplantation led to a decrease in immunity; enhancing antibodies were produced and metastases developed, which were probably derived from preexisting tumor cells in the blood and lymphoid tissues. Hence it is possible that immunotherapy applied at a moment after surgery when the quantity of antigen is insufficient to maintain immunity could support the immune reaction and prevent circulating tumor cells from forming metastases. The sequence of surgery followed by active immunotherapy is justified on two counts: the reduction of the tumor mass by surgery so that the residual tumor can be eradicated by immunotherapy; the contribution of immunotherapy to boosting the weak immune reactions when the circulating cancer cells do not furnish enough antigen to maintain the state of immunity required for their eradication.

There are more reports of experiments on the relation of chemotherapy and active immunotherapy.

One might have feared, *a priori*, that the sequential use of chemotherapy followed by immunotherapy had no justification, as many chemotherapeutic compounds are immunosuppressive (Amiel *et al.*, 1967b). In fact, this immunosuppression is transitory, and rarely prolonged after stopping chemotherapy; I have mentioned earlier how mice cured of tumors by chemotherapy were thereafter immunized against the tumor (Glynn *et al.*, 1963; Schabel *et al.*, 1966). If the animal is tolerant to the tumor, chemotherapy may well be able to break the tolerance (Orbach-Arbouys, 1968b).

In practice, the experiments made by Pouillart and Mathé (1970) on L 1210 leukemia have proved the value of this sequence of treatment. In animals given 10^6 leukemic cells immunotherapy alone was ineffective, but it became effective when it was given after a dose of 6-mercaptopurine sufficient to reduce the number of cells by 2 logs. Amiel and Bérardet (1970) have published results obtained in E ♂ G2 leukemia.

The experiments of Currie and Bagshawe (1970) are even more interesting, for they demonstrate that the timing of administration of adjuvant after chemotherapy is extremely critical. When *Corynebacterium parvum* was used alone to enhance immunological activity of mice carrying transplanted isogenic fibrosarcomas, it produced a transient inhibition of their growth. Giving this adjuvant 12 days after a single dose of cyclophosphamide produced a dramatic inhibition of tumor growth and resulted in a complete and lasting regression in up to 70% of the animals. The results were negative if the time interval was shorter (0, 3, or 6 days) and when it was longer (16 days). An earlier study by

Sokoloff *et al.* (1961) is worth recalling; he showed that the oncolytic effect of mitomycin C on several nonspecific murine tumors could be enhanced by zymosan, but this adjuvant action of yeast extract was critically dependent on the time of its administration.

Chemotherapy itself may be preceded by surgery, as has been demonstrated by Martin *et al.* (1964), who followed this combination with zymosan for the treatment of mammary adenocarcinomas in mice and demonstrated that the timing of the administration of zymosan was extremely critical. This critical time interval that separates chemotherapy and the application of immunotherapy is perhaps related to the time required for release from the immunosuppression caused by the chemotherapy. It is possible and even probable that this time varies according to the type of chemotherapy. The immunosuppressive action varies considerably from one drug to another (Amiel *et al.*, 1967b); from one dose to another: a dose of 403.4 mg. of cyclophosphamide is immunosuppressive while 134.5 mg. is not (Mathé *et al.*, 1968b); from one modality of administration to another: continuous administration is more immunosuppressive than intermittent treatment (Schneider, 1968).

It can be foreseen that small modifications of chemotherapy in the repetition of an experimental protocol combining chemotherapy and immunotherapy could lead to considerable differences in the results; this factor needs further close attention. Under certain circumstances chemotherapy can annul the effects of immunotherapy, but it is not impossible that, providing the time interval between the two treatments is well chosen, an enhancement could occur. It is known that if rabbits are treated with 6-mercaptopurine and then rested for 5 days, they produce hyperimmune responses to antigen (Chanmougan and Schwartz, 1966). A similar rebound of delayed hypersensitivity reactions has been seen after immunosuppression by cortisone (Long and Miles, 1950).

The reverse sequence of therapy, immunotherapy followed by chemotherapy, is theoretically not to be recommended; immunotherapy makes lymphocytes commence cyclic division and then they would be more susceptible to destruction by chemotherapy (most of the chemotherapeutic agents are cycle or phase dependent). Currie and Bagshawe (1970) demonstrated that *Corynebacterium parvum* as a prelude to chemotherapy by cyclophosphamide was generally ineffective. Amiel and Bérardet (1969b) have shown in E ♂ G2 leukemia that chemotherapy with methylhydrazine (a powerful immunosuppressive in mice) cancels the effects of immunotherapy (by BCG) given beforehand.

On the other hand, it does not seem to be illogical to precede immunotherapy by surgical excision or radiotherapy, as they do not have systemic effects. Haddow and Alexander (1964) demonstrated that rat sarcomas are radiosensitized by immunization of the host with irradiated autologous tumor.

III. Clinical Trials

The pressing need for clinical application of immunotherapy resulted in the first trials being made at the same time or even before studies in animals. Clinicians were struck by the extreme effectiveness of chemotherapy for the induction of a remission in acute lymphoblastic leukemia; that is, to make the disease change from a detectable state to an undetectable state (residual disease). Unfortunately, relapse was inevitable despite "maintenance chemotherapy." This constant relapse is perfectly explained by the fact that chemotherapy obeys first-order kinetics (Skipper et al., 1964) as it only destroys a certain percentage of leukemic cells and never 100%. Clinicians sought another method of therapy which could attack the residual disease and that would not obey the law of first kinetics order. The experiments, described above (Mathé, 1968), have shown precisely how the best indication for active immunotherapy was found to be the treatment of residual disease.

A. TREATMENT OF RESIDUAL DISEASE

The choice of cancers in man on which the first trials could be made were limited by the fact that knowledge of the immunology of human tumors is very small compared to experimental tumors. Hamilton-Fairley (1969) has written an excellent review of this topic. Membrane tumor-associated antigenicity and humoral or lymphocyte-mediated cytotoxic reactions have been demonstrated in Burkitt's tumor (G. Klein et al., 1966), leukemias (Doré et al., 1967; Yoshida and Imai, 1970), malignant melanomas (Lewis, 1967; Morton et al., 1968), sarcomas (Morton and Malmgren, 1968; Old, 1970; Doré et al., 1971), and neuroblastomas (Hellström et al., 1968).

We chose to treat the residual disease that is left in acute lymphoblastic leukemia after chemotherapy. This disease was chosen because the tumor volume could be estimated conveniently and immunological enhancement, which any immunological procedure might increase, is rarer or less effective in leukemias than in solid tumors.

However, this disease was suspected to be an unwise choice for a trial of active immunotherapy, because of possible immune tolerance, we were aware of its supposed existence in spontaneous leukemia of AkR mice. Nevertheless, we chose this leukemia for the following reasons: (a) this tolerance has not been proven; (b) Doré et al. (1967) and Yoshida and Imai (1970) have found, in the serum of some patients, antibodies against their own leukemic cells; (c) if this tolerance existed at the beginning of the illness, it might be possible to break it down by chemotherapy, as Orbach-Arbouys (1968b) was able to suppress tolerance to sheep red cells in rats by methotrexate, cyclophosphamide, and 6-mercaptopurine; (d) we even doubt this alleged tolerance of AkR mice toward the tumor antigens of Gross virus-induced leukemia for several reasons, the main one being the possible production of antibodies, after immunization with K36 cells, directed against AkR leukemic cells (Doré et al., 1970).

Our experiments cited above suggested that the optimum condition for immunotherapy applied to man was that the patients should be carrying the smallest number of leukemic cells possible. To achieve this, we first reduce the cell number by chemotherapy, to induce remission. Then, we try still further reduction by sequentially administering all the different forms of chemotherapeutic drugs available (Mathé et al., 1968a, 1969a, 1970a).

In our first trial, started in 1964, 30 patients, whose ages varied from 3 to 50 years, were treated in this way. They received after remission induction, a sequential complementary cell-reducing chemotherapy (one drug at a time) combined with intrathecal administration of methotrexate and meningeal radiotherapy. Four groups were formed randomly. In the first, 10 control patients did not receive any further treatment after complementary chemotherapy was stopped. In the second, 8 patients were treated by BCG (Figs. 5, 6, and 7) and received, on every fourth day and then on every eighth day, twenty cutaneous scratches, each 5 cm. long, and arranged in a square. Two milliliters of a suspension containing 75 mg./ml. of living bacteria were put into the scarifield area. In the third group, 5 patients received each week, both intradermally and subcutaneously, 4×10^7 leukemic cells, which had been obtained from a pool of allogenic donors suffering from acute lymphoblastic leukemia. These cells had been preserved at $-70°C$. in DMSO. For the first six injections, the cells were treated with a 4% formol solution to inactivate any possible virus and, for remaining injections, they were irradiated with 4000 rads in vitro. In the final group, 7 patients were given both forms of immunotherapy.

Each of the 10 patients left without treatment after chemotherapy was stopped, relapsed. The average duration of the remission was 66 days, the median lying between the seventieth and seventy-seventh day. The limits were 30 and 130 days. At the 130th day, only 9 of the 20 patients given immunotherapy had relapsed, and the difference between these two groups is highly significant ($\chi^2 = 6.18$, $P = 0.02$). Later, 4 other patients relapsed. An examination of the relapses gives rise to

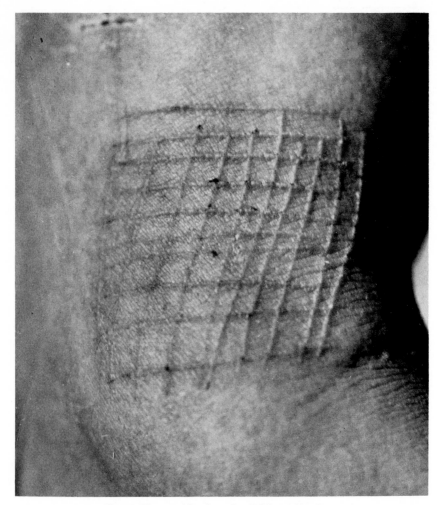

Fig. 5. The scarifications for BCG application.

the following ideas: (a) the majority of them appeared to be early: 9
before the 100th day, 5 before the 30th day, which is comparable with
the experimental observations in mice, and suggests that the number of
tumor cells left after the chemotherapy was greater than the maximum
number that could be controlled by active immunotherapy; (b) 4 of
them were late in onset. One occurred at the 210th day, another at the
324th day, and another at the 950th day (which is comparable with those
exceptional late relapses we had noted in our experiments with mice). The
fourth, which occurred at the 315th day, was in an infant in whom
the BCG treatment had been stopped 44 days previously (because of

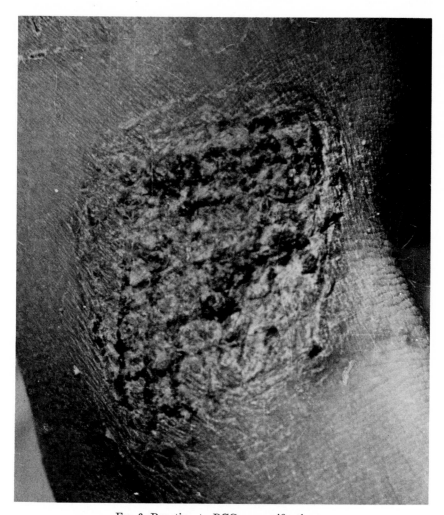

Fig. 6. Reaction to BCG on scarifications.

a severe and intractable phlyctenular keratoconjunctivitis which had required the treatment to be stopped several times). This last patient,
when considering the possibility of late relapses, answers the question
as to whether immunotherapy should be continued indefinitely. Seven
patients are still in remission more than 3 years after chemotherapy
has been terminated; in five it is more than 4 years, and in two it is
more than 5 years.

Figure 8 shows the actuarial curves, demonstrating differences between the groups submitted to immunotherapy and the control group.

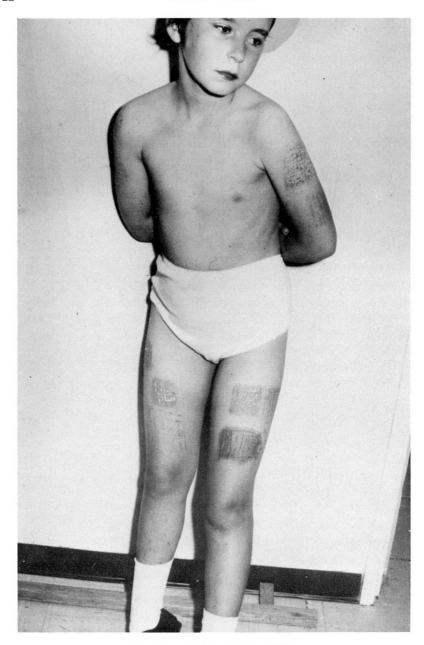

FIG. 7. A child treated by BCG.

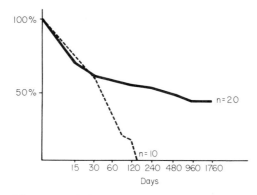

F‌IG. 8. Actuarial curves of duration of remission of patients treated or not treated by active immunotherapy after the end of chemotherapy (protocol 1). —— patients submitted to immunotherapy, --- patients without immunotherapy.

They indicate that, although the median for the remission duration in our patients given immunotherapy is of the same order as those given intensive chemotherapy (Holland and Glidewell, 1970), the shape of the curves of these two groups is quite different. That of the patients given immunotherapy tends to straighten out and continue as a plateau.

There were no significant differences between the group given BCG (5 relapses out of 8 patients; treatment had been stopped in one), that given leukemic cells alone (3 relapses in 5 patients), and the group given both these forms of immunotherapy (5 relapses in 7 patients).

The remarkable results and the failures of this trial require further discussion. With regard to the successful results, it is important to remember that the patients who underwent immunotherapy had been highly selected. That is, they all received prolonged chemotherapy, with little effect. It is possible that these patients belonged to a special category and perhaps were destined for long spontaneous remissions. However, it should be noted that the control individuals relapsed very rapidly, confirming the inefficiency of chemotherapy. In regard to the design of the trial, it is the chemotherapy that should be reviewed, in terms of the poor choice of certain drugs which rarely act against acute lymphoblastic leukemia, and in terms of sequential administration of only one drug at a time.

The protocol, which we have subsequently followed and in which we erroneously abandoned meningeal radiotherapy, confirms the ideas of the preceding discussion. The results are, in fact, disappointing, mainly because of several meningeal relapses. Nevertheless, it showed that the cumulative curve for the duration of remission had a similar form to that seen in our first trial. After a descent it flattened out into a plateau, though only a relatively small percentage of patients were left at this stage. However, this curve included all the patients who were treated according to this protocol; this comprised patients treated in the first visible phase of the disease as well as in relapse (study made in collaboration with Amiel, Schwarzenberg, Schneider, Cattan, Schlumberger and Jasmin, not published).

In a third protocol, whose results are only preliminary and have not been published, the complementary cytoreductive preimmunotherapy treatment was as intensive as possible. The chemotherapeutic drugs were given two at a time in four sequences of chemotherapy; chemotherapy using two drugs was given intrathecally and radiotherapy was given to the central nervous system. A splenectomy was carried out in patients with splenomegaly; and any enlarged lymph nodes were treated by radiotherapy. At the end of this cytoreductive therapy immunotherapy was commenced. One third of the patients received BCG, *Corynebacterium parvum*, and leukemic cells, one third the same treatment combined with a monthly injection of vincristine, and one third the same treatment combined with a continuous treatment with amantadine, an antiviral agent (Galbraith *et al.*, 1969). The preliminary results are very encouraging. In the group of patients given this therapy in the first visible phase of their leukemia, no relapse has occurred in those who received immunotherapy alone (the longest period is only 14 months). Relapses have occurred in patients given a combination of immunotherapy and chemotherapy and in those given immunotherapy and amantadine. It seems likely that this result is going to confirm the experimental findings that (a) chemotherapy administered at the same time as immunotherapy inhibits its effects (Amiel and Bérardet, 1969b); (b) amantadine is an immunosuppressive agent (Bredt and Mardiney, 1969).

A fourth protocol of therapy is starting to be used in which the action of poly-IC, a new adjuvant, on residual disease is to be studied. I describe later how poly-IC has an action on leukemia in the visible phase, providing the number of leukemic cells are still fairly low (Mathé *et al.*, 1970b).

A comparable clinical trial was carried out by Guyer and Crowther (1969) who gave patients with acute lymphoblastic leukemia a treatment with *Bordetella pertussis* vaccine (0.5 ml. being given either weekly or twice a week by intramuscular injection, in a rotating system, to the four quadrants of the body). The pertussis vaccine was given during a remission induced by intensive chemotherapy. The treated patients relapsed after 65–455 days, while the control patients relapsed after 65–215 days; half the treated cases had relapsed by 186 days whereas half the controls had relapsed by 112 days. Their observation of this partial response without the occurrence of a number of long-term remissions suggests that this form of nonspecific stimulation is not as effective as that obtained by BCG or irradiated leukemic cells and their combination. The results from this clinical trial are in good agreement with experimental data.

The Medical Research Council in Great Britain is conducting a trial on the effects of BCG, not applied by scarification but with a Heaf injection gun and coming from a source of supply different from ours. The BCG was given to patients prepared by a scheme of systemic chemotherapy close to our last protocol but without the intensive chemotherapy and radiotherapy that we have applied to the nervous system. The preliminary results indicate that the duration of remissions in patients given BCG is not greater than the controls (personal communication).

The preliminary results mentioned by Willoughby (1970), who applied to acute lymphoblastic leukemia patients, weekly intradermal BCG after intensive chemotherapy seem to be more promising.

The adjuvant effect of the different modalities of administering BCG in man needs to be studied.

Sokal et al. (1970) have treated six patients, with chronic myelocytic leukemia "under good chemotherapeutic control," with a combination of BCG and cells from a permanent culture obtained from the blood of a case of acute myeloblastic leukemia. Their survival was apparently better than that of eleven controls (not randomized) and the treatment caused "unequivocal regression of splenomegaly."

It would be interesting to try the effects of active immunotherapy on the residual disease in solid tumors; (a) either in operable tumors after surgery, or in inoperable tumors after a maximum reduction of the tumor mass by surgery and/or radiotherapy and chemotherapy; (b) or in radiosensitive tumors after the disappearance of the tumor following irradiation. The patients given immunotherapy should be compared to a control group, and the patients allocated to the two groups at random.

Bagshawe and Golding (1971) have treated women suffering from choriocarcinoma, a semiallogenic solid tumor, with intradermal injections of BCG and skin grafts from their husbands. Eight patients may have benefited from this immunization procedure and were, at the time of publication, in remission; but in no case was the evidence for remission unequivocal. In one patient, immunization alone may have been effective in eliminating residual tumor resistant to chemotherapy. These authors have noted that BCG was more effective in abrogating the prolonged acceptance of the husbands' grafts (acceptance previously described by

Mathé *et al.*, 1964; Amiel *et al.*, 1967a; Robinson *et al.*, 1963, 1967), than specific immunization procedures (skin grafts or leukocyte administration). Doniach *et al.* (1958) and Cinader *et al.* (1961) were the first to treat women with choriocarcinoma by skin grafts or leukocyte injections from their husbands; in both instances, the immunotherapy had been used in addition to conventional chemotherapy, and it was difficult to assess the benefits.

The reasons why the use of the sequence surgery or radiotherapy for tumor mass reduction followed by active immunotherapy is advised is not only the limitation of the number of cells immunotherapy can eradicate, but also the fact that large tumor masses seem to be accompanied by an "immune paralysis" as demonstrated by serological studies on sarcomas (Morton *et al.*, 1970), melanomas (Lewis, 1967), and cytological studies on experimental chemically induced tumors (Alexander, 1970).

B. Use of Active Immunotherapy in Other Conditions of Malignant Disease

It can be questioned whether active immunotherapy ought to be limited to the treatment of cancers that have been reduced to a small number of cells, in particular residual disease. Or, despite experimental findings, is it reasonable to conduct clinical trials on large tumor masses?

The exceptional, but nevertheless real, spontaneous remissions in cancer (Everson and Cole, 1966) are good reasons why we should not dismiss the potential value of immunotherapy when the tumor mass is still large. It is known that these spontaneous remissions occur more frequently in those tumors for which immune reactions have already been demonstrated: neuroblastomas (Hellström *et al.*, 1968), melanomas (Lewis, 1967), sarcomas (Morton and Malmgren, 1968; Old *et al.*, 1959).

A good number of reports of attempted "vaccination" in cancer patients can be found in the literature (von Leyden and Blumenthal, 1902; Graham and Graham, 1959); see Southam, 1961). We have not analyzed all the trials of specific active immunotherapy, for the majority of them were not based on knowledge from animal experiments or made in a sufficiently scientific fashion for their results to be of any value.

Skurkovich *et al.* (1969) gave living allogeneic leukemia cells to patients with acute leukemia, in its visible phase, whom they consider to be suffering from "immunological inertness." Plasma and "leukocytes" were also used in this therapy and a fall in the number of leukemia cells was obtained. The protocol of this trial is complex and it is difficult to draw clearcut conclusions about this study.

Krementz *et al.* (1970) have treated patients suffering from various cancers by six intradermal injections of irradiated autochthonous cultured cells over a 2-week period, with weekly injections for 6 more weeks: of the 16 patients treated, 1 has shown complete regression without recurrence for 3 years and 3 have demonstrated weak antibody titer without clinical response.

The observations of tumor regressions after spontaneous or induced infections (Coley, 1893, 1911; Pelner, 1960) or after giving various substances that can modify the reactions of the host are worthy of further attention.

Having seen that poly-IC acts as an adjuvant in mice (similar results as Braun, 1970) and accepting that in man as in mice adjuvants can only destroy a very small number of tumor cells, we have used poly-IC in acute leukemia. The patients were in the visible phase of the disease, but carrying a reduced number of leukemic cells, less than 30% of the bone marrow cells were leukemic blasts; under these conditions poly-IC caused eight remissions (Mathé et al., 1970b) (Fig. 9).

The idea of turning to such a model to test adjuvants in man is upheld by our experience of obtaining remissions by BCG injections every second day in two patients who had commenced to relapse while on BCG weekly (Fig. 10).

Recently, Morton and Eilber (1970) injected 0.05–0.20 ml. of a

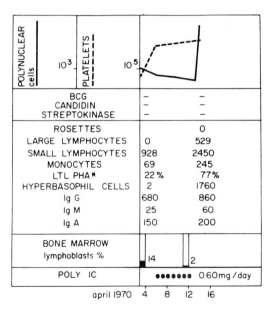

Fig. 9. Remission obtained with poly-IC in a patient with acute lymphoblastic leukemia and treated at the very beginning of a relapse.

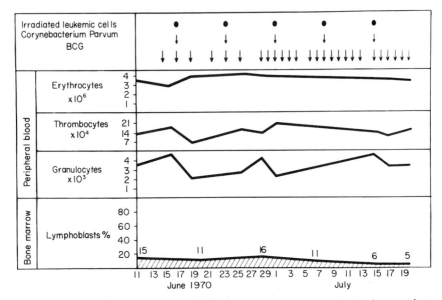

Fig. 10. Remission obtained by BCG injections every second day in a patient who had begun to relapse while on BCG weekly.

BCG suspension into cutaneous melanotic nodules and obtained not only a regression of these nodules, but also nodules into which no BCG had been injected; the titer of antibodies directed against these cells was raised.

Hadziev and Kavaklieva-Dimitrova (1969) have given BCG systematically to 71 patients with bronchial carcinoma (5–10 μg. injected intradermally every 3 to 4 days for 4 to 6 weeks, or 5 μg. twice with 1 or 2 weeks' interval between injections). The survival time was 8.8 to 22.8 months according to the therapy scheme used, while it was only 5.9 months for 85 controls (the difference is significant but they do not mention whether the patients were divided into the three groups at random). The same authors have observed apparently complete regression in skin cancers (9 to 25% according to the scheme of therapy).

The effects of giving various virus preparations have been tried. Regressions of both cutaneous and visceral lesions in malignant melanoma have been reported after injection of smallpox vaccine (vaccinia virus) (Burdick, 1960; Belisario and Milton, 1961; Burdick and Hawk, 1964; Milton and Brown, 1966; Hunter-Craig et al., 1970). The response is generally limited to the site of inoculation. It has been suggested that the action of the virus might be the result of nonspecific stimulation of the patients' immune response.

Can spontaneous immunization be sufficiently powerful in certain human cancers for it to play a therapeutic role? This hypothesis has been raised for the two forms of cancer that are curable by chemotherapy; choriocarcinoma, which is a semiallogenic tumor (see Bagshawe, 1969), and Burkitt's tumor (Burkitt, 1967). It appears reasonable from experimental data described above to consider that in these tumors, in which the immune reactions seem particularly active (Robinson *et al.*, 1967; Mathé *et al.*, 1964; Amiel *et al.*, 1967a; G. Klein *et al.*, 1966, 1967; Osunkoya, 1967), it is the spontaneous immunotherapy, probably further amplified by the cell destruction caused by chemotherapy that eradicates the last remaining cancer cells.

However, one may equally ask whether a state of active immunity would not be able to facilitate the chemotherapy in these two tumors, and if the brilliant results might not be explained by the patients' immunity? If this was the case, could immunotherapy given before the chemotherapy enhance its effect?

Clifford *et al.* (1967) have indicated that in Burkitt's tumor the results of chemotherapy appear to be related to the strength of the patient's reaction to the disease. This led them to give irradiated tumor cells combined with adjuvants before chemotherapy. The results are at least encouraging, but not definitely convincing.

As it has been demonstrated that hepatomas (Tatarinov, 1964; Stanislawski-Birencwajg *et al.*, 1967) and some tumors of the alimentary tract (Gold and Freedman, 1965; Burtin *et al.*, 1965; Druet and Burtin, 1967) carry embryonic antigens, it would certainly be important to make attempts at immunotherapy using embryonic antigens. It should be remembered that these embryonic antigens are internal and not surface antigens.

The use of active immunotherapy in patients with immunodeficiency syndromes has, up until the present, only been exceptional. There is only the report of Sokal and Aungst (1969) who claimed that they restored the immune responses and enhanced survival in advanced stage IV Hodgkin's disease.

Czajkowski *et al.* (1967) have attempted to use in man a method for making tumor cells more antigenic which they previously devised in animals. The method consisted of chemically coupling the tumor cells to a highly antigenic foreign protein (rabbit γ-globulin) with bisdiazobenzidine and reinjecting this complex back into the tumor donor. Of the 14 patients treated, 2 had been, at the time of publication, tumor free for about 4 years; biopsies of their tumors revealed necrotic changes; 3 patients had shown stabilization or slow progression of tumor. Antibodies in high titers directed toward the tumors were demonstrated in 13 of these patients.

Hatanaka *et al.* (1968) obtained similar results by treating autologous tumor cells with mercapto undecahydroduodecabrate and using them as a vaccine. Cunningham *et al.* (1969) have treated 42 patients suffering from various cancers with autologous tumor cells coupled to rabbit γ-globulin. They only obtained one objective regression and were unable to obtain evidence for delayed hypersensitivity or humoral antibodies against the tumor extract.

Ayre (1969) treated women with *in situ* carcinoma of the cervix by injections of tumor cell proteins coupled to rabbit γ-globulins with bis-diazobenzidine, and has claimed tumor regression.

C. The Special Case of Antitumor Immunotherapy from Local Delayed Hypersensitivity Reaction to Another Antigen

E. Klein (1968, 1969) has treated skin cancer in man by indirect immunotherapy from local delayed hypersensitivity reactions to other antigens. He first used 2,3,5-triethyleneimino-(1,4)benzoquinone (TEIB) as a sensitizing agent, then dichloronitrobenzene. The latter has no direct cytostatic effect. He induced a cutaneous hypersensitivity to the agent by the daily topical application on the tumor of a cream containing the agent, and it often caused the skin tumor to regress. It is remarkable that the challenging dose causes a more intense reaction at the sites involved in cutaneous neoplasms than in the normal skin. When the concentration of this challenging dose was titrated carefully, the reaction was confined to the site of neoplastic involvement, with minimal or no reaction in the adjacent normal tissues. It is not resolved whether the removal of neoplastic cells by immune challenge reaction is related to qualitative or quantitative differences in the antigenic composition of normal cells and their malignant counterpart, or to a proportionately greater access of the sensitizer to neoplastic rather than normal cells.

Similar results were obtained in mycosis fungoides by Ratner *et al.* (1968), who used 2,4-dinitrochlorobenzene and 5,2-aminoethyliso-thiuronium.

IV. Conclusions and Perspectives

Although for a long time active immunization or immunostimulation has been thought of as a procedure for the prevention of cancer, its use in the therapy of an established tumor, or active immunotherapy, has sustained a lively interest during the past few years. The main reason lies not only in the failure of other methods of therapy available today, and the great need for a complementary treatment; but also it is the mode of action of active immunotherapy, which unlike other procedures, though it can only destroy a small number of tumor cells, can kill the last remaining cell.

Experimental studies of the effects of active immunotherapy applied after the establishment of a malignant growth are increasing, and the clinical trials, which are still few, are arousing great interest.

The further development of this method of therapy is going to depend on several research programs: (a) development of our knowledge of tumor-associated antigens in human cancers and the immunological reactions that they excite, especially those that are responsible for immunological enhancement which could lead to facilitation of tumor growth, the opposite to what is wanted; (b) efforts to discover and prepare new adjuvants; screening programs should be developed as for the direct cytostatic agents; (c) preparation of specific vaccines, which requires the culture of cells in bulk and the chemical characterization and purification of tumor-associated antigens; (d) operational research designed to evaluate in animals the place of active immunotherapy in the arsenal of weapons at our disposal for the treatment of cancer, and to carry out clinical trials in man that are scientific and at the same time ethical. These clinical trials should be proposed when their results in animals are well understood; the questions that are to be tested in animals should be influenced by the problems that have been raised by the results obtained in man. Active immunotherapy illustrates the need of the closest possible collaboration between experimental research and clinical research.

REFERENCES

Abelev, G. I., Perova, S. D., Khramkova, N. I., Postnikova, Z., and Irlin, I. S. (1963). *Transplantation* **1**, 174.

Alexander, P. (1970). Personal communication.

Allison, A. C. (1964). *Life Sci.* **3**, 1415.

Amiel, J. L. (1967). *Rev. Franc. Etud. Clin. Biol.* **12**, 912.

Amiel, J. L., and Bérardet, M. (1969a). *Rev. Fr. Etud. Clin. Biol.* **14**, 685.

Amiel, J. L., and Bérardet, M. (1969b). *Rev. Fr. Etud. Clin. Biol.* **14**, 912.

Amiel, J. L., and Bérardet, M. (1970). *Eur. J. Cancer* **6**, 557.

Amiel, J. L., Méry, A. M., and Mathé, G. (1967a). *In* "Cell-Bound Immunity with Special Reference to ALS and Immunotherapy of Cancer," Vol. 1, p. 197. Univ. Liège, Liège.

Amiel, J. L., Sékiguchi, M., Daguet, G., Garattini, S., and Palma, V. (1967b). *Eur. J. Cancer* **3**, 47.

Apffel, C. A., Arnason, B. G., Twinam, C. W., and Harris, C. A. (1966). *Brit. J. Cancer* **20**, 122.

Ayre, J. E. (1969). *Oncology* **23**, 177.

Bagshawe, K. D. (1969). *In* "Choriocarcinoma," Vol. 1, p. 180. Arnold, London.

Bagshawe, K. D., and Currie, G. A. (1968). *Nature (London)* **218**, 1254.

Bagshawe, K. D., and Golding, P. R. (1971). *In* "Immunity and Tolerance in Oncogenesis," Vol. 1, Publ. Div. Cancer Research, Perugia (in press).

Balner, H., Old, L. J., and Clarke, D. A. (1962). *Proc. Soc. Exp. Biol. Med.* **109**, 58.

Belisario, J. C., and Milton, G. W. (1961). *Aust. J. Dermatol.* **6**, 113.

Berger, F. M., Fukui, G. M., Ludwig, G. J., and Rosselet, J. P. (1968). *Proc. Soc. Exp. Med. Biol.* **127**, 556.

Berman, L. D., Allison, A. C., and Pereira, H. G. (1967). *Int. J. Cancer* **2**, 539.

Biozzi, G., Stiffel, C., Halpern, B. N., and Mouton, D. (1959). *C. R. Soc. Biol.* **153**, 987.

Biozzi, G., Stiffel, C., Halpern, B. N., and Mouton, D. (1960). *Rev. Fr. Etud. Clin. Biol.* **5**, 876.

Biozzi, G., Howard, J. G., and Stiffel, C. (1965). *Transplantation* **3**, 170.

Biozzi, G., Stiffel, C., Mouton, D., Oudier, Y., and Decreusefond, C. 1968. *Immunology* **14**, 7.

Blaney, D. J., Rotte, T. C., and Stier, V. E. (1964). *Surg. Gynecol. Obstet.* **118**, 341.

Bradner, W. T., Clarke, D. A., and Stock, C. C. (1958). *Cancer Res.* **18**, 347.

Braun, W. (1970). *In* "Progress in Antimicrobial and Anticancer Chemotherapy," Vol. 1, p. 17. Univ. of Tokyo, Tokyo.

Braun, W., and Kessel, R. W. I. (1964). *In* "Bacterial Endotoxins" (M. Landy and W. Braun, eds.), Vol. 1, p. 397. Rutgers Univ. Press, New Brunswick, New Jersey.

Braun, W., and Nakano, M. (1967). *Science* **157**, 819.

Braun, W., Lampen, J. O., Plescia, O. J., and Pugh, L. (1963). *In* "Conceptual Advances in Immunology and Oncology," Vol. 1, p. 450. Harper (Hoeber), New York.

Braun, W., Nakano, M., Jeroskova, L., Yajima, Y., and Jimenez, L. (1968). *In* "Nucleic Acids in Immunology," Vol. 1, p. 347. Springer, Berlin.

Braun, W. (1970). Personal communication.

Bredt, A. B., and Mardiney, M. R. (1969). *Transplantation* **8**, 763.

Burdick, K. H. (1960). *Arch. Dermatol.* **82**, 438.

Burdick, K. H., and Hawk, W. A. (1964). *Cancer* **17**, 708.

Burkitt, D. (1967). *Cancer* **20**, 756.

Burtin, P., von Kleist, S., Rapp, W., Loisillier, F., Bonatti, A., and Grabar, P. (1965). *Presse Med.* **73**, 2599.

Chanmougan, D., and Schwartz, R. S. (1966). *J. Exp. Med.* **124**, 363.

Cinader, B., Haylay, M. A., Rider, W. D., and Warwick, O. H. (1961). *Can. Med. Assn. J.* **84**, 306.

Clifford, P., Singh, S., Sternjwärd, J., and Klein, G. (1967). *Cancer Res.* **27**, 2578.

Coley, W. B. (1893). *Amer. J. Med.* **105**, 487.

Coley, W. B. (1911). *Surg., Gynecol. Obstet.* **13**, 174.

Cruse, J. M. (1967). *Z. Immunitaetsforsch., Allerg. Klin. Immunol.* **132**, 196.

Cudkowicz, G. (1968). *In* "Proliferation and Spread of Neoplastic Cells," Vol. 1. Williams & Wilkins, Baltimore, Maryland.

Cunningham, T. J., Olson, K. B., Laffin, R., Horton, J., and Sullivan, J. 1969. *Cancer* **24**, 932.

Currie, G. A., and Bagshawe, K. D. (1970). *Brit. Med. J.* **1**, 541.

Czajkowski, N. P., Rosenblatt, M., Cushing, F. R., Vazquez, J., and Wolf, P. L. (1966). *Cancer* **19**, 739.

Czajkowski, N. P., Rosenblatt, M., Wolf, P. L., and Vazquez, J. (1967). *Lancet* **2**, 905.

David, J., and Burkitt, D. (1968). *Brit. Med. J.* **4**, 288.

Deichman, E. I., and Kluchareva, T. E. (1964). *Nature (London)* **202**, 1126.

Denham, S., Grant, C. K., Hall, J. G., and Alexander, P. (1970). *Transplantation* **9**, 366.

Doniach, I., Crookston, J. H., and Cope, T. I. 1958. *J. Obstet. Gynaecol. Brit. Emp.* **65**, 553.

Donner, M., Oth, D., and Burg, C. (1970). *Abstr. Int. Cancer Congr., 10th, 1970* Vol. 1, p. 190.

Doré, J. F., Motta, R., Marholev, L., Hrsak, Y., Colas de la Noue, H., Seman, G., de Vassal, F., and Mathé, G. (1967). *Lancet* **2**, 1396.

Doré, J. F., Schneider, M., and Mathé, G. (1969). *Eur. J. Clin. Biol. Res.* **14**, 1003.

Doré, J. F., Ajuria, E., and Mathé, G. (1970). *Eur. J. Clin. Biol. Res.* **15**, 81.

Doré, J. F. *et al.* (1971). Unpublished data.

Druet, P. H., and Burtin, P. (1967). *Eur. J. Cancer* **3**, 327.

Dubost, R. J., and Schaedler, R. W. (1957). *J. Exp. Med.* **105**, 703.

Eddy, B. E. (1965). *In* "Slow, Latent and Temperate Virus Infections" (D. C. Gajdusek, C. J. Gibbs, Jr., and M. Alpers, eds.), Vol. 1, p. 369, N.I.N.D.B. Monogr. No. 2. Washington.

Eddy, B. E., Grubbs, G. E., and Young, R. D. (1964). *Proc. Soc. Exp. Biol. Med.* **117**, 575.

Emerson, J. D., and Emerson, G. M. (1965). *Fed. Proc., Fed. Amer. Soc. Exp. Biol.* **24**, 495.

Everson, T. C., and Cole, W. H. (1966). *In* "Spontaneous Regression of Cancer," Vol. 1, p. 164. Saunders, Philadelphia, Pennsylvania.

Fenyö, E. M., Klein, E., Klein, G., and Swiech, K. (1968). *J. Nat. Cancer Inst.* **40**, 69.

Ferrer, J. F. (1966). *Fed. Proc., Fed. Amer. Soc. Exp. Biol.* **25**, 614.

Ferrer, J. F., and Mihich, E. (1968). *Cancer Res.* **28**, 1116.

Finger, H., Emmerling, P., and Schmidt, H. (1967). *Experientia* **23**, 591.

Finney, J. W., Byers, E. F., and Wilson, R. H. (1960). *Cancer Res.* **20**, 351.

Floersheim, G. L. (1967). *Nature (London)* **216**, 1235.

Foley, E. J. (1953). *Cancer Res.* **13**, 835.

Fowler, G. A. (1969). Vol. 1, Monograph No. 9. Cancer Res. Inst., New York.

Freund, J. (1953). *In* "The Nature and Significance of the Antibody Response" (A. M. Pappenheimer, ed.), Vol. 1. Columbia Univ. Press, New York.

Freund, J., Lipton, M., and Thompson, G. E. (1955). *J. Exp. Med.* **101**, 591.

Galbraith, A. W., Oxford, J. S., Schild, G. C., and Watson, G. I. (1969). *Lancet* **2**, 1026.

Gershon, R. K., Carter, R. L., and Kondo, K. (1968). *Science* **159**, 646.

Glynn, J. P., Humphreys, S. R., Trivers, G., Bianco, A. R., and Goldin, A. (1963). *Cancer Res.* **23**, 1008.

Glynn, J. P., Halpern, B. L., and Fefer, A. (1969). *Cancer Res.* **29**, 515.

Gold, T., and Freedman, S. O. (1965). *J. Exp. Med.* **122**, 467.

Goldner, H., Girardi, A. J., and Hilleman, M. R. (1965). *Virology* **27**, 225.

Graham, J. B., and Graham, R. M. (1959). *Surg., Gynecol. Obstet.* **109**, 131.

Graham, J. B., and Graham, R. M. (1962). *Surg., Gynecol. Obstet.* **114**, 1.

Guyer, R. J., and Crowther, D. (1969). *Brit. Med. J.* **4**, 406.

Haddow, A., and Alexander, P. (1964). *Lancet* **1**, 452.

Hadziev, S., and Kavaklieva-Dimitrova, J. (1969). *Folia Med. Neer.* **11**, 8.

Halpern, B. N., Prevot, A. R., Biozzi, G., Stiffel, C., Mouton, D., Morard, J. C., Bouthillier, Y., and Decreusefond, C. (1964). *J. Reitculoendothel. Soc.* **1**, 77.

Hamilton-Fairley G. (1969). *Brit. Med. J.* **2**, 467.

Hatanaka, H., Sano, K., and Nagai, M. (1968). *Proc. Jap. Cancer Ass.* **27**, 284.

Hayat, M., and Mathé, G. (1971). *C. R. Acad. Sci.* **272**, 170.

Hellström, I. E., Hellström, K. E., Pierce, G. E., and Bill, A. H. (1968). *Proc. Nat. Acad. Sci. U. S.* **60**, 1231.

Hirano, M., Sinkovics, J. G., Shullenberger, C. C., and Howe, C. D. (1967). *Science* **158**, 1061.

Hiu, I. J., Amiel, J. L., and Jollès, P. (1969). *Rev. Fr. Etud. Clin. Biol.* **14**, 508.

Holland, J. F., and Glidewell, O. (1970). *In* "Advances in the Treatment of Acute (Blastic) Leukaemia" (G. Mathé, ed.), Vol. 1, p. 95. Springer, Berlin.

Hunter-Craig, I., Newton, K. A., Westbury, G., and Lacey, B. W. (1970). *Brit. Med. J.* **2**, 512.

Jerne, N. K., Nordin, A. A., and Henry, C. C. (1963). *In* "Cell-bound Antibodies" (B. Amos and H. Koprowski, eds.), Vol. 1, p. 109. Wistar Inst. Press, Philadelphia, Pennsylvania.

Johnson, A. G., Cone, R. E., Han, I., Johnson, H. G., Schmidtke, J. R., and Stout, R. D. (1970). *In* "Developmental Aspects of Antibody Formation and Structure" (J. Sterzl, ed.), Vol. 1. Academic Press, New York.

Jollès, P., Samour, D., and Lederer, E. (1962). *Arch. Biochem. Biophys., Suppl.* **1**, 283.

Jung Koo Youn, Barski, G., and Hupper, J. (1968). *C. R. Acad. Sci. Ser. D.* **267**, 816.

Kaliss, N. (1966). *Ann. N. Y. Acad. Sci.* **129**, 155.

Klein, E. (1968). *N. Y. State J. Med.* **68**, 900.

Klein, E. (1969). *Cancer Res.* **29**, 2351.

Klein, G. (1966a). *Annu. Rev. Microbiol.* **20**, 223.

Klein, G. (1966b). *In* "Viruses Inducing Cancer" (W. D. Burdette, ed.), Vol. 1, p. 323. Univ. of Utah Press, Salt Lake City, Utah.

Klein, G., Clifford, P., Klein, E., and Stjernswärd, J. (1966). *Proc. Nat. Acad. Sci. U. S.* **55**, 1628.

Klein, G., Klein, E., and Clifford, P. (1967). *Cancer Res.* **27**, 2510.

Kline, I., Gang, M., Tyrer, D. D., Mantel, N., Venditti, J. M., and Goldin, A. (1968). *Chemotherapy* **13**, 28.

Kobayashi, H., Sendo, F., Kaji, H., Shirai, T., Saito, H., Takeichi, N., Hosokawa, M., and Kodama, T. (1970). *J. Nat. Cancer Inst.* **44**, 11.

Krementz, E. T., Samuels, M., Wallace, J. H., and Benes, E. N. (1970). *Abstr. Int. Cancer Congr., 10th, 1970* Vol. 1, p. 202.

Kronman, B. S., Wepsic, H. T., Churchill, W. H., Jr., Zbar, B., Borsos, T., and Rapp, H. J. (1970). *Science* **168**, 257.

Lamensans, A., Stiffel, C. Mollier, M. F., Laurent, M., Mouton, D., and Biozzi, G. (1968). *Rev. Fr. Etud. Clin. Biol.* **13**, 773.

Lemonde, P., and Clode-Hyde, M. (1966). *Cancer Res.* **26**, 585.

Levy, J. P. (1969). *Actual. Hematol.* 200.

Lewis, M. G. (1967). *Lancet* **2**, 921.

Lewis, M. G., Ikonopisov, R. L., Nairn, R. C., Phillips, P. M., Hamilton-Fairley. G., Bodenham, D. C., and Alexander, P. (1969). *Brit. Med. J.* **3**, 547.

Lhéritier, D. D. *et al.* (1971). To be published.

Lin, J. S. L., and Murphy, W. H. (1969). *Cancer Res.* **29**, 2163.

Lindenmann, J., and Klein, P. A. (1967). *J. Exp. Med.* **126**, 93.

Long, D. A., and Miles, A. A. (1950). *Lancet* **1**, 492.

Macieira-Coelho, A., Brouty-Boyé, D., Thomas, M. T., and Gresser, I. (1971). *J. Cell Biol.* (in press).

Martin, D. S., Hayworth, P., Fugmann, R. A., English, R., and McNeill, H. W. (1964). *Cancer Res.* **24**, 652.

Martyré, M. C., and Halle-Pannenko, O. (1968). *Rev. Fr. Etud. Clin. Biol.* **13**, 1010.

Mathé, G. (1967). *C. R. Acad. Sci.* **264**, 2702.

Mathé, G. (1968). *Rev. Fr. Etud. Clin. Biol.* **13**, 881.

Mathé, G. (1969). *Brit. Med. J.* **4**, 7.

Mathé, G., and Bernard, J. (1956). *C. R. Soc. Biol.* **150**, 1768.

Mathé, G., Dausset, J., Hervet, E., Amiel, J. L., Colombani, J., and Brulé, G. (1964). *J. Nat. Cancer Inst.* **33**, 193.

Mathé, G., Amiel, J. L., Schwarzenberg, L., Schneider, M., Cattan, A., Schlumberger, J. R., Hayat, M., and de Vassal, F. (1968a). *Rev. Fr. Etud. Clin. Biol.* **13**, 454.

Mathé, G., Schneider, M., and Schwarzenberg, L. (1968b). *Rev. Fr. Etud. Clin. Biol.* **13**, 695.

Mathé, G., Amiel, J. L., Schwarzenberg, L., Schneider, M., Cattan, A., Schlumberger, J. R., Hayat, M., and de Vassal, F. (1969a). *Lancet* **1**, 697.

Mathé, G., Pouillart, P., and Lapeyraque, F. (1969b). *Brit. J. Cancer* **23**, 814.

Mathé, G., Amiel, J. L., Schwarzenberg, L., Schneider, M., Cattan, A., Hayat, M., de Vassal, F., and Schlumberger, J. R. (1970a). *In* "Advances in the Treatment of Acute (Blastic) leukaemia" (G. Mathé ed.), Vol. 1, p. 109. Springer, Berlin.

Mathé, G., Amiel, J. L., Schwarzenberg, L., Schneider, M., Hayat, M., de Vassal, F., Jasmin, C., Rosenfeld, C., Sakouhi, M., and Choay, J. (1970b). *Eur. J. Clin. Biol. Res.* **15**, 671.

Mathé, G., Pouillart, P., and Lapeyraque, F. (1971). *Experientia* (in press).

Mihich, E. (1969). *Cancer Res.* **29**, 2345.

Milton, G. W., and Brown, M. M. L. (1966). *Aust. N. Z. J. Surg.* **35**, 286.

Möller, E. (1965). *Science* **147**, 873.

Möller, G. (1964). *Nature (London)* **204**, 846.

Möller, G., and Möller, E. (1966). *Ann. N. Y. Acad. Sci.* **129**, 735.

Morton, D. L., and Eilber, F. R. (1970). Personal communication.

Morton, D. L., and Malmgren, R. A. (1968). *Science* **162**, 1279.

Morton, D. L., Malmgren, R. A., Holmes, E. C., and Ketcham, A. S. (1968). *Surgery* **64**, 233.

Morton, D. L. *et al.* (1970). Personal communication.

Nauts, H. C., Swift, W. E., and Coley, B. L. (1946). *Cancer Res.* **6**, 205.

Neveu, T., Branullec, A., and Biozzi, G. (1964). *Ann. Inst. Pasteur, Paris* **106**, 771.

Old, L. J. (1970). Personal communication.

Old, L. J., and Boyse, E. A. (1964). *Annu. Rev. Med.* **15**, 167.

Old, L. J., Clarke, D. A., and Benacerraf, B. (1959). *Nature (London)* **184**, 291.

Orbach-Arbouys, S. (1968a). *Rev. Fr. Etud. Clin. Biol.* **13**, 1013.

Orbach-Arbouys, S. (1968b). *Rev. Fr. Etud. Clin. Biol.* **13**, 1014.

Orbach-Arbouys, S. (1968c). *Rev. Fr. Etud. Clin. Biol.* **13**, 1017.

Osunkoya, B. O. (1967). *In* "The Treatment of Burkitt Tumour" (J. H. Burchenal and D. Burkitt, eds.), U.I.C.C. Monogr. Ser. No. 8, Vol. 1, p. 204. Springer, Berlin.

Parr, I. (1971). Personal communication.

Pelner, L. (1960). *J. Amer. Geriat. Soc.* **8**, 378.

Peries, J., Chaut, J. C., Canivet, M., and Boiron, M. (1966). *Nature (London)* **209**, 738.

Pouillart, P., and Mathé, G. (1970). Unpublished data.

Prehn, R. T. (1968). *Cancer Res.* **28**, 1326.

Prevot, A. R. (1965). *Pathol. Biol.* **13**, 321.

Ratner, A. C., Waldorf, D. S., and Van Scott, E. J. (1968). *Cancer* **21**, 83.

Rauscher, F. J., Fink, M. A., and Kvader, J. P. (1963). *J. Nat. Cancer Inst.* **30**, 654.

Regelson, W. (1967). *Advan. Exp. Med. Biol.* **1**, 315.

Regelson, W., and Munson, A. E. (1971). *Ann. N. Y. Acad. Sci.* (to be published).

Regelson, W., Munson, A., and Wooles, W. (1971). To be published.

Robinson, E., Shulman, J., Ben-Hur, N., Zuckerman, M., and Neuman, Z. (1963). *Lancet* **2**, 300.

Robinson, E., Ben-Hur, N., Zuckerman, H., and Neuman, Z. (1967). *Cancer Res.* **27**, 1202.

Schabel, F. M., Skipper, H. E., Laster, W. R., Jr., Trader, M. W., and Thompson, S. A. (1966). *Cancer Chemother. Rep.* **50**, 55.

Schneider, M. (1968). *Rev. Fr. Etud. Clin. Biol.* **13**, 877.

Schoenberg, M. D., and Moore, R. D. (1960). *Cancer Res.* **20**, 1505.

Sedallian, J. P., and Triau, R. (1968). *Lyon Med.* **220**, 101.

Shilo, M. (1960). *In* "Reticuloendothelial Structure and Function" (J. H. Heller, ed.), Vol. 1, p. 155. Ronald Press, New York.

Sjögren, H. O., and Hellström, I. (1965). *Exp. Cell Res.* **40**, 208.

Skipper, H. E., Schabel, F. M., and Wilcox, W. S. (1964). *Cancer Chemother. Rep.* **35**, 3.

Skurkovich, S. V., Kisljak, N. S., Machoniva, L. A., and Begunenko, S. A. 1969. *Nature (London)* **223**, 509.

Smith, L. H., and Woodruff, M. F. A. (1968). *Nature (London)* **219**, 197.

Sokal, J. E., and Aungst, C. W. (1969). *Cancer* **24**, 128.

Sokal, J. E., Aungst, C. W., and Grace, J. T. (1970). *Abstr. Int. Congr. Haematol. 13th.* Vol. 1, p. 278.

Sokoloff, B., Toda, Y., Fuyisawa, M., Enomoto, K., Saelhof, C. C., Bird, L., and Miller, C. (1961). *Growth* **25**, 249.

Southam, C. M. (1961). *Cancer Res.* **21**, 1302.

Stanislawski-Birencwajg, M., Uriel, J., and Grabar, P. (1967). *Cancer Res.* **27**, 1990.

Stevens, J. E., and Willoughby, D. A. (1967). *Nature (London)* **215**, 967.

Stück, B., Old, L. J., and Boyse, E. A. (1964). *Nature (London)* **202**, 1016.

Svet-Moldavsky, G. J., and Hamburg, V. P. (1964). *Nature (London)* **202**, 303.

Talmage, D. W., and Pearlman, D. S. (1963). *J. Theor. Biol.* **5**, 321.

Tatarinov, U. S. (1964). *Vop. Med. Khim.* **10**, 90.

von Leyden, E., and Blumenthal, F. (1902). *Deut. Med. Wochenschr.* **28**, 637.

Weiss, D. W., Bonhag, R. S., and de Ome, K. B. (1961). *Nature (London)* **190**, 889.

Weiss, D. W., Bonhag, R. S., and Leslie, P. (1966). *J. Exp. Med.* **124**, 1039.

White, R. G. (1967). *Int. Arch. Allergy Appl. Immunol.* **32**, 49.

Williams, A. C., and Klein, E. (1970). *Cancer* **25**, 450.

Willoughby, M. L. N. (1970). *Arch. Dis. Childhood* **45**, 600.

Wissler, R. W., Craft, K., Kesden, D., Polisky, B., and Dzoza, K. 1968. *In* "Advance in Transplantation" (J. Dausset and F. T. Rapaport, eds.), Vol. 1, p. 308. Munksgaard, Copenhagen.

Yoshida, T. O., and Imai, K. (1970). *Eur. J. Clin. Biol. Res.* **15**, 61.

Zbar, B., Wepsic, H. T., Borsos, T., and Rapp, H. J. (1970). *J. Nat. Cancer Inst.* **44**, 473.

THE INVESTIGATION OF ONCOGENIC VIRAL GENOMES IN TRANSFORMED CELLS BY NUCLEIC ACID HYBRIDIZATION

Ernest Winocour

Department of Genetics, Weizmann Institute of Science, Rehovot, Israel

I. Introduction

Polyoma virus, simian virus 40 (SV40), and some human adenoviruses induce tumors when inoculated into newborn rodents. In cells growing in tissue culture, these DNA-containing oncogenic viruses induce two types of response. In one type of response—known as the productive infection—the virus replicates and the cell is killed. In the second type of response, the infection is abortive in the sense that the replication of infectious virus and consequent cytopathic effects do not occur to a measureable extent. The progeny of the abortively infected cells display altered growth properties. When these new properties are stably inherited throughout many cell generations, the cells are considered to be transformed. The neoplastic potential of such transformed cells can be demonstrated by their ability to grow into tumors when implanted into

37

animals of the appropriate strain. This process of cell transformation by oncogenic viruses has been intensively studied in recent years as a model system for investigating the mechanisms of viral carcinogenesis (see reviews by Defendi, 1966; Sachs, 1967; Black, 1968; Dulbecco, 1969; Schlesinger, 1969; Crawford, 1969; Winocour, 1969; Green, 1970).

A central issue that has dominated our thinking on the possible mechanisms of viral carcinogenesis concerns the presence, the state, and the role of viral genetic material in the transformed cell. Naturally occurring production of infectious virus is an extremely rare event in most transformed cells. However, several lines of evidence have pointed to, or established the persistence of viral genes in all transformed cells and their descendants. The transformed cells display new antigenic determinants which are specific to the virus which induces the transformation. For example, the sera of animals bearing virus-induced tumors contain antibodies which react, by complement fixation or immunofluorescence, with a new antigen, (the "T-antigen") that appears in the nuclei of all transformed cells, all abortively infected cells, and all productively infected cells (Huebner et al., 1963; Black et al., 1963; Pope and Rowe, 1964; Habel, 1966). The T-antigens induced by polyoma virus, SV40, and adenoviruses do not cross-react immunologically; but T-antigens induced by the same virus in different host species do cross-react. The T-antigens are not related to viral structural proteins. Although there is no unequivocal proof that T-antigens are in fact viral *coded* products, their specificity with respect to the infecting virus makes this a strong possibility. Another antigenic marker characteristic of transformed cells is the transplantation antigen which is demonstrated by the rejection of transformed cell implants in animals preimmunized with the same transformed cells or with the respective transforming virus (Habel, 1961; Sjögren et al., 1961). This antigen, too, is not related to any virion component and is specific to the virus which induced the transformation. Hence, specific antigenic "fingerprints" induced by the virus persist in the transformed cell.

A second line of evidence which has established the presence of a viral genome is the demonstration that under certain conditions, infectious virus can be recovered from some transformed cells. Gerber and Kirschstein (1962) and Sabin and Koch (1963) were the first to report the recovery of infectious virus when SV40-transformed cells were cultivated together with permissive cells (cells of a species which readily supports viral multiplication). Subsequently, it was shown that the recovery of infectious virus was enhanced by cell fusion (Harris and Watkins, 1965) between SV40-transformed cells and permissive cells (Gerber, 1966; Koprowski et al., 1967; Watkins and Dulbecco,

1967). A "spontaneous" activation of infectious virus production, which was enhanced by cell fusion with permissive cells, has been found in a line of rat cells transformed by polyoma virus (Fogel and Sachs, 1969). It was also found that infectious virus production, in this line of cells, could be activated by X-irradiation (Fogel and Sachs, 1969), mitomycin C, and UV-irradiation (Fogel and Sachs, 1970). Activation of virus production has been shown to occur following temperature shift in a line of mouse cells transformed by a thermosensitive mutant of polyoma virus (Vogt, 1970). No infectious virus has been recovered from adenovirus-transformed cells by cell fusion or any other technique. Thus, the recovery of infectious virus has been demonstrated principally in SV40-transformed cells and in two lines of polyoma-transformed cells. The reason for the failure to recover infectious virus in most polyoma-transformed cells, and in all adenovirus-transformed cells, is not known. One possible explanation is that many of these cells may have been transformed by defective virus particles; another possible reason is that transforming virus, although fully infectious initially, may end up as a defective genome in the transformed cells.

The third line of evidence for the persistence of viral genes in the transformed cells is based upon the chemical identification, by means of nucleic acid hybridization techniques, of virus-specific nucleotide sequences in the genome of the transformed cell. Several important advantages can be derived from the use of this approach. The viral genome can be identified irrespective of whether it is defective or not; information can be obtained on the physical state and intracellular location of the viral genome; and information can be obtained on the transcription (and hence the expression) of the viral genes. In this review, we will survey the knowledge that has been obtained so far, by the use of the nucleic acid hybridization techniques, on the location, state, and functioning of viral genes in cells transformed by polyoma virus, SV40, and adenoviruses. The primary purpose of this survey is not encyclopedic, but rather to accentuate those aspects which we believe are relevant to an understanding of the role of the viral genes in the transformed cells, and which appear to us to be promising areas for future research.

The basis for nucleic acid hybridization techniques was established in 1961 when it was shown that hybrid complexes could be formed between different single-stranded DNA molecules (Schildkraut et al., 1961) or between single-stranded DNA and RNA molecules (Hall and Spiegelman, 1961) provided there was a sufficient degree of complementarity (homology) between the base sequences of the interacting polynucleotide chains. The reader is referred to reviews by Thomas (1966), Walker (1969), and McCarthy and Church (1970) for a discussion of the theoretical aspects of these reactions. In most of the experiments to be discussed here, the hybridization technique used is that devised by Gillespie and Spiegelman (1965; see also Gillespie, 1968). In essence, this method consists of immobilizing single-stranded DNA on a nitro-cellulose filter and incubating the DNA filter with radioactive single-stranded DNA or RNA in solution, under temperature and salt conditions which favor the formation of specific hybrid complexes. The amount of complex formed is measured by counting the amount of radioactive DNA or RNA which is bound to the DNA on the filter.

II. Viral DNA Sequences in the DNA of Transformed Cells

In this section we describe first the types of hybridization procedures that have been developed for the identification of viral DNA in the transformed cell genome. We then discuss the information that has been obtained by these techniques on the amount, location, and state of the viral DNA in the transformed cell.

A. HYBRIDIZATION PROCEDURES FOR THE DETECTION OF VIRAL DNA SEQUENCES IN TRANSFORMED CELLS

Hybridization techniques for the detection of viral-specific nucleotide sequences in the cellular genome must be endowed with a high degree of sensitivity. A mammalian cell contains, on the average, 10^{-5} μg. of DNA. A molecule of SV40 or polyoma DNA weighs 5×10^{-12} μg. (calculated from a molecular weight of 3×10^6 daltons). Hence, one molecule of viral DNA per transformed cell would represent only one part in 2×10^6 parts of cell DNA. For the adenoviruses (molecular weight of the DNA = $\sim 23 \times 10^6$ daltons) one molecule of viral DNA per transformed cell would represent one part in 260,000 parts of cell DNA. Table I summarizes the types of hybridization reactions used for the detection of viral genomes in transformed cells. The sensitivity of the procedure is dependent upon the specific activity of the radioactive component and the background level of "hybridization" to the DNA of control cells.

The most commonly used procedure exploits radioactive, complementary RNA (cRNA) that is synthesized *in vitro* using viral DNA as a primer for the DNA-dependent RNA polymerase (reaction 1, Table I). Filters containing single-stranded immobilized DNA (Gillespie and Spiegelman, 1965) derived from transformed cells, or control cells, are incubated with a solution of the radioactive viral cRNA in 0.9 M NaCl at 65–67°C. for 18 to 30 hours. The filters are then washed, treated with RNase to remove nonspecifically bound viral cRNA, and counted for the amount of radioactive cRNA which remains complexed to the

TABLE I
HYBRIDIZATION REACTIONS FOR THE DETECTION OF VIRAL DNA IN THE DNA
OF TRANSFORMED CELLS

Reaction number	Hybridization between:		References
	Radioactive RNA or DNA in solution	Nonradioactive DNA on filters[a]	
1.	Synthetic cRNA (made from viral DNA)[b]	Transformed cell DNA Control cell DNA[c]	Winocour (1965); Reich et al. (1966); Westphal and Dulbecco, (1968); Sambrook et al. (1968); Tai and O'Brien (1969); Green et al. (1971); A. S. Levine et al. (1970).
2.	Viral DNA	Transformed cell DNA Control cell DNA[c]	Axelrod et al. (1964); zur Hausen and Schulte-Holthausen (1970).
3.[d]	Transformed cell DNA Control cell DNA[c]	Viral DNA	Aloni (1967); (Section II,B,2, this review).

[a] Gillespie and Spiegelman (1965) procedure. In the techniques used by Winocour (1965) and A. S. Levine et al. (1970) both the radioactive cRNA and the nonradioactive DNA were in solution; the resulting hybrid complexes were isolated by filtration through a nitrocellulose filter (Nygaard and Hall, 1964, procedure).

[b] Complementary RNA synthesized in vitro off a DNA template by a DNA-dependent RNA polymerase. The reaction may be written: radioactive ATP, UTP, CTP, GTP $\xrightarrow[\text{DNA template}]{\text{RNA polymerase}}$ radioactive cRNA. The enzyme is usually of bacterial origin. Using ^{3}H-labeled nucleoside triphosphate, cRNA of high specific activity (5×10^6 cpm/ μg.) can be obtained.

[c] DNA from normal cells or from cells transformed by a virus (or agent) other than that being investigated.

[d] This hybridization reaction is best carried out in two stages (see Section II,B,2).

DNA on the filter. The presence of viral genomes in the transformed cell should result in an increased level of hybridization between viral cRNA and transformed cell DNA. The sensitivity of the procedure is calibrated by reconstruction experiments which measure the ability of radioactive viral cRNA to hybridize with control DNA containing known amounts of added viral DNA (in a range of proportions from 1 part viral DNA in 2×10^5 to 2×10^6 parts of control DNA). The above procedure can be extremely sensitive, mainly owing to the very high specific activity of the radioactive viral cRNA. However, a serious problem arises from the fact that there is a variable loss of immobilized DNA (and consequently of hybrid complex) from the filter during the

incubation at 65–67°C. The amount of viral cRNA in solution is greatly
in excess of the possible amounts of viral DNA present in the transformed cell DNA immobilized on the filter. Hence, relatively small
variations in the amounts of transformed and control cell DNA's immobilized on the filter will produce significant differences in the amounts
of radioactive cRNA bound. The total amount of DNA remaining on
the filter at the end of the hybridization reaction must therefore be
measured and the amounts of cRNA bound "normalized" to a constant
amount of DNA. The variable loss of DNA from the filter may be
reduced by hybridizing at low temperatures in the presence of formamide (Bonner *et al.*, 1967). A more precise control of the amount of
DNA in the reaction has been obtained by A. S. Levine *et al.* (1970)
using hybridization between ^{3}H-labeled SV40-cRNA and ^{14}C-labeled
transformed cell DNA in aqueous solution (Nygaard and Hall, 1964).
It should be noted that the hybridization techniques based upon reaction
1 in Table I are dependent on the assumption that all viral DNA
sequences are transcribed by the RNA polymerase during the *in vitro*
synthesis of cRNA.

The DNA-DNA hybridization procedures (reactions 2 and 3, Table I)
are independent of any assumptions made concerning the quality and
nature of *in vitro* synthesized cRNA. Reaction 3 has the added advantage
that variations in the amount of viral DNA on the filter (and variable
loss from the filter) do not seriously affect the results since the amount
of viral DNA on the filter is greatly in excess of the amount of viral
DNA sequences likely to be present in the transformed cell DNA fragments in solution. The lack of routine nuclease digestion procedures, for
the elimination of mismatched regions in the DNA-DNA duplex, is the
main disadvantage of the DNA-DNA hybridization procedures. This
problem can be partly overcome through the use of short fragments of
radioactive DNA.

The results of all hybridization procedures for the detection of viral
genomes in transformed cells are relative to those obtained in the control
reactions. Thus, the background level of "hybridization" to control DNA
is a crucial factor. Exceptional care must obviously be taken to ensure
that the viral DNA is completely free of cellular DNA contamination.
Rigorous purification of the virus is not by itself sufficient since during
the replication of polyoma virus, host cell DNA fragments are enclosed
within a proportion of the particles (pseudovirions) (Winocour, 1967,
1968, 1969; Kaye and Winocour, 1967; Michel *et al.*, 1967). Pseudovirions also appear during the replication of SV40 in *some* host cell
species (Trilling and Axelrod, 1970; A. J. Levine and Teresky, 1970).
The purification of polyoma and SV40 DNA's must therefore include

steps for the removal of any encapsidated host DNA. Most of these procedures take advantage of the supercoiled configuration (form 1) of polyoma and SV40 DNA (see Crawford, 1969). The linear host DNA is effectively removed by velocity sedimentation techniques, preferably in alkaline gradients (Vinograd *et al.*, 1963); or by equilibrium centrifugation in cesium chloride density gradients supplemented with ethidium bromide (Radloff *et al.*, 1967); or by methylated albumin-kieselguhr chromatography of the DNA after a brief heat-treatment which selectively denatures host cell DNA, in contrast to supercoiled viral DNA (Sheinin, 1966). A special problem exists in the case of SV40 DNA where there is evidence indicating that some of the supercoiled DNA molecules may contain host DNA in covalent linkage. This problem will be discussed further in Section II,C.

B. The Number and State of the Viral Genomes

1. *SV40-Transformed Mouse Cells*

The presence of SV40-specific sequences in the DNA of three lines of mouse 3T3 cells transformed by SV40 (Table II) has been investigated by Westphal and Dulbecco (1968) using radioactive SV40-cRNA. The level of hybridization of SV40 ^{3}H-cRNA to these DNA's was 1.4 to 3-fold greater than the level of hybridization to the control DNA (the nontransformed parent 3T3 cell line or 3T3 cells transformed by polyoma virus). Although the levels of increased homology to transformed cell DNA (relative to control DNA) were not always large, they were consistently obtained in a large number of replicate hybridization reactions. From reconstruction experiments, Westphal and Dulbecco (1968) estimated that the SV40-transformed 3T3 mouse lines contained 7–44 viral DNA equivalents per cell. The presence of only four viral DNA equivalents per SV40-transformed mouse 3T3 cell has been reported by A. J. Levine *et al.* (1970) using a modified hybridization procedure with a high degree of sensitivity.

The location and state of the SV40 DNA in SV40-transformed 3T3 cells (clone SV3T3-47) has been studied by Sambrook *et al.* (1968). The DNA from SV40-transformed cells, and the DNA from polyoma-transformed 3T3 cells as a control, were fractionated according to various criteria and tested for their ability to hybridize with SV40-cRNA. The main results obtained can be summarized as follows: (a) The SV40 DNA in the transformed cells does not exist in a supercoiled form since the fraction which hybridizes with SV40 cRNA bands with linear DNA in a cesium chloride–ethidium bromide gradient; (b) chromosomes isolated from metaphase SV40-transformed cells contain DNA which hybridizes

TABLE II

NUMBER OF VIRAL DNA EQUIVALENTS IN THE DNA OF CELLS TRANSFORMED
BY SV40, POLYOMA VIRUS, AND ADENOVIRUSES

Trans-forming virus	Cell line	Recovery of infectious virus[a]	No. of viral DNA equivalents	References
SV40	Hamster: T-1-1-7	+	100	Aloni (1967) and see Section II,B,2, this review.[b]
	T-1-1-2	+	100	
	T-6	+	100	
	T-11	+	100	
	T-1-1-7	+	20	Reich et al. (1966)[c]
	T-2-2	+	20	
	T-5	+	20	
	BHK(A8)	?	20	
	T-1-1-7	+	64	Tai and O'Brien (1969)[d]
	H50	−	58	Westphal and Dulbecco (1968)[c]
	H50	−	9	A. S. Levine et al. (1970)[e]
	2675	+	5	
	1808	−	2	
	Mouse: SV3T3-47	+	20	Westphal and Dulbecco (1968)[c]
	SV3T3-56[f]	−	7	
	SVPy. 3T3-11[g]	+	44	
	SV3T3 479	+	4	A. S. Levine et al. (1970)[e]
Polyoma	Mouse: SVPy. 3T3-11[g]	−	10	Westphal and Dulbecco (1968)[c]
	Hamster: Py. 8(BHK)	−	7	
Adeno 12	Hamster	−	53–60	Green et al. (1971)[c]
Adeno 2	Rat	−	22–30	

[a] By the technique of cell fusion with permissive cells (Koprowski et al., 1967; Watkins and Dulbecco, 1967).

[b] The hybridization procedure was the two-stage DNA-DNA hybridization procedure described in Section II,B,2.

[c] DNA-cRNA hybridization in which the tumor and control DNA's (immobilized on filters) were hybridized with radioactive cRNA synthesized from viral DNA.

[d] Same method as (c) but hybridization was at room temperature in the presence of formamide.

[e] Same method as (c) but hybridization of the cRNA and the DNA was carried out in solution.

[f] These 3T3 mouse cells were transformed by nitrous acid-treated SV40.

[g] Mouse 3T3 cells transformed by both SV40 and polyoma. This "double-transformed" line displays both SV40 and polyoma-specific T-antigens (Todaro et al., 1965).

with SV40 cRNA; (c) high molecular-weight DNA isolated from SV40-transformed cells by alkali treatment followed by alkaline sucrose gradient sedimentation (110 S region of the gradient) hybridized with SV40 cRNA. In each case, the level of hybridization was about 2.5 times greater than that obtained with DNA from polyoma-transformed 3T3 cells which was isolated or fractionated in an identical manner. From reconstruction experiments, the SV40-transformed cells were found to contain 20 viral DNA equivalents. If these were joined end-to-end in linear array, the resulting complex of molecular weight 60×10^6 daltons would be expected to sediment in the 50 S region of the alkaline sucrose gradient. Supercoiled complexes, which have a fast sedimentation rate in alkaline sucrose gradients, were excluded by the CsCl–ethidium bromide centrifugation experiment. On the basis of these factors, Sambrook *et al.* (1968) conclude that the state of the SV40 DNA in the transformed cell is linear and linked (in an alkali-stable form) to chromosomal DNA.

2. SV40-Transformed Hamster Cells

The presence of SV40 DNA in SV40-transformed hamster cells has been investigated by Aloni (1967) using a DNA-DNA hybridization reaction (reaction 3, Table I). ^{32}P-DNA was extracted from randomly labeled transformed cells and fragmented by sonic vibration into small segments of molecular weight ca. 5×10^5 daltons; after denaturation, the ^{32}P-DNA fragments were tested for their ability to hybridize with SV40 DNA immobilized on filters (relative to the ability of ^{32}P-DNA fragments from control cells). Since the proportion of viral DNA fragments in the population of DNA fragments from the transformed cell was expected to be very small (1 in 2×10^6 to 1 in 2×10^4 for transformed cells containing 1–100 viral DNA copies) very high inputs of ^{32}P-DNA were used in these reactions. Out of 50×10^6 cpm of ^{32}P-DNA, only 25 cpm to 2500 cpm can be expected to be in viral DNA sequences, assuming 1–100 viral DNA copies per tranformed cell (and assuming random ^{32}P-labeling). The requirement for high radioactive inputs to the reaction resulted, as expected, in high background levels of radioactive DNA bound to filters containing control DNA or no DNA. This difficulty was overcome by carrying out the hybridization reaction in two stages. In stage 1, large amounts of ^{32}P-DNA from SV40-transformed cells or control cells were hybridized with SV40 DNA on a filter; the bound ^{32}P-DNA was then eluted (by heating the filter in a boiling solution of 0.015 M NaCl) and tested for its ability to rehybridize with SV40 DNA or control DNA (step 2). The reconstruction experiment in Table III shows that 58–71% of the ^{14}C-SV40 DNA present in the original mixture (input to stage 1) was recovered by

TABLE III

RECOVERY OF ^{14}C-SV40 DNA IN THE TWO-STAGE DNA-DNA HYBRIDIZATION METHOD[a]

| | | Stage 2: rehybridization | | % recovery of ^{14}C-SV40 DNA |
| | | cpm bound to filter | | |
Mixture in stage 1 hybridization	DNA on filter	^{32}P	^{14}C	
1. ^{32}P-mouse DNA + ^{14}C-SV40 DNA	SV40	253	283	71
(60 × 10^6 cpm) (400 cpm)	Polyoma	164	0	
	None	127	0	
2. ^{32}P-mouse DNA + ^{14}C-SV40 DNA	SV40	300	600	60
(60 × 10^6 cpm) (1000 cpm)	Polyoma	152	0	
	None	153	0	
3. ^{32}P-mouse DNA + ^{14}C-SV40 DNA	SV40	412	1732	58
(60 × 10^6 cpm) (3000 cpm)	Polyoma	172	0	
	None	143	0	

[a] Three equal samples of ^{32}P-mouse DNA (60 × 10^6 cpm; 10^5 cpm/μg.) were mixed with 400 cpm, 1000 cpm, and 3000 cpm of ^{14}C-SV40 DNA (10^4 cpm/μg.). After fragmentation and denaturation, each of the three mixtures was incubated with one SV40 DNA filter (stage 1); the radioactive DNA was then eluted and rehybridized (stage 2) with filters containing 10 μg. SV40 DNA, 10 μg. polyoma DNA, or no DNA. The experiment was carried out exactly as described in Table IV. On a radioactive count basis (^{14}C: ^{32}P) the three starting mixtures contained, respectively, 13, 30, and 100 viral genome equivalents. The data are taken from Aloni (1967).

rehybridization to SV40 DNA in stage 2. The ratio of viral DNA to cellular DNA in the population of radioactive DNA fragments incubated in stage 2 is thus increased enormously compared to the ratio in the original incubation mixture of stage 1. Table IV summarizes the results of experiments to detect viral-specific sequences in the DNA of SV40-transformed hamster cells using the two-stage DNA-DNA hybridization method. Four different lines of SV40-transformed hamster cells were tested; hamster cells transformed by polyoma virus, or by the chemical carcinogen dimethylnitrosamine, or by X-irradiation, served as controls. It will be noted that the fraction of the stage 2 input which was bound to SV40 DNA was significantly higher for DNA derived from each of the four SV40-transformed cell lines (8.9–11.1%) compared to the fraction bound to SV40 DNA for DNA from the four control cell lines (2.3–4.6%). There was thus a significantly increased level of homology between SV40 DNA and the DNA of SV40-transformed cells. From reconstruction experiments in which mixtures containing various proportions of ^{3}H-cell DNA and ^{3}H-viral DNA were subjected to the two-stage DNA-DNA

TABLE IV

SV40-Transformed Hamster Cells: Detection of Viral DNA Base Sequences by Means of a Two-Stage DNA-DNA Hybridization Test[a]

³²P-DNA from hamster cells transformed by:	Stage 1: hybridization		Stage 2: rehybridization			
	Input cpm × 10⁻⁶	cpm bound to SV40 DNA filter × 10⁻³	Input cpm × 10⁻³	cpm bound to filter with:		Percent of input which binds specifically to SV40 DNA
				SV40 DNA	Polyoma DNA	
SV40; cell lines;						
T-1-1-2	55	45	12.0	1238	115	9.15
T-1-1-7	51	29	5.9	703	46	11.10
T-6	35	41	7.6	760	83	8.90
T-11	43	27	6.7	716	90	9.35
Polyoma; cell lines;						
LP-11	19	22	6.7	400	91	4.60
SP-2	5	7	1.1	45	14	3.00
Dimethylnitrosamine	18	26	5.8	320	90	4.00
X-irradiation	14	9	1.7	100	60	2.30

[a] Hamster cells transformed by SV40 (Black, 1966) polyoma virus, the chemical carcinogen dimethylnitrosamine (Huberman et al., 1968), and X-irradiation (Borek and Sachs, 1966) were labeled with ³²P (1.0 mC/plate; specific activity 75 C/mg. P) for 4 days. The ³²P nucleic acids were extracted by the SDS-phenol procedure (Dulbecco et al., 1965), fragmented by sonic vibration, and dialyzed against 0.3 N KOH for 12 hours at room temperature and against 3 × SSC (5 changes) for 24 hours. By this procedure ³²P-RNA was removed and the ³²P-DNA was denatured. The specific activity of each of the ³²P-DNA preparations was 7–8 × 10⁵ cpm/μg. DNA. In stage 1 hybridization, each of the hamster ³²P-DNA's was incubated (60°C., 24 hours) with 10 μg. of denatured SV40 DNA (component 1) immobilized on a nitrocellulose membrane filter. At the end of incubation, the filters were washed extensively in 3 × 10⁻³ M tris buffer, pH 9.4 (Warnaar and Cohen, 1966) and the amount of ³²P-DNA bound was determined. For stage 2 (rehybridization) the bound ³²P-DNA was eluted from each SV40 DNA filter by boiling each filter individually for 5 minutes in 2 ml. of 0.01 × SSC. Essentially 100% of the ³²P-DNA was eluted into the solution by this step. The ³²P-DNA samples were then rehybridized with filters containing 10 μg. of SV40 DNA, or 10 μg. of polyoma DNA. See Aloni et al. (1969) and Table V for fuller details of the DNA-DNA hybridization technique. In the final column, the percentage values were calculated from

$$100 \times \frac{\text{cpm bound to SV40 DNA} - \text{cpm bound to polyoma DNA}}{\text{stage 2 input cpm}}$$

The data are from Aloni (1967).

hybridization procedure, a 2-fold increase in hybridization over the controls (cell DNA with no added virus DNA) was obtained at a ratio of 1 part virus DNA per 20,000 parts of cell DNA. From this, it would appear that the four lines of SV40-transformed hamster cells contain approximately 100 viral DNA equivalents per cell. The data in Table IV also show that SV40 DNA (form 1) will bind ^{32}P-DNA from the control cells to a greater extent compared to polyoma DNA. This phenomenon will be discussed further in Section II,C.

The presence of SV40 DNA in SV40-transformed hamster cells has also been investigated by the SV40 cRNA–cell DNA hybridization procedure (Reich et al., 1966; Westphal and Dulbecco, 1968; Tai and O'Brien, 1969; A. S. Levine et al., 1970). Values of from 2 to 64 viral DNA equivalents per cell have been reported (Table II). It will be noted from Table II that the values reported by A. S. Levine et al. (1970) are considerably lower than those reported by other workers. The reason for this is not clear. Information on the location and state of the SV40 DNA in transformed hamster cells has not been reported so far.

3. Polyoma-Transformed Mouse and Hamster Cells

Using hybridization reactions between polyoma cRNA and polyoma-transformed mouse and hamster cell DNA, Westphal and Dulbecco (1968) report low levels of hybridization, corresponding to 5–10 viral DNA equivalents per cell (Table II). An early attempt (Winocour, 1965) to detect polyoma DNA in the DNA of two polyoma-induced transplantable mouse tumors produced negative results; the calibration experiments indicated that the level of polyoma DNA, if present in these tumors, must· be less than 20 viral DNA equivalents per cell. Using a DNA-DNA hybridization procedure (reactions 2, Table I) Axelrod et al. (1964) reported that radioactive polyoma DNA fragments were bound by polyoma mouse tumor DNA immobilized in agar (Bolton and McCarthy, 1962) to a greater extent compared to the fraction bound by control DNA. The data reported on the relationship between the input of viral DNA per unit of immobilized cell DNA, and the amount of viral DNA bound per unit of immobilized cell DNA, suggest that the homology to polyoma tumor cell DNA was not due to the presence of random cell DNA fragments in the viral DNA preparation. It is difficult, however, to interpret the results quantitatively since no calibration experiments were reported.

4. Adenovirus-Transformed Rat and Hamster Cells

Using radioactive cRNA, synthesized from the appropriate adenovirus DNA template, Green and his associates (1971) have studied the presence and number of viral DNA copies in various adenovirus-transformed rat and hamster cells. All the transformed cells possessed a large number of viral DNA equivalents; 53–60 in the case of adenovirus 12-transformed hamster cells, 22–30 in adenovirus 2-transformed rat cells (Table II). Green et al. (1971) also report that the transformed cell DNA which hybridizes with adenovirus cRNA is localized in the cellular chromosomes.

5. *Burkitt Lymphoma Cells and the Epstein-Barr Virus*

A herpes-type virus has been detected in some tissue culture lines of cells, derived originally from Burkitt lymphomas (Epstein et al., 1964). This DNA-containing virus, now known as the Epstein-Barr virus (EBV) has been partially purified (A. Weinberg and Becker, 1969; Schulte-Holthausen and zur Hausen, 1970). Although the role of EBV in the etiology of Burkitt lymphomas has not been established, immunological evidence points to a relationship (Klein et al., 1968). In some of the cell lines established from Burkitt lymphomas, no EBV can be detected by electron microscopy and immunofluorescent techniques (Epstein et al., 1966). The possibility that the DNA of one of these "virus-free" cell lines (The Raji line) might contain base sequences homologous to EBV-DNA has recently been investigated (zur Hausen and Schulte-Holthausen, 1970). Using DNA-DNA hybridization (reaction 2, Table I), these authors found that the binding between radioactive EBV-DNA and Raji cell DNA was 4-fold greater than the binding between radioactive EBV-DNA and the DNA of human KB cells, or hamster cells. A larger number of "virus-free" Burkitt lymphoma cell lines and a larger number of control cell lines will have to be tested before the significance of these hybridization tests can be evaluated.

C. THE HOMOLOGY BETWEEN SV40 DNA AND CELL DNA

As mentioned above, one of the crucial factors affecting the sensitivity of the nucleic acid hybridization procedures for the study of viral genomes in transformed cells is the background level of apparent hybridization to the DNA of normal cells. Using DNA-DNA hybridization tests, Aloni et al. (1969) found that significant levels of SV40 DNA were bound by normal monkey DNA. In contrast, there was no detectable binding between SV40 DNA and chicken DNA, bacteriophage T4 DNA, and *Escherichia coli* DNA. (Some of these results are summarized in Table V.) There is a considerable body of evidence which shows that the binding of SV40 DNA to monkey cell DNA is not due to contamination of the viral DNA preparations by cell DNA. For example, SV40 DNA still binds to monkey cell DNA after it has been subjected to a variety of procedures

TABLE V

DNA-DNA Hybridization Tests Between Cellular DNA and SV40 DNA[a]

³H-DNA in solution	DNA on filter	cpm bound to filter	% of input bound
1. Monkey cell (BS-C-1)	Monkey (10 μg.)	2976	21.4
14,000 cpm/reaction	SV40 (10 μg.)	971	7.0
(= 0.5 μg.)	Polyoma (10 μg.)	12	0.09
	Escherichia coli (10 μg.)	9	0.06
	None	8	0.06
2. SV40	SV40 (10 μg.)	12,800	85
15,000 cpm/reaction	Monkey (50 μg.)	750	5
(= 0.1 μg.)	*Escherichia coli* (50 μg.)	12	0.08
	None	10	0.07

[a] DNA-DNA hybridization was carried out as described by Aloni *et al.* (1969). Briefly, nitrocellulose membrane filters carrying the denatured immobilized DNA (Gillespie and Spiegelman, 1965) were first preincubated for 6 hours in a solution of 3 × SSC containing 0.04% bovine serum albumin (Denhardt, 1966) and then incubated at the same temperature with the radioactive, fragmented, denatured DNA (M.W. = ∼ 700,000 daltons). At the end of incubation the filters were washed extensively with 0.003 M tris-HCl buffer, pH 9.4 (Warnaar and Cohen, 1966) and assayed for the amount of radioactive DNA bound. The SV40 DNA (form I) was purified by MAK chromatography in experiment 1 (Gershon *et al.*, 1966) and by sedimentation in alkaline sucrose gradients (Sambrook and Shatkin, 1969) in experiment 2. The data in experiment 1 are taken from Aloni *et al.* (1969); those in experiment 2 are from Lavi and Winocour (1970).

which specifically select for the supercoiled component (form 1) (Aloni *et al.*, 1969; Lavi and Winocour, 1970) ; and SV40 DNA duplexes, reassociated from single-stranded fragments after 30 minutes incubation at 60°C, showed, upon subsequent denaturation, the same capacity to bind to monkey DNA as unfractionated SV40 DNA fragments (under the same conditions of DNA concentration, ionic strength, and time at 60°C, monkey DNA fragments did not reassociate to a detectable extent).

A question may arise concerning the specificity of the homology detected by DNA-DNA hybridization between SV40 DNA and cell DNA. Conceivably, very short sequences of bases, randomly distributed in the SV40 genome, might by chance be homologous to parts of the mammalian cell genome. However, preliminary experiments (Lavi and Winocour, 1970) indicate that this is unlikely. As shown in Table VI, the proportion of SV40 DNA fragments which binds to monkey DNA is related to the size of the SV40 DNA fragments in the reaction. The binding of the ⅕th and ¹⁄₁₅th molecular weight fragments (about 1000 and 300 base pairs long, respectively) was very sharply reduced compared to that of the complete genome (about 5000 base pairs). A further reduction in size to

TABLE VI

Size of SV40 DNA Fragments and the Percentage Bound by Monkey DNA[a]

³H-SV40 DNA in solution	cpm incubated	DNA on filter	cpm bound to filter as percentage of input	percent bound, monkey
				SV40
Single-stranded circles	10,000	SV40 (10 µg.)	87	17.2
(complete genome of		Monkey (50 µg.)	15	
~ 5000 base pairs)		None	0.1	
⅕th M.W. fragments	10,460	SV40	85	4.7
(~ 1000 base pairs)		Monkey	4	
		None	0.1	
$\frac{1}{15}$th M.W. fragments	10,704	SV40	77	2.5
(~ 300 base pairs)		Monkey	1.9	
		None	0.1	
$\frac{1}{50}$th M.W. fragments	14,500	SV40	71	2.1
(~ 100 base pairs)		Monkey	1.5	
		None	0.1	
< $\frac{1}{50}$th M.W. fragments (< 100 base pairs)	12,200	SV40	75	2.5
		Monkey	1.9	
		None	0.1	

[a] Single-stranded (circular) SV40 DNA was obtained by treating supercoiled SV40 DNA with dilute pancreatic DNase (5×10^{-5} µg./ml.) under conditions where 60% of the double-stranded molecules received a single random cut. The single-stranded circular molecules were then isolated by sedimentation in alkaline sucrose gradients (Sambrook and Shatkin, 1969). The ⅕th and $\frac{1}{15}$th molecular weight fragments were obtained by subjecting supercoiled SV40 DNA to different periods of sonic vibration; the $\frac{1}{50}$th and < $\frac{1}{50}$th molecular weight fragments were obtained by treating the sonic-disrupted fragments with dilute pancreatic DNase (5×10^{-3} µg./ml.) for various times. Fractionation according to size was carried out in 5–20% neutral sucrose gradients (containing 1 M NaCl) calibrated with 20 S SV40 DNA (form 1) and 4 S tRNA markers. DNA-DNA hybridization was carried out as described in Table V. The data are from Lavi and Winocour (1970).

$\frac{1}{50}$th and to < $\frac{1}{50}$th of the genome (< 100 bases) *produced no further change in the proportion of fragments bound.* If the homology to cell DNA was due to the presence of short complementary sequences, randomly distributed throughout the SV40 genome, we would expect the proportion bound to cell DNA to be affected only when very small fragments (well below 300 bases long) are incubated. The results shown in Table VI suggest that the sequences in SV40 DNA which are complementary to cell DNA are of the order of 300 bases long; and that these complementary stretches are not distributed at random in the SV40 DNA molecule. It has not, so far, been possible to determine if *every*

SV40 DNA molecule contains a stretch of sequences homologous to cell DNA. The presence of the cell homologous sequences might be confined to "defective" SV40 DNA molecules which acquired a small segment of host DNA during replication.

Results which are at variance with those described above have been obtained by A. S. Levine *et al.* (1970). Using cRNA synthesized from SV40 DNA (by a bacterial RNA polymerase) these authors found that the level of hybridization to monkey cell DNA was no higher than the level of hybridization to mycoplasma or *Escherichia coli* DNA. One possible reason for the lack of detectable homology between SV40 cRNA and monkey DNA may be that the bacterial RNA polymerase does not transscribe (or transcribes poorly) the cell DNA homologous sequences that are present in *some* SV40 DNA molecules. Whatever the explanation is, it is clear from the work of A. S. Levine *et al.* (1970) that SV40 cRNA can be prepared which shows an insignificant level of background homology to cell DNA; this cRNA is therefore a valuable reagent for the detection of SV40 DNA sequences in the transformed cell DNA.

The significance of the cell DNA homologous sequences found in some SV40 DNA molecules requires further investigation. Nevertheless, it is tempting to postulate that the integration of such molecules into the host DNA may be facilitated, or enhanced, by the stretch of homologous sequences. Supercoiled polyoma DNA displays only a very small degree of binding to rodent DNA (barely 2-fold over the degree of binding to the bacterial DNA used as a control; Aloni *et al.*, 1969). It has been suggested that both the higher transformation frequencies obtained with SV40, and the larger number of viral DNA equivalents in the DNA of SV40-transformed cells (cf. polyoma transformed cells; Table II) may be due to an enhanced probability for integration which is related to the more abundant prevalence of cell DNA-virus DNA homologous sequences in SV40 DNA (Winocour, 1970).

D. The Integration of the Viral DNA

Can one obtain any direct evidence for integration of viral DNA shortly after the infection of the cells? This problem has been studied by Doerfler (1968, 1971) using adenovirus 12 and baby hamster kidney (BHK) cells. The interaction between adenovirus 12 and BHK cells leads to an abortive infection which gives rise to a small proportion of transformed cells (see Schlesinger, 1969). The strategy employed was to infect BHK cells (previously grown in medium with 5-bromodeoxyuridine) with ^{3}H-thymidine labeled adenovirus 12; the intracellular DNA of the infected cell was then analyzed by equilibrium centrifugation in alkaline cesium chloride density gradients. In such gradients the bromouracil-substituted BHK cell DNA can be separated from adenovirus 12 DNA. Doerfler found that 30% of the cell-associated ^{3}H-label had shifted into the density region of the cell DNA. Three explanations for this density shift were considered: (a) viral ^{3}H-DNA was degraded to mononucleotides and the ^{3}H-TMP was reutilized in cellular DNA synthesis, (b) viral DNA replicated in the presence of 5-bromodeoxy-uridine and consequently acquired a higher buoyant density sufficient to shift it into the density region of the cell DNA, (c) viral DNA became covalently linked (integrated) with cellular DNA. Evidence against possibilities (a) and (b) was obtained from the following experiments. After fragmentation, the ^{3}H-DNA isolated from the density region characteristic of cell DNA shifted to an intermediate density position; the ^{3}H-DNA, from the cellular DNA region of the density gradient, hybridized predominently to viral DNA and only to a minor extent with cellular DNA; the shift of the ^{3}H-label into the density region characteristic of cellular DNA was not affected when DNA synthesis, in the infected cell complex, was strongly inhibited ($> 96\%$) by cytosine arabinoside. In addition, it was shown that adenovirus 12 DNA does not replicate in BHK cells. Therefore, it was concluded that the shift of the ^{3}H-label into the density region of cell DNA resulted from the integration of adenovirus 12 DNA (or fragments thereof) into BHK cell DNA (Doerfler, 1968, 1971). The mechanism by which the "integration event" occurs has yet to be explored; but it is significant that it can proceed in the absence of cellular DNA synthesis. Experiments of a similar nature have been carried out by zur Hausen and Sokol (1969) on Nil-2 Syrian hamster cells infected with ^{3}H-thymidine-labeled adenovirus 12. In Nil-2 cells, it was found that a substantial fraction of the absorbed ^{3}H-adenovirus was degraded after infection and that part of the viral DNA degradation products were reutilized for cellular DNA synthesis. Nevertheless, evidence was obtained by DNA-DNA hybridization analysis of the ^{3}H-labeled DNA in the cellular DNA region of the density gradient that some viral DNA (probably small fragments) was inserted into cellular DNA.

III. Transcription of the Viral Genome in the Transformed Cells

In the preceding sections we have discussed the evidence for the continuous presence of viral DNA in transformed cells. We now turn to the transcription of the viral genome with particular reference to the identification and control of viral gene activity.

A. THE CODING POTENTIAL OF ONCOGENIC VIRUS DNA

On the basis of the molecular weights of polyoma, SV40, and adeno-virus DNA's, an estimate can be made of the number of average-sized (20,000–50,000 daltons) polypeptides that can be coded for by the viral

DNA. This estimate ranges from 3 to 8 for polyoma or SV40 DNA and 24 to 60 for adenovirus DNA (Table VII).

Since the major viral coat proteins are not synthesized in the transformed cell, we may next enquire as to the proportion of the viral genome required for the synthesis of the viral capsid structure. Studies on the polyoma capsid (Thorne and Warden, 1967; Fine *et al.*, 1968; Kass, 1970) indicate that it contains one major species of polypeptide of molecular weight 45,000–50,000. Some evidence of a low molecular weight (around 13,000) minor polypeptide component has also been obtained (Fine *et al.*, 1968). From the complementation analysis of

TABLE VII

CODING POTENTIAL OF ONCOGENIC DNA VIRUSES

	Polyoma or SV40	Adenovirus
M.W.[a]	3×10^6	23×10^6
No. of base pairs[b]	4,700	36,000
No. of amino acids[c]	1,600	12,000
M.W. of total number of amino acids	160,000	1,200,000
No. of polypeptides[d] (of M.W. 20,000–50,000)	3 to 8	24 to 60

[a] See Crawford (1969); Schlesinger (1969); Green *et al.* (1971).

[b] Taking the average molecular weight of a nucleotide as 320.

[c] At a coding ratio of 3 nucleotides to 1 amino acid.

[d] Equivalent to the number of viral cistrons. Polyoma capsid protein contains a single major polypeptide component of molecular weight 45,000–50,000 and possibly one low-molecular weight minor component. Complementation analysis of polyoma temperature-sensitive mutants points to the existance of two cistrons which are involved in the synthesis of viral structural components (Eckhart, 1969; Di Mayorca *et al.*, 1969).

temperature-sensitive polyoma mutants (Eckhart, 1969; Di Mayorca *et al.*, 1969), two of the four complementation groups appear to be involved in the synthesis of viral structural proteins (Di Mayorca *et al.*, 1969). Thus, approximately one-third of the polyoma viral genome is required to code for viral capsid protein and this fraction may involve two distinct viral cistrons. The studies of Anderer *et al.* (1967) on the SV40 capsid proteins suggest the presence of three distinct polypeptides with a total molecular weight of about 50,000. Again, approximately one-third of the viral genome would be required for the synthesis of the SV40 capsid structure. On the basis of these figures, the number of polyoma and SV40 viral genes left for involvement in the transformation process is limited. The adenovirus virion proteins present a much more complex picture (see Schlesinger, 1969). At least nine polypeptide components have been distinguished by gel electrophoresis (Maizel *et al.*, 1968a,b). From the total molecular weights of the virion polypeptides it can be estimated that approximately one third of the adenovirus DNA is required for their synthesis.

B. THE QUANTITY, LOCATION, AND SIZE OF VIRAL mRNA IN TRANSFORMED CELLS

By hybridization experiments between purified viral DNA and labeled cellular RNA, virus-specific RNA has been detected in rodent cells transformed by polyoma virus, SV40, and the adenoviruses (Tables VIII–X). The quantity of polyoma or SV40-specific RNA found in transformed cells is small. It represents only a fraction of a percent of the cellular RNA species labeled during 3–98 hours (Table VIII). The detection of this small amount of viral RNA can, however, be greatly enhanced by means of two successive hybridization steps (Aloni *et al.*, 1968). In this procedure, the radioactive RNA which binds to viral DNA in step 1 is eluted and rehybridized to a second sample of viral DNA in step 2. Under these conditions, 62% of the radioactive RNA in the second hybridization reaction can be shown to bind to SV40 DNA (Table IX). Considerably larger amounts of virus-specific RNA have been detected in adenovirus-transformed cells (Table VIII). Using

TABLE VIII

AMOUNT OF VIRUS-SPECIFIC RNA IN CELLS TRANSFORMED BY SV40, POLYOMA VIRUS, AND ADENOVIRUSES

Transforming virus	Transformed cells	Labeling time (hours)	Cell fractions	Percent of total labeled RNA which is virus-specific	Reference
SV40	Mouse 3T3	6	Whole cells	0.01	Aloni *et al.* (1968)
		96	Whole cells	0.003	
SV40	Mouse 3T3	3	Nuclear	0.002–0.02	Lindberg and
			Polyribosomes	0.02–0.04	Darnell (1970)
Polyoma	Mouse 3T3	4	Whole cells	0.005–0.017	Benjamin (1966)
	Hamster	4	Whole cells	0.003	
	Rat	4	Whole cells	0.002–0.015	
Adenovirus-12	Hamster	3	Nuclear	0.20–0.27	Fujinaga and
		3	Polyribosomes	0.27	Green (1967)
		3	Whole cells	0.13–0.19	
Adenovirus-12	Hamster	0.5	Polyribosomes	1.3	Fujinaga and Green (1966)

TABLE IX
REHYBRIDIZATION OF VIRUS-SPECIFIC RNA ISOLATED FROM MOUSE 3T3 CELLS
TRANSFORMED BY SV40[a]

First step hybridization: ^{32}P-RNA from 3T3 (SV40) mouse cells			Second step hybridization: ^{32}P-RNA eluted from SV40 DNA filter in step 1		
DNA on filter	cpm bound	cpm bound as % of input	DNA on filter	cpm bound	cpm bound as % of input
SV40 (5 μg.)	13,760	0.0088	SV40 (10 μg.)	4010	62
None	2,688	0.0017	Polyoma (10 μg.)	57	0.8
			3T3 cell (3 μg.)	160	2.5
			none	71	1.1

[a] Data from Aloni et al. (1968). Mouse 3T3 cells transformed by SV40 were labeled with ^{32}P for 22 hours. The ^{32}P-RNA was extracted and (step 1) incubated with filters containing SV40 DNA or no DNA. After incubation at 66°C. for 24 hours, the filters were treated with RNase, washed, and counted for the amount of ^{32}P-RNA bound. In step 2, the ^{32}P-RNA bound to the SV40 DNA filter was eluted (the filter was boiled for 3 minutes in 0.01 × SSC to dissociate the hybrid), purified by filtration through a series of blank filters and tested for its ability to rehybridize with a second SV40 DNA filter or filters containing control DNA's.

short labeling periods, it has been estimated that some 2–5% of the labeled RNA in the polyribosomes is virus-specific (Fujinaga and Green, 1966) and it has been suggested that viral genes may in fact be preferentially transcribed in the adenovirus-transformed cells (Green et al., 1971). Virus-specific RNA has been detected both in the nuclear and cytoplasmic fractions. The association of the virus-specific RNA with cytoplasmic polyribosomes has been demonstrated for SV40-transformed cells (Lindberg and Darnell, 1970), and for adenovirus-transformed cells (Fujinaga and Green, 1967) and thus this criterion for a functional messenger RNA has been satisfied (in the following discussion, the terms virus-specific RNA and viral messenger RNA, or mRNA, are used synonymously.

The size of the viral mRNA molecules in SV40-transformed mouse cells has recently been studied by Lindberg and Darnell (1970). Labeled RNA from the nuclear and cytoplasmic fractions was sedimented in a sucrose gradient; various fractions from the gradient were then tested for their ability to hybridize with SV40 DNA. SV40-specific sequences were detected in a variety of RNA molecular species—in polyribosomal RNA sedimenting at 6–30 S, in nuclear RNA sedimenting at 30–45 S, and in nuclear RNA sedimenting faster than 45 S. Use of a disaggregating agent did not alter the sedimenting pattern of the RNA species containing sequences complementary to SV40 DNA. Although discrete size classes of SV40 mRNA species were not obtained, it is interesting to note the existence of large RNA molecules which contain SV40-specific sequences. Double-stranded SV40 DNA has a molecular weight of 3×10^6 daltons. A transcript of one complete genome (~ 5000 bases) would be expected to sediment at about 28 S. Hence, the large nuclear RNA molecules which contain virus-specific sequences and which sediment at > 45 S, contain a considerably larger number of bases than that present in the SV40 genome. The Lindberg and Darnell experiments can be interpreted in several ways. The SV40 mRNA associated with cytoplasmic polyribosomes may be cleaved from a larger nuclear precursor molecule. The large SV40-specific nuclear RNA could arise either from the transcription of several integrated viral genes in tandem array or from the transcription of integrated viral DNA and contiguous cell DNA. In fact, the demonstration that large nuclear RNA molecules from transformed cells contain cell DNA-complementary sequences covalently linked to viral-specific sequences would be elegant proof of the chromosomal integration of viral genes. Green *et al.* (1971) have also reported that some adenovirus 2-specific RNA in adeno 2-transformed cells is larger than the transcript of a complete adenovirus 2 genome. It is also interesting to note that virus-specific RNA molecules larger than the transcript of the complete viral genome have recently been detected in cells productively infected with SV40 (R. A. Weinberg and Winocour, 1970) and polyoma virus (Hudson *et al.*, 1970).[1]

C. The Proportion of the Viral Genome Transcribed

The evidence to be discussed in this section indicates that in most transformed cells only a part of the viral genome is transcribed into RNA. In the following section we will consider which part of the viral genome undergoes transcription in such cases.

The numerical fraction of the viral genome transcribed in productively infected cells serves as a reference in the estimation of the fraction transcribed in the transformed cells. The proportion of the viral genome transcribed in productively infected cells can be estimated from RNA-DNA hybridization-saturation experiments. Increasing amounts of labeled RNA are hybridized with a known, constant amount of viral DNA until all sites available for hybridization on the DNA are saturated. The amount of DNA saturated with RNA can be calculated from the specific activity of the viral mRNA. If 50% of the amount of viral DNA in the hybridization test is saturated with viral mRNA then, on the basis that transcription is asymetric, 100% of the viral genome is transcribed. In productively infected cells, DNA-RNA saturation

---

[1] *Note added in proof:* Tonegawa *et al.* (1971) have presented additional evidence for the occurrence of large SV40-specific RNA molecules in the nuclei of productively infected monkey cells and in the nuclei of transformed mouse cells.

experiments have indicated that essentially the entire polyoma genome
(M. A. Martin and Axelrod, 1969a) and the entire SV40 genome (Aloni
et al., 1968; M. A. Martin and Axelrod, 1969b) are transcribed. The
DNA-RNA hybridization-saturation method depends, however, on
knowing the specific activity of the viral mRNA in the productively
infected cells. This can only be estimated in a general way from the
specific activity of all the species of RNA synthesized in the cell. A
novel way out of this difficulty has been devised by Fujinaga *et al.*
(1968). In this method, the denatured viral DNA is first hybridized with
saturating amounts of radioactive RNA from infected cells and then
challenged with radioactive viral DNA in a subsequent DNA-DNA
hybridization test. If the viral mRNA contains sequences complementary
to the entire viral genome, the subsequent challenge of the RNA-DNA
complex with radioactive viral DNA will be inhibited by 50%. The
results of this method are thus independent of assumptions made as
to the precise specific activity of the viral mRNA. With adenovirus 2

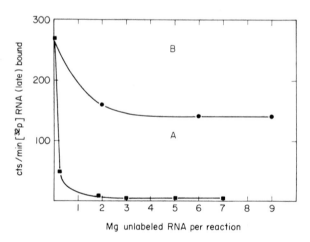

Mg unlabeled RNA per reaction

Fig. 1. Hybridization competition between ³²P-RNA from SV40-infected monkey
(BS-C-1) cells and unlabeled RNA from SV40-transformed mouse 3T3 cells. Curve
A: each reaction mixture contained one SV40 DNA filter, one blank filter, 5×10^6
cpm ($= 30$ μg.) of ³²P-RNA extracted from BS-C-1 cells labeled from 2–72 hours
postinfection, and increasing amounts of unlabeled RNA extracted from BS-C-1
cells at 72 hours postinfection (control experiment for full competition). Curve B:
each reaction mixture contained one SV40 DNA filter, one blank filter, 5×10^6 cpm
($= 30$ μg.) of ³²P-RNA extracted from BS-C-1 cells labeled from 2 to 72 hours postinfection, and increasing amounts of unlabeled RNA extracted from SV40-trans-
formed mouse 3T3 cells. The amount of ³²P-RNA bound to the blank filters has
been subtracted from the values plotted for the amounts bound to the SV40 DNA
filter. The amount of ³²P-RNA bound to SV40 DNA in the absence of unlabeled
RNA was 270 cpm (this is a saturation level). (From Aloni *et al.*, 1968).

and adenovirus 12 productively infected cells, it was found that 80–100% of the viral genome was transcribed (Green *et al.*, 1971).

Knowing the numerical fraction of the genome transcribed in productively infected cells, the fraction transcribed in transformed cells can then be estimated by competitive hybridization between the two viral mRNA's. An example of this type of test is shown in Fig. 1. The data indicate that only about one third of the sites on SV40 DNA which bind mRNA from productively infected cells, bind mRNA from transformed cells and hence that only about one third of the SV40 genome is transcribed in the transformed cell. Table X summarizes the estimates reported by various workers of the fraction of the viral genome transcribed in cells transformed by polyoma virus, SV40, and adenovirus 2. Complete transcription of the viral genome has been demonstrated in one case; that of mouse Balb c cells transformed by SV40 (M. A. Martin and Axelrod, 1969b). Since SV40 DNA and coat protein are not synthesized in these cells, it would appear that the control of viral gene activity must be exerted at some point beyond the transcription process. In all the other transformed cells examined, the transcription of the viral genome appeared to be restricted.

From Table X it can be seen that there is considerable variation in the reported levels of SV40 DNA transcription in mouse 3T3 cells (29–66%, excluding special cases such as 3T3 cells transformed by both SV40 and polyoma or by UV-inactivated SV40). It is unlikely that this degree of variation can be ascribed to differences in hybridization techniques. The cultural conditions under which the transformed cells were grown (such as cell density) might affect the level of transcription. The transcription of the SV40 genome may also vary in different clonal isolates of the transformed 3T3 cell population. It will also be noted from Table X that the transcription is severely restricted in some cases. In one polyoma-induced, transplantable mouse tumor, only 20% of the viral genome was found to be transcribed (M. A. Martin and Axelrod, 1969a); in adenovirus 2-transformed rat cells, only 4–10% of the viral genome was transcribed (Fujinaga and Green, 1970). It should be noted, however, that infectious virus has not been recovered, by the cell-fusion technique, from the polyoma and adenovirus-transformed cells listed in Table X. Hence, the "restriction" on transcription might well be due to the presence of only part of the viral DNA in these cells. In SV40-transformed mouse 3T3 cells, this argument cannot be applied since infectious virus has been recovered from cells in which only one third of the viral genome was detectably transcribed. Viral gene activity in these cells may therefore be controlled, at least in part, at the level of transcription. It is also important to note that Sauer and Kidwai (1968)

TABLE X

PROPORTION OF THE VIRAL GENOME TRANSCRIBED IN TRANSFORMED CELLS

Virus	Transformed cells	Recovery of infectious virus[a]	Percent of viral genome transcribed[b]	Reference
SV40	Mouse 3T3 (SV-10/1)[c]	+	31–37	Aloni et al. (1968)
	Mouse 3T3	+	29	Oda and Dulbecco (1968)
	Mouse 3T3	+	40	Sauer and Kidwai (1968)
	Monkey AGMK[d]	+	80	Sauer and Kidwai (1968)
	Monkey AGMK[e]	−	80	Sauer and Kidwai (1968)
	Mouse Balb c(SV-T2)	+	100	M. A. Martin and Axelrod (1969b)
	Mouse 3T3 (SV-Py-11)	+	82	M. A. Martin and Axelrod (1969b)
	Mouse 3T3 (SV-935c)	±	66	M. A. Martin and Axelrod (1969b)
	Mouse 3T3 (SV-UV-15-5)[f]	−	30	M. A. Martin and Axelrod (1969b)
	Mouse 3T3 (SV-UV-30-1)[f]	−	38	M. A. Martin and Axelrod (1969b)
Polyoma	Hamster tumor	−	40	M. A. Martin and Axelrod (1969b)
	Mouse tumor	−	20	M. A. Martin and Axelrod (1969a)
Adenovirus 2	Rat embryo	−	4–10	Fujinaga and Green (1970)

[a] Infectious virus recovered by the technique of cell fusion with permissive cells (Koprowski et al., 1967; Watkins and Dulbecco, 1967).

[b] The figures refer to the percentage amount of homology with the viral RNA present in productively infected cells. Since in productively infected cells the entire viral genome is transcribed (that is, 50% of the double-stranded viral DNA), the figures also indicate the percent of the viral *genome* transcribed in transformed cells.

[c] The information in brackets is the line, or clone designation (where given by the authors).

[d] Derived from African Green Monkey kidney (AGMK) cells. Although these cells cannot be successfully superinfected with SV40, they yield infectious virus after fusion with sensitive cells.

[e] A clonal derivative of SV40-transformed AGMK cells which does not yield infectious virus after fusion with sensitive cells.

[f] Transformed by UV-irradiated virus.

found the same level of viral genome transcription (80%) in two lines of SV40-transformed monkey (AGMK) cells although infectious virus was recovered only from the parent line and not from the clonal derivative of the parent line (Table X).

We are therefore faced with a highly variable pattern of viral DNA transcription in different transformed cells. The factors which give rise to this variability are unknown. In SV40-transformed cells, the control of viral gene activity appears to be exerted both at the level of transcription and at some point beyond the transcription process. We have also noted previously that, on the basis of size, the SV40 or polyoma genome may contain only 3–8 genes. If, in some transformed cells, mRNA is transcribed from only 20 to 30% of the viral genome, then only 1 or 2 viral genes would appear to be involved in the maintenance of the transformed state. By the same calculation, only 1–5 adenovirus 2 genes seem to be required for the maintenance of the transformed phenotype induced by this virus (Green et al., 1971).

D. The Common Sequences in Viral mRNA's from Productively Infected and Transformed Cells

Where viral genome transcription is restricted in the transformed cell (relative to productively infected cells) it is of interest to determine *which* sections of the viral genome are transcribed. During the productive infection of monkey cells by SV40, two classes of virus-specific RNA have been distinguished on the basis of hybridization competition (Aloni et al., 1968); Sauer and Kidwai, 1968; Oda and Dulbecco, 1968) and base composition (Aloni et al., 1968). Class I appears before the onset of virus DNA replication ("early" viral mRNA); class II appears after the onset of viral DNA replication ("late" viral mRNA). "Early" viral RNA can be obtained in small quantities from the infected cells before the onset of viral DNA replication. Larger quantities of "early" viral RNA can be obtained by treating infected cells with inhibitors of viral DNA replication (Carp et al., 1969); or by infecting cells with "hybrid" virus such as the E46+ recombinant adeno-SV40 (enclosed in a adeno-7 capsid) which expresses only "early" SV40 functions (Oda and Dulbecco, 1968). The isolation of "late" RNA, free of "early" RNA, is a much more difficult problem. The difficulty is that "early" RNA persists late in the infectious cycle. The temporal relationship cannot, therefore, be used as the sole basis for the isolation of "late" RNA. Recently, R. A. Weinberg and Winocour (1970) showed that there are two distinct types of SV40 mRNA's in the cytoplasm of productively infected cells, sedimenting at 16 S and 19 S. When viral DNA replication was inhibited (by treating the infected cells with low levels of actinomycin

D or with cytosine arabinoside) the 19 S species of viral homologous RNA was found to accumulate relative to the 16 S species. This result suggests that the 16 S species is a "late" viral mRNA and that the 19 S species is an "early" viral mRNA. Thus, it may be possible to isolate "late" viral mRNA, free of "early" viral mRNA, on the basis of size.

Hybridization competition experiments between viral mRNA from transformed cells, "early" mRNA from productively infected cells, and "early + late" mRNA from productively infected cells, have indicated that "early" viral genes predominate in the transformed cell (Oda and Dulbecco, 1968; Fujinaga and Green, 1970). "Early" viral mRNA from productively infected cells and viral mRNA from transformed cells are not, however, completely identical; differences in base composition have been detected (Aloni et al., 1968); some "early" mRNA sequences are not present in transformed cells (Oda and Dulbecco, 1968; Fujinaga and Green, 1970); and some sequences present in SV40-transformed cells are not found in the "early" RNA from productively infected cells (Oda and Dulbecco, 1968). In adenovirus 2-transformed cells, all the viral sequences transcribed are present also in the "early" viral mRNA from productively infected cells (Fujinaga and Green, 1970).

E. Is There a Common Viral Gene Expression in Cells Transformed by Different Oncogenic DNA Viruses?

In view of the relatively small number of viral genes transcribed in transformed cells, the question arises as to the possible presence of a viral "oncogene" which the tumor viruses may hold in common. The evidence available to date does not support the concept of a common viral "oncogene." There is no significant homology between the viral mRNA's found in cells transformed by different viruses. For example, 3T3 mouse cells transformed by polyoma contain no RNA which detectably hybridizes with SV40 DNA (Benjamin, 1966) and SV40-transformed 3T3 cells contain no RNA which detectably hybridizes with polyoma DNA (Benjamin, 1966; Aloni et al., 1968). 3T3 cells transformed by *both* SV40 and polyoma contain species of RNA which will hybridize with both viral DNA's (Benjamin, 1966). No significant homology between polyoma and SV40 DNA's has been observed (Winocour, 1965). The human adenoviruses can be divided into three families on the basis of the degree of their oncogenicity for rodent cells (see Green et al., 1971). Members of the same family share 70–100% of their DNA base sequences in common. Members of different families share 9–35% of their DNA base sequences. Despite some degree of cross-homology between members of different families, the viral mRNA's in cells transformed by *members of different families show no detectable cross-homology* (Fujinaga *et al.*, 1969; Green *et al.*, 1971). Thus, in this case, too, the evidence does not support the concept of a common viral "oncogene."

IV. Discussion and Conclusions

A. The State of the Viral Genome in Transformed Cells

The nucleic acid hybridization experiments described in Section II have supplied evidence that viral DNA persists in the transformed cell and its descendents. Is this viral DNA integrated into chromosomal DNA or does it exist as an extrachromosomal, self-replicating entity? The experiments of Sambrook *et al.* (1968) (see Section II,B,1), on the state of the SV40 DNA in transformed mouse 3T3 cells favor the chromosome integration hypothesis. Benjamin (1968) found no evidence, by DNA-DNA hybridization, for the presence of polyoma-specific base sequences in the *mitochondrial* DNA of polyoma-transformed mouse cells. Further confirmation of the chromosomal location of viral genes may arise out of current studies on the giant nuclear RNA from transformed cells if it should be shown that such molecules contain both cell-specific and virus-specific sequences in covalent linkage.

There is no *a priori* reason to assume that the state of the viral genome is identical in all transformed cells; or that it is irreversibly fixed in any one line of transformed cells. Under some conditions, the genome may be released from its site on the chromosome and be converted into an extrachromosomal, self-replicating form. Autonomously replicating, extrachromosomal entities are known in bacteria (Freifelder, 1968; Ikeda and Tomizawa, 1968; Matsubara and Kaiser, 1968). In this respect, it would be of interest to determine the state of the viral genome in transformed cells which are "exceptional" in the sense that virus production can be activated by temperature shift (Vogt, 1970) or mitomycin C and UV treatment (Fogel and Sachs, 1970). Polyoma-transformed cells which have lost some characteristics of the transformed phenotype ("revertants") have been described (Rabinowitz and Sachs, 1968; Pollack *et al.*, 1968). The loss of transformed properties in these "revertant" cells is not associated with a loss of the viral genome (Rabinowitz and Sachs, 1968). Perhaps a change in the state (or transcription) of the viral genome is involved in the reversion process.

The nucleic acid hybridization experiments (Section II,B) have also indicated that multiple copies of the viral genome are present in most transformed cells. The results of these experiments are expressed in terms of viral DNA equivalents since there is no way of knowing how many (if any) of the multiple copies are *complete* viral DNA copies (the recovery of infectious virus by the cell-fusion technique can be interpreted in two ways: either that at least one of the copies is complete or else that a variety of incomplete copies functionally complement each other). One may enquire as to how these multiple copies are distributed in the cellular genome. Some evidence suggesting that the viral genomes are distributed over many chromosomes has been obtained from studies on the loss of the SV40 T-antigen from somatic hybrids between mouse cells and SV40-transformed human cells (Weiss, 1970). During passage in culture, the hybrid cells tend to lose the SV40-transformed human parent chromosomes. The presence or absence of T-antigen in the hybrid cells can therefore be correlated with the number of human chromosomes. It was observed that loss of the T-antigen in the hybrid cells occurred only after most of the human chromosomes had been lost. This result argues quite strongly that the SV40-determinants involved, directly or indirectly, in the synthesis of T-antigen must have been distributed over a large number of the human chromosomes.

One may next enquire as to the distribution of the viral genomes in any given chromosome. The possibility that two or more viral genomes are arranged in tandem has been raised by some authors. The polyoma viral DNA that is synthesized as a result of a temperature shift, in 3T3 cells transformed by a thermosensitive mutant of polyoma, is unusual in that a proportion of the newly made DNA consists of closed-circular oligomeric forms (Cuzin et al., 1970). These oligomeric forms could arise from the excision of genomes arranged in tandem. The observations of Lindberg and Darnell (1970) on the giant nuclear RNA which contains SV40-specific sequences, may also point to tandem array of viral genomes. It is worthy of note here that recent studies on eukaryotic genomes suggest that a significant fraction of the DNA is repetitious (Britten and Kohne, 1968) and consists of tandemly repeated sequences (Thomas et al., 1970). Callan (1967), on the basis of cytological studies with lampbrush chromosomes, has suggested that there are multiple copies of each gene arranged in tandem. The tandem array of integrated viral genes would not therefore be a unique occurrence in the eukaryotic genome. It remains to be determined whether or not this type of arrangement is essential for the functioning of the genes. The question of highly specific sites for viral gene integration also remains unanswered at the present time. Perhaps future improvements in the sensitivity of the techniques for performing hybridization directly on cytological preparations (Gall and Pardue, 1969; Pardue and Gall, 1969; Jones, 1970) will supply precise answers to this question.

Little is known about the nature of the integration event whereby viral DNA is inserted into chromosomal DNA (and which presumably occurs shortly after infection). The technique developed by Doerfler (see Section II,D) for demonstrating the covalent insertion of adenovirus 12 DNA into hamster cell DNA has yet to be extended and applied to polyoma and SV40-infected cells. Once a convenient, routine method can be devised for measuring the amount of viral DNA inserted into cell DNA, it should be possible to obtain information on the metabolic conditions necessary for this event to take place. As noted before, the covalent linkage of adenovirus 12 DNA and hamster cell DNA does not appear to require cell or viral DNA duplication (Doerfler, 1970). The "integration event" may therefore be the result of an early viral function. It may also occur, to some degree, in all cells infected with tumor viruses, irrespective of the final outcome of the infection— whether lytic or nonlytic leading to transformation.

B. Transcription and Functioning of the Viral Genome

A central issue in viral carcinogenesis is concerned with the functioning of the viral genes and their role in the maintenance of the neoplastic state. It might be argued that transcription of the viral genes, and synthesis of viral gene products, are not absolutely essential for the maintenance of the neoplastic state. This argument would be based on the hypothesis that the integrated viral DNA acts indirectly—either at the time of integration or continuously throughout the succeeding generations of tumor cells—by altering the physical arrangement of cellular genes such that the expression of the cellular genome is modified. This hypothesis appears unlikely in view of recent results which suggest that some expressions of the transformed phenotype are thermosensitive in cells transformed by thermosensitive mutants of polyoma virus (Dulbecco and Eckhart, 1970) and Rous sarcoma virus (G. S. Martin, 1970). Furthermore, as we have discussed in Section III,B, viral genes in the transformed cell are transcribed and the virus-specific RNA becomes associated with cytoplasmic polyribosomes.

We have drawn attention, in Section III,C, to the variable extent to which the viral genomes are transcribed in cells transformed by SV40, polyoma virus, and adenoviruses. The viral mRNA in one line of SV40-transformed mouse cell is indistinguishable, by hybridization-competition experiments, from the viral mRNA in productively infected cells (M. A. Martin and Axelrod, 1969b). Yet viral DNA and viral coat proteins (the "late" functions) are not synthesized in these cells. Clearly, in this case, the control of viral gene activity is exerted at some point beyond transcription. A novel form of control is suggested by the experiments of Lindberg and Darnell (1970) which indicate that cytoplasmic viral mRNA may be cleaved from larger nuclear precursor molecules; thus control of viral gene activity may be exerted during transportation of mRNA out of the nucleus, ensuring that only viral mRNA of a particular size reaches cytoplasmic ribosomes in a metabolically stable form. Future studies on this possible control mechanism will be facilitated by a new method which has recently been developed for isolating undegraded viral mRNA molecules (R. A. Weinberg and Winocour, 1970).

The cases of highly restricted viral genome transcription, described in Sections III,C and III,D, are interesting from the point of view of the *minimum* viral gene activity that may be required for the maintenance of the transformed state. The hybridization-competition experiments indicate that the genes transcribed are predominently "early" viral genes. Which early consequences of the virus infection in productively infected cells are expressed in transformed cells? The T-antigens are expressed early during the lytic cycle of infection (Rapp *et al.*, 1965; Sabin, 1966); and they continue to be synthesized in the transformed cells. Unfortunately, however, nothing is known about their function. Another early consequence of the infection of resting cells by the DNA-containing tumor viruses is the stimulation of host cell DNA synthesis (Dulbecco *et al.*, 1965; Winocour *et al.*, 1965; Weil *et al.*, 1965; Gershon *et al.*, 1965, 1966; Ben-Porat *et al.*, 1966; Hatanaka and Dulbecco, 1966; Henry *et al.*, 1966; Kit, 1967; Branton and Sheinin, 1968; Shimojo and Yamashita, 1968; Strohl, 1969). It has been shown that this consequence of the viral infection can be induced by the viral DNA alone (Rozenblatt and Winocour, 1971) and that it involves not only the stimulation of host DNA synthesis but also the stimulation of histone synthesis (Shimojo and Kaplan, 1969; Hancock and Weil, 1969; Winocour and Robbins, 1970). In SV40-infected mouse cells exposed to X-irradiation prior to infection, the virus was found capable of inducing the progression of the irradiated cells through the cell cycle into mitosis (Winocour and Robbins, 1970). Thus, an early viral function may affect the control of cell multiplication. Since transformed cells display new growth properties (see Sachs, 1967; Clarke *et al.*, 1970), it is tempting to speculate that these are controlled by an "early" viral gene.

C. DNA AND RNA TUMOR VIRUSES: A COMMON MECHANISM OF ACTION?

The recent exciting studies with the RNA tumor viruses indicate that there is a common basic feature in the mode of action of both DNA-containing and RNA-containing tumor viruses. Temin (1964a) was the first to propose that the genome of the RNA tumor virus may integrate into the cellular genome by means of a complementary DNA intermediate. An important factor which led to this hypothesis was the demonstration that the replicative and transforming capabilities of Rous sarcoma virus were transiently sensitive, shortly after infection, to inhibitors of DNA synthesis (Temin, 1964b; Bader, 1964; Vigier and Goldé, 1964). Nucleic acid hybridization experiments have suggested that tumor virus RNA shows a degree of homology to normal cell DNA (Harel et al., 1966; Baluda and Nayak, 1970) and an increased degree of homology to the DNA of cells transformed by the RNA virus (Temin, 1964c; Baluda and Nayak, 1970). Now it has been shown that many oncogenic RNA viruses contain, within the virion, an enzyme system which synthesizes a DNA copy from the viral RNA template (Temin and Mizutani, 1970; Baltimore, 1970; Spiegelman et al., 1970a,b; Rokutanda et al., 1970). An eminently suitable candidate for the DNA "provirus" intermediate thus exists. It is a comforting thought that the biology of the RNA and DNA tumor viruses has a basic common feature and that tumor virologists are unlikely to be faced with the awkward task of formulating a fundamentally different mechanism to account for the oncogenic action of the RNA viruses.

ACKNOWLEDGMENT

Some of the research cited was supported by grant DRG-1060 from the Damon Runyon Memorial Fund for Cancer Research.

REFERENCES

Aloni, Y. (1967). Thesis, Weizmann Institute of Science, Rehovot, Israel.
Aloni, Y., Winocour, E., and Sachs, L. (1968). *J. Mol. Biol.* 31, 415–429.
Aloni, Y., Winocour, E., Sachs, L., and Torten, J. (1969). *J. Mol. Biol.* 44, 333–345.
Anderer, F. A., Schlumberger, H. D., Koch, M. A., Frank, H., and Eggers, H. J. (1967). *Virology* 32, 511–523.
Axelrod, D., Habel, K., and Bolton, E. T. (1964). *Science* 146, 1466–1468.
Bader, J. P. (1964). *Virology* 22, 462–468.
Baltimore, D. (1970). *Nature (London)* 226, 1209–1211.
Baluda, M. A., and Nayak, D. P. (1970). *Proc. Nat. Acad. Sci. U. S.* 66, 329–336.
Benjamin, T. L. (1966). *J. Mol. Biol.* 16, 359–373.
Benjamin, T. L. (1968). *Virology* 36, 685–687.
Ben-Porat, T., Cato, C., and Kaplan, A. S. (1966). *Virology* 30, 74–81.
Black, P. H. (1966). *J. Nat. Cancer Inst.* 37, 487–493.
Black, P. H. (1968). *Annu. Rev. Microbiol.* 22, 391–426.
Black, P. H., Rowe, W. P., Turner, H. C., and Huebner, R. J. (1963). *Proc. Nat. Acad. Sci. U. S.* 50, 1148–1156.
Bolton, E. T., and McCarthy, B. J. (1962). *Proc. Nat. Acad. Sci. U. S.* 48, 1390–1397.
Bonner, J., Kung, G., and Bekhor, I. (1967). *Biochemistry* 6, 3650–3653.
Borek, C., and Sachs, L. (1966). *Nature (London)* 210, 276–278.
Branton, P. E., and Sheinin, R. (1968). *Virology* 36, 652–661.
Britten, R. J., and Kohne, D. E. (1968). *Science* 161, 529–540.
Callan H. G. (1967). *J. Cell. Sci.* 2, 1–7.
Carp, R. I., Sauer, G., and Sokol, F. (1969). *Virology* 37, 214–226.

Clarke, G. D., Stoker, M. G. P., Ludlow, A., and Thornton, M. (1970). *Nature (London)* **227**, 798–801.

Crawford, L. V. (1969). *Advan. Virus Res.* **14**, 89–152.

Cuzin, F., Vogt, M., Dieckmann, M., and Berg, P. (1970). *J. Mol. Biol.* **47**, 317–333.

Defendi, V. (1966). *Progr. Exp. Tumor Res.* **8**, 125–188.

Denhardt, D. T. (1966). *Biochem. Biophys. Res. Commun.* **23**, 641–646.

Di Mayorca, G., Callender, J., Marin, G., and Giordano, R. (1969). *Virology* **38**, 126–133.

Doerfler, W. (1968). *Proc. Nat. Acad. Sci. U. S.* **60**, 636–643.

Doerfler, W. (1970). *J. Virol.* **6**, 652–666.

Dulbecco, R. (1969). *Science* **166**, 962–968.

Dulbecco, R., and Eckhart, W. (1970). *Proc. Nat. Acad. Sci. U. S.* **67**, 1775–1781.

Dulbecco, R., Hartwell, L. H., and Vogt, M. (1965). *Proc. Nat. Acad. Sci. U. S.* **53**, 403–410.

Eckhart, W. (1969). *Virology* **38**, 120–125.

Epstein, M. A., Achong, B. G., and Barr, Y. M. (1964). *Lancet* **1**, 702–703.

Epstein, M. A., Achong, B. G., Barr, Y. M., Zajac, B., Henle, G., and Henle, W. (1966). *J. Nat. Cancer Inst.* **37**, 547–559.

Fine, R., Mass, M., and Murakami, W. T. (1968). *J. Mol. Biol.* **36**, 167–177.

Fogel, M., and Sachs, L. (1969). *Virology* **37**, 327–334.

Fogel, M., and Sachs, L. (1970). *Virology* **40**, 174–177.

Freifelder, D. (1968). *Cold Spring Harbor Symp. Quant. Biol.* **33**, 425–434.

Fujinaga, K., and Green, M. (1966). *Proc. Nat. Acad. Sci. U. S.* **55**, 1567–1574.

Fujinaga, K., and Green, M. (1967). *J. Virol.* **1**, 576–582.

Fujinaga, K., and Green, M. (1970). *Proc. Nat. Acad. Sci. U. S.* **65**, 375–382.

Fujinaga, K., Mak, S., and Green, M. (1968). *Proc. Nat. Acad. Sci. U. S.* **60**, 959–966.

Fujinaga, K., Piña, M., and Green, M. (1969). *Proc. Nat. Acad. Sci. U. S.* **64**, 255–262.

Gall, J. G., and Pardue, M. L. (1969). *Proc. Nat. Acad. Sci. U. S.* **63**, 378–383.

Gerber, P. (1966). *Virology* **28**, 501–509.

Gerber, P., and Kirschstein, R. L. (1962). *Virology* **18**, 582–588.

Gershon, D., Hausen, P., Sachs, L., and Winocour, E. (1965). *Proc. Nat. Acad. Sci. U. S.* **54**, 1584–1592.

Gershon, D., Sachs, L., and Winocour, E. (1966). *Proc. Nat. Acad. Sci. U. S.* **56**, 918–925.

Gillespie, D. (1968). *Methods Enzymol.* **12**, Part B, 641–668.

Gillespie, D., and Spiegelman, S. (1965). *J. Mol. Biol.* **12**, 829–842.

Green, M. (1970). *Annu. Rev. Biochem.* **39**, 701–756.

Green, M., Parsons, J. T., Pina, M., Fujinaga, K., Caffier, H., and Landgraf-Leurs, I. (1971). *Cold Spring Harbor Symp. Quant. Biol.* **35**, 803–818.

Habel, K. (1961). *Proc. Soc. Exp. Biol. Med.* **106**, 722–725.

Habel, K. (1966). *Cancer Res.* **26**, 2018–2024.

Hall, B. D., and Spiegelman, S. (1961). *Proc. Nat. Acad. Sci. U. S.* **47**, 137–146.

Hancock, R., and Weil, R. (1969). *Proc. Nat. Sci. U. S.* **63**, 1144–1150.

Harel, L., Harel, J., Lacour, F., and Huppert, J. (1966). *C. R. Acad. Sci.* **263**, 616–619.

Harris, H., and Watkins, J. F. (1965). *Nature (London)* **205**, 640–646.

Hatanaka, M., and Dulbecco, R. (1966). *Proc. Nat. Acad. Sci. U. S.* **56**, 736–740.

Henry, P., Black, P. H., Oxman, M. N., and Weissman, S. M. (1966). *Proc. Nat. Acad. Sci. U. S.* **56**, 1170–1176.

Huberman, E., Salzberg, S., and Sachs, L. (1968). *Proc. Nat. Acad. Sci. U. S.* **59**, 77–82.

Hudson, J., Goldstein, D., and Weil, R. (1970). *Proc. Nat. Acad. Sci. U. S.* **65,** 226–233.

Huebner, R. J., Rowe, W. P., Turner, H. C., and Lane, W. T. (1963). *Proc. Nat. Acad. Sci. U. S.* **50,** 379–389.

Ikeda, H., and Tomizawa, J. (1968). *Cold Spring Harbor Symp. Quant. Biol.* **33,** 791–798.

Jones, K. W. (1970). *Nature (London)* **225,** 912–915.

Kass, S. J. (1970). *J. Virol.* **5,** 381–387.

Kaye, A. M., and Winocour, E. (1967). *J. Mol. Biol.* **24,** 475–478.

Kit, S. (1967). *In* "The Molecular Biology of Viruses" (S. J. Colter and W. Paranchych, eds.), pp. 495–525. Academic Press, New York.

Klein, G., Pearson, G., Henle, G., Henle, W., Diehl, V., and Niederman, J. C. (1968). *J. Exp. Med.* **128,** 1021–1030.

Koprowski, H., Jensen, F. C., and Steplewski, Z. (1967). *Proc. Nat. Acad. Sci. U. S.* **58,** 127–133.

Lavi, S., and Winocour, E. (1970). Unpublished experiments.

Levine, A. J., and Teresky, A. K. (1970). *J. Virol.* **5,** 415–457.

Levine, A. S., Oxman, M. N., Henry, P. H., Levine, M. J., Diamandopoulos, G. T., and Enders, J. F. (1970). *J. Virol.* **6,** 199–207.

Lindberg, U., and Darnell, J. E. (1970). *Proc. Nat. Acad. Sci. U. S.* **65,** 1089–1096.

McCarthy, B. J., and Church, R. B. (1970). *Annu. Rev. Biochem.* **39,** 131–150.

Maizel, J. V., White, D. O., and Scharff, M. D. (1968a). *Virology* **36,** 115–125.

Maizel, J. V., White, D. O., and Scharff, M. D. (1968b). *Virology* **36,** 126–136.

Martin, G. S. (1970). *Nature (London)* **227,** 1021–1023.

Martin, M. A., and Axelrod, D. (1969a). *Science* **164,** 68–70.

Martin, M. A., and Axelrod, D. (1969b). *Proc. Nat. Acad. Sci. U. S.* **64,** 1203–1210.

Matsubara, K., and Kaiser, A. D. (1968). *Cold Spring Harbor Symp. Quant. Biol.* **33,** 769–775.

Michel, M. R., Hirt, B., and Weil, R. (1967). *Proc. Nat. Acad. Sci. U. S.* **58,** 1381–1388.

Nygaard, A. P., and Hall, B. D. (1964). *J. Mol. Biol.* **9,** 125–142.

Oda, K., and Dulbecco, R. (1968). *Proc. Nat. Acad. Sci. U. S.* **60,** 525–532.

Pardue, M. L., and Gall, J. G. (1969). *Proc. Nat. Acad. Sci. U. S.* **64,** 600–604.

Pollack, R. E., Green, H., and Todaro, G. J. (1968). *Proc. Nat. Acad. Sci. U. S.* **60,** 126–133.

Pope, J. H., and Rowe, W. P. (1964). *J. Exp. Med.* **120,** 121–128.

Rabinowitz, Z., and Sachs, L. (1968). *Nature (London)* **220,** 1203–1206.

Radloff, R., Bauer, W., and Vinograd, J. (1967). *Proc. Nat. Acad. Sci. U. S.* **57,** 1514–1521.

Rapp, F., Butel, J. S., Feldman, L. A., Kitahara, T., and Melnick, J. L. (1965). *J. Exp. Med.* **121,** 935–944.

Reich, P. R., Black, P. H., and Weissman, S. M. (1966). *Proc. Nat. Acad. Sci. U. S.* **56,** 78–85.

Rokutanda, M., Rokutanda, H., Green, M., Fujinaga, K., Ranjit, K. R., and Gurgo, C. (1970). *Nature (London)* **227,** 1026–1028.

Rozenblatt, S., and Winocour, E. (1971). *Virology* **43,** 300–303.

Sabin, A. B. (1966). *Proc. Nat. Acad. Sci. U. S.* **55,** 1141–1148.

Sabin, A. B., and Koch, M. A. (1963). *Proc. Nat. Acad. Sci. U. S.* **50,** 407–417.

Sachs, L. (1967). *Curr. Top. Develop. Biol.* **2,** 129–150.

Sambrook, J., and Shatkin, A. J. (1969). *J. Virol.* **4,** 719–726.

Sambrook, J., Westphal, H., Srinivasan, P. R., and Dulbecco, R. (1968). *Proc. Natl. Acad. Sci. U. S.* **60**, 1288–1295.

Sauer, G., and Kidwai, J. R. (1968). *Proc. Nat. Acad. Sci. U. S.* **61**, 1256–1263.

Schildkraut, C. L., Marmur, J., and Doty, P. (1961). *J. Mol. Biol.* **3**, 595–617.

Schlesinger, R. W. (1969). *Advan. Virus Res.* **14**, 1–61.

Schulte-Holthausen, H., and zur Hausen, H. (1970). *Virology* **40**, 776–779.

Sheinin, R. (1966). *Virology* **28**, 621–632.

Shimojo, H., and Kaplan, A. S. (1969). *Virology* **37**, 690–694.

Shimojo, H., and Yamashita, T. (1968). *Virology* **36**, 422–433.

Sjögren, H. O., Hellström, I., and Klein, G. (1961). *Cancer Res.* **21**, 329–337.

Spiegelman, S., Burny, A., Das, M. R., Keydar, J., Schlom, J., Travnicek, M., and Watson, K. (1970a). *Nature (London)* **227**, 563–567.

Spiegelman, S., Burny, A., Das, M. R., Keydar, J., Schlom, J., Travnicek, M., and Watson, K. (1970b). *Nature (London)* **227**, 1029–1031.

Strohl, W. A. (1969). *Virology* **39**, 653–665.

Tai, H. T., and O'Brien, R. L. (1969). *Virology* **38**, 698–701.

Temin, H. M. (1964a). *Nat. Cancer Inst., Monogr.* **17**, 557–570.

Temin, H. M. (1964b). *Virology* **23**, 486–494.

Temin, H. M. (1964c). *Proc. Nat. Acad. Sci. U. S.* **52**, 323–329.

Temin, H. M., and Mizutani, S. (1970). *Nature (London)* **226**, 1211–1213.

Thomas, C. A. (1966). *Progr. Nucl. Acid Res. Mol. Biol.* **5**, 315–337.

Thomas, C. A., Hamkalo, B. A., Misra, D. N., and Lee, C. S. (1970). *J. Mol. Biol.* **51**, 621–632.

Thorne, H. V., and Warden, D. (1967). *J. Gen. Virol.* **1**, 135–137.

Todaro, G. J., Habel, K., and Green, H. (1965). *Virology* **27**, 179–185.

Tonegawa, S., Walter, G., Bernardi, A., and Dulbecco, R. (1971). *Cold Spring Harbor Symp. Quant. Biol.* **35**, 823–831.

Trilling, D. M., and Axelrod, D. (1970). *Science* **168**, 268–271.

Vigier, P., and Goldé, A. (1964). *Virology* **23**, 511–519.

Vinograd, J., Bruner, R., Kent, R., and Weigle, J. (1963). *Proc. Nat. Acad. Sci. U. S.* **49**, 902–910.

Vogt, M. (1970). *J. Mol. Biol.* **47**, 307–316.

Walker, P. M. B. (1969). *Progr. Nucl. Acid Res. Mol. Biol.* **9**, 307–326.

Warnaar, S. O., and Cohen, J. A. (1966). *Biochem. Biophys. Res. Commun.* **24**, 544–558.

Watkins, J. F., and Dulbecco, R. (1967). *Proc. Nat. Acad. Sci. U. S.* **58**, 1396–1403.

Weil, R., Michel, M. R., and Ruschmann, G. L. (1965). *Proc. Nat. Acad. Sci. U. S.* **53**, 1468–1476.

Weinberg, A., and Becker, Y. (1969). *Virology* **39**, 312–321.

Weinberg, R. A., and Winocour, E. (1970). Unpublished experiments.

Weiss, M. C. (1970). *Proc. Nat. Acad. Sci. U. S.* **66**, 79–86.

Westphal, H., and Dulbecco, R. (1968). *Proc. Nat. Acad. Sci. U. S.* **59**, 1158–1165.

Winocour, E. (1965). *Virology* **25**, 276–288.

Winocour, E. (1967). *Virology* **31**, 15–28.

Winocour, E. (1968). *Virology* **34**, 571–582.

Winocour, E. (1969). *Advan. Virus Res.* **14**, 153–200.

Winocour, E. (1970). *Proc. Int. Symp. Tumor Viruses, 2nd,* No. 183, pp. 113–117.

Winocour, E., and Robbins, E. (1970). *Virology* **40**, 307–315.

Winocour, E., Kaye, A. M., and Stollar, V. (1965). *Virology* **27**, 156–169.

zur Hausen, H., and Schulte-Holthausen, H. (1970). *Nature (London)* **227**, 245–248.

zur Hausen, H., and Sokol, F. (1969). *J. Virol.* **4**, 256–263.

VIRAL GENOME AND ONCOGENIC TRANSFORMATION: NUCLEAR AND PLASMA MEMBRANE EVENTS

Georges Meyer

Research Department of the Regional Cancer Center of Marseilles,
13, Marseilles, France

I. Introduction

A. General Properties of Virus-Cell Interaction

The interaction of mammalian cells and oncogenic viruses can be a useful model for the elucidation of the steps of malignant transformation. Events in the nucleus and plasma membrane seem particularly important in this model. In fact, the early phases of this interaction—the genetic events and the first-appearing antigenic events—are localized in the nucleus. The relationship of a cell with neighboring cells, with different tissues, and finally with the whole organism seems to be mediated by the plasma cell membrane. The cytoplasmic changes during transformation have been fully described by Kit (1968) in a recent issue of this review. We shall not discuss them further.

If it were possible to determine a relationship between the different events occurring during carcinogenesis by viruses, the understanding of the mechanism of carcinogenesis and of the immune reaction by host could be elucidated. It is particularly important to know if the nuclear events and/or the membrane modifications are the main mechanisms which lead to cancerous transformation. To be sure to avoid as many ambiguities as possible, we shall recall established facts, especially the characteristics of a transformed cell and the proofs of viral genome and host cell interaction. In the first section we shall deal with the nature of oncogenic viruses, the properties of the different fractions of the viral genome, and the interaction of the viral genome and the target cell. In the second section we shall try to study the modification of the nucleus during the transformation of the cell and particularly, the chromosome modifications, the antigenic modifications, and the regulation of the expression of the viral genome. In the third section we will be concerned with the modifications of the cell surface in relation to viral transformation, morphological changes, especially ultrastructural aspects of the very important new antigens present on the plasma membrane, and the relationship of these facts with the new behavior of the cell. Perhaps in a general discussion we might try to relate these findings with the hypothesis of the cell transformation phenomenon.

Our purpose is not the enumeration of all the reactive viruses and the different animal cells, inasmuch as several excellent reviews on transformation by these various viruses exist (Habel, 1963; Dulbecco, 1963; Enders, 1965; Defendi, 1966; Rapp and Melnick, 1966; Black, 1968), but in Table I we report the viruses as well as the target cells that are pertinent to our argument. We will mainly discuss DNA virus-directed transformation. In fact, thoughts concerning RNA virus transformation are at this moment in total revolution after Temin and Mizutani's discovery (1970) that RNA tumor viruses can act as templates for the synthesis of DNA. This case, which has been confirmed by several laboratories (Rokutanda et al., 1970; Spiegelman et al., 1970), shows that the RNA viruses may act in a manner similar to that of the DNA viruses. It is too early to establish a definitive comparison between both types of viruses from these recent results and this problem could probably be better reviewed in the next issue.

The exhibition of a differential behavior according to the cell type infected is the major characteristic of these viruses: either there is a complete lytic cycle with production of infectious particles and subsequent lysis of the cell in the "permissive cells," or an incomplete cycle without production of virus particles, thus resulting in the cure of the cell (this is abortive infection or abortive transformation) or in a perma-

TABLE I

SOME ONCOGENIC VIRUSES AND THEIR HOST CELLS

Virus	Natural host	Cancerizable host	Permissive cells	Transformable cells	Cell lines used
Polyoma	Mouse	Hamster, mouse, rat, guinea pig, rabbit	Mouse embryo	Hamster, Mouse, Rat	BHK21/C13 3T3
SV40	Green monkey	Hamster	Green monkey kidney (GMK)	Hamster, Mouse, Human cells, Green monkey	BHK21 3T3 WI38 AGMK
Adenoviruses	Human	Hamster	Human cells WI38	Hamster	BHK21
Rous	Chicken	Chicken	Chicken	Chicken, Hamster	BHK21

nent transformation with phenotypic and genotypic modifications of the cell (this is transformation). In some cases this transformation is compatible with little virus production; it is the case of nondefective Rous virus-transformed chicken cells (see Hanafusa, 1969, for a general review) or polyoma virus-transformed rat cells (Fogel and Sachs, 1969, 1970). We can call this state a "productive" transformation.

B. Viral Genome

1. *Isolation of the Virus and of Its DNA*

It is the viral genome consisting only of DNA or RNA which carries the information necessary both for the virus reproduction and for the cell transformation (Di Mayorca *et al.*, 1959). First experiments showed that the nucleic acid fraction extracted from mouse embryo cells infected with polyoma virus was again infectious. Further experiments after purification of the virus showed that the fractions obtained by density centrifugation were also infectious (Table II). In a similar way, it was demonstrated that crude extracts of tumors could initiate a tumor when injected into a suitable host. After purification of the virus by density gradient centrifugation, it was demonstrated that only full particles could transform the susceptible cells. Empty particles or particles containing mouse DNA instead of viral DNA (pseudovirions demonstrated by Michel *et al.*, 1967; Winocour, 1968; Cramer *et al.*, 1967) could neither give rise to productive infection nor transform the cells. However, this viral genome must have a well-defined physical state to be able either to infect or to transform a cell. This has been demonstrated by the fractionation of the viral DNA into several fractions. After purification of the virus, its nucleic acid could be easily extracted and studied. Extraction was done with phenol and the different fractions were separated by density gradient centrifugation in sucrose or CsCl solutions. This method allowed the separation of two major components (Crawford, 1964): a fast band and a slower one with sedimentation coefficients of 21 S and 15.5 S respectively.

In fact, these fractions were not homogeneous and more recently four fractions have been described (Weil and Vinograd, 1963; Blackstein *et al.*, 1969). Fraction I, which is the faster band, comprises 80–90% of the DNA (Weil and Vinograd, 1963). It has recently been proved that fraction I itself was not homogeneous (Thorne *et al.*, 1968; Blackstein *et al.*, 1969); two subfractions can be shown—Ia, with a molecular weight of 3×10^6, corresponds to fraction I of Weil and Vinograd; Ic and Id were obtained by serial passages of a polyoma virus strain on mouse embryo cells; their amount increased with the number of passages. They

TABLE II

Properties of the Different Fractions of SV40 or Polyoma Virus Particles

Virus	Nature of the fraction	Density (CsCl gradient)	Biological properties			References
			Hemagglutination	Infectious power	Transforming power	
Polyoma	Full particles	1.32	+	+	+	Abel and Crawford (1963)
Polyoma	Empty particles	1.29	+	−	−	Abel and Crawford (1963)
Polyoma	Pseudovirions	1.315	+	−	−	Michel et al. (1967) Winocour (1968) Cramer et al. (1967)
SV40	Full particles	1.32	+	+		Crawford and Black (1964)
SV40	Empty particles	1.29	+	−		Crawford and Black (1964)
SV40	Pseudovirions	1.32	+	−		Trilling and Axelrod (1970)

have a molecular weight of 1.5 to 2.2 $\times$ 10^6 and they are located in the slower part of the fast band in equilibrium density gradient centrifugation. These molecules are in general defective; fraction II, which is slower than fraction I and comprises 1–20% of the DNA; fraction III which had been for a long time confused with fraction II and has been identified only recently. Several observations suggest that this fraction might be derived from host cell DNA (Michel *et al.*, 1967) and would therefore be mouse DNA.

Denaturation and renaturation studies of these DNA fractions with different agents led to the conclusion that each one of these fractions corresponded to a different type of polyoma DNA, i.e., that each fraction had a different molecular configuration. Fraction I consists of closed circular DNA helixes which are in a supercoiled form; fractions Ic and Id have the same configuration. Fraction II is an open circular form derived from fraction I by a single strand break. Fraction III is a linear form (Vinograd *et al.*, 1965). Similar results have been obtained for simian virus 40.

2. Properties of the Different Fractions of the DNA

Table III shows infectious and transforming ability of each fraction. The viral DNA alone has transforming ability which has been confirmed by several authors. Fractions I and II equally transform a tissue culture (Crawford *et al.*, 1964). Fraction I retains its transforming ability even when heated, unlike fraction II (Abel and Crawford, 1963). Nevertheless, the transforming ability of fraction I is about ten times that of fraction II (Bourgaux *et al.*, 1965).

Fraction III has also been studied. It seems that its transforming ability is very low and this may be due to a small amount of contamination by fraction II (Bourgaux *et al.*, 1965). The transforming abilities of fractions Ic and Id have not yet been reported.

On the whole, it is evident that the DNA of oncogenic viruses has infective and transforming properties, though some conditions must be fulfilled in order for it to exert this action. On the one hand, the DNA must be able to cross the membrane of the cell it has to transform; on the other hand, it has to be under the supercoiled or coiled configuration to transform the recipient cell. In polyoma virus as well as SV40, the size of the viral genome is sufficient to accomodate six to ten small genes. Some functions of these genes have been identified; one-third of the genetic information codes for the proteins present in the viral particle.

Other functions coded for by the viral genome are the induction of

TABLE III
Some Properties of the Different Fractions of the
DNA of Polyoma or SV40

Fraction	Physical properties			Biological properties	
	φ(CsCl)	S	Configuration	IP[a]	TA[b]
Polyoma virus[c]					
I (1,2,3,4,6,7) or Ia (5)	1709 gm./cm.³	20.3 ± 0.45 M.W. 3 × 10⁶	Double-stranded cyclic coiled form	+	+
Ic-Id (5)		M.W. 2.2 × 10⁶ 1.5 × 10⁶	Double-stranded cyclic coiled form	−	?
II (1,2,3,4)	1709 gm./cm.³		Open circular form	+	+
III (1,2,3)	1702 gm./cm.³		Linear form	−	
Simian virus 40					
I (8)	21.2	M.W. 3.2 × 10⁶	Double-stranded coiled form	+	+
II (8)	16.1		Linear	+	+

[a] Infectious power.

[b] Transforming ability.

[c] 1, Weil and Vinograd (1963); 2, Bourgaux et al. (1965); 3, Crawford et al. (1964); 4, Dulbecco and Vogt (1963); 5, Blackstein et al. (1969); 6, Thorne (1968); 7, Thorne et al. (1968); 8, Crawford and Black (1964).

cellular DNA synthesis and the induction of virus-specific antigens, T-antigen, TSTA, and/or surface antigens.

3. DNA Functions Studied with Temperature-Sensitive Mutants

The isolation and study of temperature-sensitive mutants of polyoma virus have been means for the identification of different functions of the viral genome. This has been carried out independently by Eckhart (1969a) and Di Mayorca et al. (1969). The results they obtained differed in that Eckhart found three complementation groups and Di Mayorca et al. found four groups. This can be easily explained by the fact that they isolated different mutants. Eckhart studied six temperature-sensitive mutants of polyoma virus. The mutants were obtained by treatment of wild-type virus by nitrous acid and plated on mouse embryo cells at 31.5°C. The virus so produced was then tested for its plating efficiency at 31.5°C. and 38.5°C.; the mutants selected showed a 10-fold or higher plating efficiency at 31.5°C. compared to 38.5°C. Six temperature-sensitive mutants and among them, the *Ts-a* mutant isolated by Fried

(1965a,b) were studied for their transforming ability and were complemented one with another. The results showed that the six mutants fell into three classes on the basis of complementation and transformation tests at the nonpermissive temperature. Class I (2 mutants): the mutants of this class are able to synthesize infectious viral DNA but not mature virus particles. They transform normally at the nonpermissive temperature. Class II (3 mutants): these mutants (among them is the *Ts-a* of Fried) are defective in the synthesis of infectious viral DNA. They are also defective in transformation at the nonpermissive temperature. Class III (1 mutant): this mutant is defective in the synthesis of infectious viral DNA but transforms normally at the nonpermissive temperature.

Di Mayorca *et al.* (1969) also isolated many temperature-sensitive mutants of polyoma virus and subjected them to a genetic analysis. Following the complementation experiments there are at least four com-

TABLE IV

TEMPERATURE-SENSITIVE MUTANTS OF POLYOMA VIRUS: COMPLEMENTATION GROUPS ACCORDING TO ECKHART (1969a) AND DI MAYORCA *et al.* (1969)

Class	Induction of cellular DNA synthesis	Synthesis of mature virus particles	Synthesis of infectious viral DNA	Transformation
I Di Mayorca	+	−	−	−
II Eckhart	NT excepted for *Ts-a* (+)	−	−	−
II Di Mayorca	+	−	+	+
I Eckhart	NT	−	+	+
III Di Mayorca	+	−	+	+
III Eckhart	NT	−	−	+

plementation groups (Table IV). Group I: the mutants belonging to this group were found to be mutated in a gene involved in the synthesis of viral DNA. They do, however, promote cellular DNA synthesis. The *Ts-a* mutant belongs to this complementation group. These mutants are temperature-sensitive for transformation. However, cells transformed by these mutants at the permissive temperature do not revert to the normal when shifted to the nonpermissive temperature. The mutation appears, therefore, to affect a function necessary for the initiation but not for the maintenance of the transformed state. Groups II and III: the mutants belonging to these groups synthesize viral DNA at the nonpermissive temperature but do not synthesize any antigenic determinant of the protein(s) of the virion. The synthesis of the viral proteins would therefore be under the control of two genes. Group IV contains a mutant which does not complement at all.

Class II of Eckhart and group I of Di Mayorca *et al.* (1969) are the same since they both contain the *Ts-a* mutant. The *Ts-a* function has been further investigated by Vogt (1970) and by Cuzin *et al.* (1970) in the case of 3T3 cells transformed at the nonpermissive temperature by this *Ts-a*. The *Ts-a* function would be implicated in both the infectious cycle and the transformation process.

This last mutant is particularly interesting in the study of the initiation of host cell DNA synthesis. In all cases of lytic, abortive, or transforming cycles, the infection of the cell by oncogenic DNA viruses is followed by cell DNA synthesis. Gershon *et al.* (1965) demonstrated by nitrous acid inactivation that this activation was dependent on a viral function. They also showed that the rate of inactivation of the DNA-inducing ability of the virus was similar to that of the cell-transforming ability. The relative target size of this function was found to be one fourth of the target size necessary for replication. Using the *Ts-a* mutant of polyoma virus, Fried (1970) demonstrated that induction of cell DNA synthesis and transformation could be dissociated although the rates of inactivation of both functions are very similar. In fact, the *Ts-a* mutant is temperature sensitive for transformation but not for the induction of cell DNA synthesis.

C. Cell-Virus Interactions

1. *The Lytic Cycle*

When some cell types are infected with papova viruses, the infection leads to the synthesis of progeny virus and to a concomitant death of the cell; that is why this infection is called "lytic." In the case of polyoma virus, the lytic cycle proceeds in two distinct phases (Weil *et al.*, 1965). Phase I corresponds to early events which take place before replication of the viral DNA occurs; they are therefore under the dependence of the infecting DNA. This phase is characterized by the synthesis of viral-specific messenger RNA, by the appearance of the T-antigen, and by the initiation of cellular DNA synthesis, which is perhaps the most important event. The transition between phases I and II is achieved by synthesis of the viral DNA.

The viral DNA is then used as a template for transcription in messenger RNA—late messenger RNA—which is produced in great amounts. This late RNA corresponds to the synthesis of late proteins, in particular the capsid proteins. It has been shown (Aloni *et al.*, 1968) that early mRNA and late mRNA are different.

After adsorption (Crawford, 1962) the virus penetrates into the cell and is uncoated in the cytoplasm; the viral DNA is rapidly found in the nucleus of the cell where it is in close association with the cell chromosomes. Recent experimental results (Hudson *et al.*, 1970) suggest that at least one viral DNA molecule would be integrated into the cell DNA; a small fraction of viral-specific messenger RNA would be transcribed from the integrated DNA (early messenger RNA).

During this phase the synthesis of the T-antigen also occurs (Takemoto *et al.*, 1966). The first new virus-specific antigen observed is located in the nucleus and has been demonstrated by immunofluorescence. A genuine burst of synthesis of different enzymes whose activity is required for the synthesis of the pyrimidine deoxyribonucleotides and of DNA, a thymidine kinase (Basilico *et al.*, 1969; Sheinin, 1966a) and a DNA polymerase for example (Dulbecco *et al.*, 1965), then occurs. It seems now that all or nearly all these enzyme syntheses are the result of a viral function activating a group of cellular genes which were previously inactive or partially repressed, since the cultures are in general confluent or nearly confluent and the DNA synthesis is then inhibited. Under certain conditions, it has been demonstrated that the characteristics of some enzymes were different from those of noninfected cells. This occurs, for example, in a DNA polymerase induced by SV40 (Kit *et al.*, 1967b). The enzyme would be coded by the viral genome. The SV40 genome also seems to code for a thymidine kinase. All these enzymes lead to the replication of the cell chromosomal DNA, but this is not followed by mitosis. At the same time, the replication of the viral DNA takes place. Recent results of Cuzin *et al.* (1970), studying 3T3 cells transformed by the *Ts-a* mutant of polyoma virus point out the possibility that another function of the viral genome, the *Ts-a* function, is needed for the initiation of the replication of the viral DNA.

Immediately after the onset of viral DNA synthesis, increased amounts of viral-specific RNA are synthesized, presumably messenger RNA (Benjamin, 1966). This late messenger RNA is composed of large molecules of RNA (polycistronic messenger RNA) which carry most or all of the genetic information coded by a strand of viral circular DNA (Hudson *et al.*, 1970). The viral messenger RNA is then transferred to the cytoplasm of the cell where it presumably directs the synthesis of the viral proteins (capsid proteins) which are apparently transferred to the nucleus where they can be demonstrated. However, Hare (1970) recently showed another polyoma strain (3049 strain, with the CyC + character), characterized by a cytoplasmic accumulation of capsid antigen (in the case of a lytic infection) which is then followed by the gradual appearance of polyoma virions in the nucleus. The viral proteins apparently migrate from the cytoplasm to the nucleus where maturation of the virus occurs. Polyoma virions are formed in the nucleus and the viral capsid may be either a fully infectious particle or an empty particle, or it may contain mouse cellular DNA instead of polyoma DNA; no enzyme is needed for the assembling of the DNA and the proteins. Once the viruses are mature, the cell is lysed and releases the progeny particles into the medium, even if some viruses remain attached to plasma membrane ghosts (Césarini et al., 1966).

The other virus-cell relationship leads to an abortive or stable transformation of the cell. Definitions of transformation are numerous. The most complete seems to be the one given by Black (1968): "transformation is defined as a heritage change in the properties of a cell subsequent to virus infection which is manifested by the loss of the regulatory restraints of its growth potential. The transformation is most frequently accompanied by a loss of contact inhibition of movement or mitosis; changes in morphology, glycolytic rate, karyotype, and the acquisition of malignant potential may also accompany the transformation. Some of these changes may occur in stages with the eventual progression toward a more autonomous state."

The fact that a cell presents transformed characters in vitro does not necessarily mean that this cell produces a tumor in vivo; tumor formation involves complex interactions with the immunological system of the host. Abortive transformation does not correspond to the above definition of transformation but this condition could also be called "abortive infection" and it really carries out the transition between infectious cycle and transformation.

2. The Abortive Cycle

The description "abortive infection" or "abortive transformation" varies from one author to another and especially according to the characters used to display this phenomenon. Infection of permissive cells resulted in the production of virus and the subsequent cell death. On the other hand, when nonpermissive cells are infected at high input multiplicity, a certain fraction of the cells is stably transformed; 1–5% in the case of hamster cells infected with polyoma virus, 5% in the case of rat cells transformed by polyoma virus (Sheinin, 1966b), and 45% for 3T3 cells transformed by SV40 (Todaro and Green, 1966). In 1966, Sheinin observed an abortive infection in the case of rat embryo cells infected by polyoma virus in which she noted a stimulation of DNA synthesis. Also in 1966, Sauer and Defendi demonstrated an abortive infection in human diploid cell cultures infected with SV40. Stimulation of DNA synthesis and the production of complement-fixing antigen occurred in these cells. In these experiments, abortive infection was characterized either by the activation of DNA synthesis or by production of complement-fixing antigen. The appearance in almost 80% of the cells of the nuclear or "T"-antigen (Meyer *et al.*, 1967b) and the presence of changes in the surface membrane as revealed by immunofluorescence (Lhérisson *et al.*, 1967) have also been demonstrated in BHK21 cells infected with polyoma virus. Kinetics of appearance of both antigens and their possible significance will be discussed later.

The abortive cycle was also shown using another transformation criterion. The growth of most normal cells is anchorage dependent; in general they do not grow in suspension (Stoker *et al.*, 1968). The transformation of a cell into a tumor cell may result in the loss of this dependence, so that numerous transformed cells are able to grow in suspension. When hamster cells, i.e., BHK21 cells, are infected with polyoma virus, they exhibit, a few days after exposure to the virus, a general change in the arrangement of the culture (Defendi and Lehman, 1965). This change is reversible and after 6 or 7 days most of the cells return to growth characteristic of normal cells, except the few percent which undergo a definite transformation. Normal BHK21 cells do not grow in a suspension medium containing methylcellulose. On the contrary, polyoma-transformed cells do, as do BHK21 cells heavily infected with polyoma virus (1250 PFU/cell) (Stoker, 1968). Most of the infected BHK21 cells undergo a few cell divisions, form clones, and then return to normal growth. In the same conditions, mock-infected cells undergo only one or two divisions but do not form clones. Nonpermissive cells, infected at high input multiplicity with polyoma virus, undergo a temporary change. This temporary change is evidenced by the acquisition of at least one of the characteristics of transformation: the ability to grow in suspension, which is acquired for a few cell divisions and lost again. After infection by the virus, the major part of the cells undergo a nonpermissive infection and begin a transforming cycle. This transformation, however, becomes stable only in a small percentage of the cells. The question that arises is to discover why some cells undergo transformation and why others return to a normal state. We know that this cannot be due to a lack of penetration since infection does take place. Later we will discuss if this is due to a lack of competence of the cells or of the virus.

3. *The Productive Transformation*

Productive transformation is illustrated by cells transformed by Rous virus which continue to synthesize the virus and a special case of cells transformed by polyoma virus (Fogel and Sachs, 1969, 1970).

Rat embryo muscle cell cultures have been infected either with a small plaque (SP) or a large plaque (LP) strain of polyoma virus, the transformed cell lines isolated, and the activation of virus synthesis studied in cells transformed by both strains of virus. The cell lines were cloned in the presence of antipolyoma virus antiserum. The results showed that there was no detectable virus synthesis in any of the clones isolated from the SP polyoma-transformed line. However, the results were different in the case of the clones arising from LP-transformed cells. In this experiment, 92 out of 100 clones continued to produce virus-synthesizing cells, the virus produced being the LP type.

In rat embryo muscle cells transformed by polyoma virus of the LP strain, there is a new kind of cell-virus relationship since the cells are transformed but continue to produce virus. This activation is spontaneous. Furthermore, this ability for spontaneous activation is transmitted to the progeny clones although segregation of some clones having lost this spontaneous activation can be seen. This spontaneous activation occurs in about 1 in 10^4 cells as demonstrated by immunofluorescent staining for polyoma virion antigen. The virus production by virus-yielding clones varied from 5×10^3 to 10^5 PFU per 10^6 cells.

Different treatments which were known to be successful in the induction of the production of infectious SV40 were used to try to activate virus synthesis in the LP polyoma virus-transformed cells. These treatments were: X-irradiation; fusion of LP-transformed and normal mouse cells with UV-inactivated Sendaï virus; UV-irradiation; and addition of mitomycin C to the culture medium.

These treatments proved to be successful in activating virus synthesis. In the case of X-irradiation, the frequency of virus-synthesizing cells in the clones with spontaneous activation was increased about 100-fold, with X-ray doses ranging from 200 to 5000 r. The fusion of the transformed cells with normal mouse cells also resulted in the activation of virus synthesis, as can be judged by the presence of polyoma virion antigen in the multinucleated cells. Similarly, UV-irradiation and mitomycin C induced virus synthesis in two clones with spontaneous activation. The optimum dose of UV light induced about a 200-fold difference in the yield of virus.

Finally, the infection of rat embryo muscle cells with LP polyoma virus leads to the transformation of a small fraction of the cells. However, one can isolate some clones showing a "spontaneous activation" of the production of polyoma virus, and this without any treatment. Out of these clones, numerous others can be induced by a variety of treatments to produce more virus by increasing the number of virus-producing cells. This type of virus-cell relationship seems to be rather a rare event after polyoma virus transformation. However, the "noninductible" character may be due to the production of defective viral genomes which could also explain the conversion of the mitomycin C-inductible character to the noninductible one. This way of production of polyoma virus in a cell type different from the mouse embryo cells usually used may allow the production of virus without its usual "mouse DNA" contaminant (pseudovirions) and prove useful when trying to determine if mouse DNA enclosed in polyoma viral capsids may play any role by a kind of "transduction" phenomenon (Weil and Hancock, 1970).

4. The Transformation

In fact, the virus-host cell relationship in which we are the most interested is the stable transformation. It is this problem with which we will deal now. Among virus-cell events, the first one that comes to mind is the maintenance in the cell of genetic information of viral origin. Therefore, it is necessary to prove the persistence of at least a fraction of the viral genome in the cell; this persistence can be easily demonstrated when it is possible to rescue the viral genome by coculture or hybridization. An indirect proof of the persistence of the viral genome in the cell is the acquisition of new antigenic properties differing from those of the normal cell; these antigenic modifications are virus specific. They are the acquisition of the T-antigen and of the tumor-specific transplantation antigen (TSTA) and/or surface antigens.

It became more evident that the viral genome was present in the transformed cell and in a complete form when it was demonstrated that SV40-transformed cells (and, therefore, nonpermissive cells) could be induced to produce infectious virus when fused or cultured with permissive cells: in this case with green monkey kidney cells (Gerber, 1966). Induction experiments have been successful only in the case of SV40; all induction experiments failed in the case of adenoviruses and polyoma virus. However, as we have seen in the case of productive transformation, polyoma-transformed rat cells can produce infectious virus.

a. *Rescue of the Viral Genome by Coculture and Cellular Hybridization*. The obvious proof of the presence of the viral genome in the transformed cell is its rescue in the form of infectious virus. This rescue can be achieved by various methods. The analogy of transformation with lysogenization of host bacteria by temperate phages suggested the use of different kinds of inducers which worked successfully in the phage system. Exposure of the tumors in animals to X-irradiation, cortisone, or starvation; or in tissue culture exposure to X- or UV-irradiation, nutritional deficiencies, superinfection with cytolytic or other oncogenic viruses, and growth on a sensitive feeder layer have all been tried. The only way of rescuing virus from transformed cells was the contact or fusion of these cells with permissive ones which could be done, either by cocultivation of the transformed cells with permissive indicator cells and subsequent hybrid formation, or by treatment by UV-inactivated Sendaï virus which brings about the fusion of the cells and the formation of heterokaryons of a mixture of transformed cells and permissive indicator cells. In a few cases the treatment of mitomycin C was successful. The first experiments with the UV-irradiation procedures used in the case of lysogenic bacteria were failures.

The first but only partial proof was obtained *in vivo* by Svoboda *et al.* (1963) who studied the virus-tumor relationship in the XC rat tumor produced by Rous virus. He observed that intact cells of XC tumor injected into chicks gave rise to Rous virus-containing sarcomas. Sabin and Koch (1963) for the first time used mixed cultures between nonpermissive and permissive cells infected with SV40. They obtained a very low virus production at a nonsignificant rate. Black *et al.* (1963) conducted similar experiments. Gerber (1966) modified this technique by carrying out mixed cultures in the presence of UV-inactivated Sendaï virus. He specified the conditions required for a successful experiment: the viability of the tumor cells seems to be essential, since prolonged UV-irradiation, heat, and sonic vibration abolished both cell viability and virogenicity, while similar treatments of intact SV40 had no significant effect on its infectivity. Payne and De Vries (1967) proved that production of infectious SV40 might be induced by fusion of the tumor cells with indicator cells in which the virus normally undergoes productive replication. The proportion of cultures yielding infectious SV40 increased when tumor cells were mixed with indicator cells and then exposed to UV-inactivated parainfluenza virus, type 3 (Okada, 1962). The heterokaryons contained nuclei with and without T-antigen. Viral antigen indicative of SV40 production was seen in a few cells 24 hours after fusion. These cells were frequently heterokaryons. Two to 4 days later with the second cycle of virus replication, viral antigen was mainly present in mononucleate indicator cells. At the same time Koprowski *et al.* (1967) estimated that SV40 may be present with a full complement of genetic material necessary for its synthesis in at least a fraction of the transformed cell population, although it may be unable, before fusion, to express its late function, such as synthesis of viral coat. For example, 3T3 cells transformed by SV40 do not produce infectious virus but contain functioning viral genes; in fact, they synthesize virus-specific messenger-RNA and proteins. Watkins and Dulbecco (1967) showed

that when these 3T3 cells were fused with *Cercopithecus* kidney cells
(BSC, an SV40 susceptible line allowing viral multiplication), the infectious virus was produced in heterokaryons. They established a quantitative relationship between the participation of indicator cells in heterokaryons and the capacity of these heterokaryons to produce SV40.
Lack of expression could be attributed either to the presence of a
specific repressor of viral functions in the transformed cells or to the
lack of a factor required for the expression of these functions (Cassingena
and Tournier, 1968). These authors suggested that somatic hybrids between monkey kidney cells and SV40-transformed hamster cells could
be obtained with a fall in temperature, the percentage of virogenic
heterokaryons depending upon the temperature. This fact can be used
to rescue the virus without interferon. Watkins and Dulbecco (1967)
observed that virus production required cytoplasmic fusion but not
nuclear fusion. Out of 83 mouse kidney lines transformed by UV-irradiated SV40, 5 lines have yielded virus by all techniques used, including
treatment of cell mixture with UV-inactivated Sendai virus (Dubbs and
Kit, 1969).

Failure to rescue SV40 from nonyielding lines could be due either
to a defect of viral genes essential for replication of viral components
or for viral maturation from the integrated state; or to the production
by the transformed cells of a substance incompatible with SV40 replication (repressor or interferon); or to a failure of transformed cells to
fuse with the permissive monkey kidney cells. In order to prove that
the failure in production could be due to the presence of a defective
virus, Knowles *et al.* (1968) achieved the fusion of SV40-transformed
cells, either permissive or nonpermissive, and showed that nonproductive
cell strains could become productive after complementation between
them. On the other hand, all attempts to detect the presence of an infectious viral genome by mixed culture with sensitive cells or by chemical
induction have failed in the case of polyoma virus or adenovirus 12-
transformed cells (Gerber, 1964; Burns and Black, 1969). Fusion of a
polyoma-transformed BHK21 cell line (Py 19) with 3T3 cells also
failed to induce polyoma virus (Watkins and Dulbecco, 1967). In an
experiment in which a 3T3 cell line, doubly transformed by SV40 and
polyoma virus, was fused with BSC cells or with 3T3 cells, SV40 was recovered while polyoma virus was not. In both cases, cocultivation and fusion of the transformed cells with highly sensitive "indicator" cells were
insufficient to assure the rescue of this virus in its infectious form. One
cannot explain this failure but can only postulate that polyoma virus
integrated into the cell genome may be defective and unable to secure
the synthesis of complete infective virions. Gershon and Sachs (1963)

studied the properties of a somatic hybrid between polyoma-transformed mouse cells and could not obtain viral synthesis. The induction of complete virus has been demonstrated at least for SV40 and for Rous virus. Proof is still lacking for polyoma virus and for the adenoviruses. The results of the different authors are summarized in Table V.

b. *Other Evidence for the Persistence of the Viral DNA in Transformed Cells.* The hypothesis put to test was that the viral DNA persisted in the transformed cell in a form which could be rescued under certain conditions. Several attempts were therefore made in order to evidence an integrated viral genome in the cells stably transformed and propagated in tissue culture or in the animal. Such an integrated viral genome was hard to prove in the middle of the genetic information of the cell since a molecule of viral DNA contributes a very small

TABLE V

METHODS OF VIRAL RESCUE

References	Transformed cells	Permissive cells	Method	Virus
Svoboda *et al.* (1963)	Rat tumor (XC)	Chicks	Inoculation *in vivo* Rous sarcoma	Rous
Sabin and Koch (1963)	Transformed Hamster cells	BS-C-1 (*Cercopithecus* kidney cells)	Association of tumor cells with sensitive indicator cells	SV40
Black *et al.* (1963)	Hamster kidney cells	Primary African green monkey kidney cells (AGMK)	Mixed culture	SV40
Gerber (1966)	Hamster tumor cells (ependydoma induced by SV40)	AGMK cells	Mixed culture with inactivated Sendai virus	SV40
Payne and De Vries (1967)	Hamster tumors induced by SV40	BS-C-1	Mixed culture with inactivated Sendai virus	SV40
Koprowski *et al.* (1967)	Green monkey kidney GMKVaE W18 Va 2 W98 Va E.	AGMK (Hamster embryo)	Mixed culture with inactivated Sendai virus	SV40
Watkins and Dulbecco (1967)	SV40-transformed cells (SV3T3), BHK (Py19)	AGMK 3T3	Mixed culture with inactivated Sendai virus	SV40 Py
Cassingena and Tournier (1968)	SV40-transformed Syrian hamster cells: clone 2TS V5	BS-C-1	Fusion with UV-inactivated Sendai virus or temperature action	SV40

fraction of information compared to the total DNA of the cell (about one part in 2×10^6). Techniques sensitive enough to detect this DNA had to be devised. Experiments have been made using the nucleic acid hybridization procedure of Gillespie and Spiegelman (1965) which involves the immobilization of heat-denatured DNA on nitrocellulose membrane filters and the subsequent adjunction of the RNA or DNA put to test and labeled with radioactive compounds. In the case of DNA-RNA hybridization, the unpaired RNA is eliminated by ribonuclease treatment.

If the viral DNA is integrated in the genome of the transformed cell, the persistence of the transformed state being somehow linked to the presence and the expression of the viral DNA, this viral DNA may be transcribed. Several authors looked for such a virus-specific RNA in either polyoma virus, SV40, or adenovirus-transformed cells and evidenced a fraction of messengerlike RNA able to hybridize specifically with the purified DNA of the transforming virus. Once it was demonstrated that the viral DNA could be evidenced in the transformed cell, the physical state of this integrated viral DNA was investigated. Different authors also tried to determine the chromosomes in which this DNA was integrated, i.e., to try to determine the specific integration site of the DNA of the virus.

Another indication in favor of integration can be afforded by the action of interferon. The virus-cell interaction is sensitive to interferon in the early phase of interaction and the development of the first events can be inhibited. As soon as the transformation is achieved, the viral genome becomes insensitive to interferon, indicating that it may be under another form and probably integrated in the host cell genome.

c. *Presence of Virus-Specific RNA in Transformed Cells.* The presence of virus-specific RNA complementary to virus DNA has been well evidenced in lytic infection of mouse embryo cells by polyoma virus (Benjamin, 1966), for SV40 by Reich et al. (1966) and Aloni et al. (1968), and for adenovirus 12 by Fujinaga et al. (1968). Benjamin (1966), using mouse embryo cells infected with polyoma virus, demonstrated viral-specific RNA at different stages of infection with a hybridization technique between purified polyoma DNA immobilized on a filter and ^{32}P pulse-labeled RNA of the infected cells. He showed that RNA was synthesized shortly after infection and referred to this RNA as early RNA. This RNA is synthesized only in small quantities. Later, after the synthesis of cellular DNA had stopped, viral-specific RNA was synthesized in higher quantities, this being late RNA, which differs from the early RNA. In order to find out whether the maintenance of the transformed state is accompanied by the synthesis of viral-specific RNA, Benjamin also tested a number of cell lines for the presence of viral-specific RNA. He showed that there existed, in virus-free polyoma-transformed cells, a small fraction of the total RNA which was able to hybridize with polyoma DNA. Using RNA extracted either from normal cells or from spontaneously malignant cells or from mutant cells selected by their enhanced ability to grow in agar, no hybridizable RNA could be detected. Furthermore, there was no cross hybridization between RNA extracted from polyoma or SV40-transformed cells, but the RNA extracted from cells doubly transformed by polyoma and SV40 was able to hybridize with both types of DNA. It was possible to estimate roughly the amount of virus-specific RNA per cell. The calculated values vary from one to five half-polyoma DNA equivalents per cell and they are probably underestimated. It was not demonstrated if this DNA acted as messenger RNA or if a corresponding protein was implicated in the maintenance of the transformed state.

In a similar manner, Fujinaga and Green (1966) demonstrated virus-specific RNA in polyribosomes of both tumor cells and cells transformed by adenovirus 12. The viral DNA, although present in very small amounts in the transformed cells, may be more efficiently transcribed than the bulk of cell DNA. One might expect to find viral-specific RNA in the cytoplasmic polyribosomes of the cell. Different experiments have shown that a pulse label (120 to 180 minutes) of ^{3}H-uridine labeled almost preferentially the messenger RNA. In fact, the data obtained showed 2–5% of the labeled RNA in the polyribosomes as complementary to adenovirus 12 DNA. The fractionation of polyribosomes according to their size and the subsequent search for virus-specific RNA in the polyribosomes showed that viral-specific RNA was present in both larger and smaller polyribosomes. The specificity of these reactions was also demonstrated by the fact that polysomal messenger RNA complementary to adenovirus 12 DNA could be detected only in tumor cells and in transformed cells. When polyoma-transformed hamster cells, untransformed BHK21 cells, KB cells, or 3T3 cells doubly transformed by polyoma and SV40 viruses (SVPy3T3) were used, the percentage of radioactivity bound was very low (0.03–0.09%) compared with the percent of hybridized RNA in adenovirus-transformed and tumor cells.

d. *Characterization of an Integrated Viral Genome.* Different attempts have been made to detect an integrated viral genome in the case of hereditarily transformed cells or tumor cells. The early experiments were not very successful (Axelrod *et al.*, 1964) as they only showed by the DNA-agar technique a greater affinity of viral DNA for the DNA extracted from transformed cells compared to DNA extracted from normal cells. Winocour (1965a,b) tried to detect an integrated polyoma genome by hybridization between synthetic polyoma RNA synthesized using polyoma DNA as a primer for the DNA-dependent RNA polymerase of *E. coli*, and different DNA's extracted from polyoma tumors (polyoma-induced virus-free mouse or hamster tumors). This method, although it allowed the detection of 10 parts of polyoma DNA per 10^6 parts heterologous DNA, failed to demonstrate a difference in the RNA-binding abilities of DNA extracted from mouse and hamster tumors, corresponding normal tissue, or benzopyrene-induced tumors. The results showed that the cell lines tested did not contain virus-specific nucleotide sequences at the level of 10 parts in 10^6 which would be equivalent to approximately 20 copies of the viral genome per tumor cell. Further experiments by Winocour (1967) testing mouse synthetic RNA (synthesized using mouse DNA as template for the DNA-dependent RNA polymerase of *E. coli*) for its ability to hybridize with purified polyoma DNA or DNA of other viruses, showed a degree of complementarity between mouse RNA and polyoma DNA which was not exhibited by the DNA of other viruses such as Shope papilloma virus or vaccinia virus. This apparent homology between polyoma DNA and mouse synthetic RNA was finally shown to be restricted to the slower sedimenting component of polyoma DNA and was explained by the random encapsidation of mouse DNA during the production of the virus. Similar results of Michel *et al.* (1967) were in favor of the presence in the virus population of a fraction of viral capsids containing mouse DNA instead of viral DNA and giving rise to a population of "pseudovirions."

The experiments of Winocour which failed to evidence the presence of viral DNA in polyoma-induced tumor cells, focused attention on the two major technical difficulties which had to be overcome. The first one was the preparation of pure viral DNA not contaminated by cellular DNA. The improvement of a hybridization technique sensitive enough to allow the detection of one molecule of viral DNA per cell, i.e., one part of viral DNA in 2×10^6 parts of cell DNA, was the second requirement. This was accomplished by Westphal and Dulbecco (1968) using the technique of Gillespie and Spiegelman (1965) employing cellular DNA immobilized on nitrocellulose filters and RNA synthesized *in vitro* using purified component I DNA of polyoma or SV40 as template for the DNA-dependent RNA polymerase of *E. coli*. The sensitivity of the technique enabled less than five molecules of viral DNA per cell to be detected. Except for one of the cell lines tested which produced SV40 by fusion (SV3T3-47), it was not known if the complete viral molecules were present, which had allowed the estimation of the number of copies of viral DNA per cell. All the results were then expressed as the number of viral equivalents per cell. The results of hybridization experiments with cell lines of different origins and transformed either by SV40 or by polyoma virus or even by both viruses, indicated the presence of viral DNA equivalents in the different cell lines. The number of these equivalents varied in the cell lines tested from 7 (SV3T3-156) to 60 (H50 cell line) in SV40-transformed mouse cell lines, and from 5 (Py3T3-6) to 7 (Py8, a polyoma-transformed derivative of BHK21/C13 isolated in agar) and 10 (for SVPy3T3-11). The SVPy3T3-11 cell line doubly transformed by SV40 and polyoma virus contains about forty SV40 and ten polyoma DNA equivalents per cell. There seems to be no correlation between the number of equivalents of viral DNA per cell and any biological property of the cell since cell lines with a high average number of viral equivalents per cell are not "more" transformed. Their ability to produce infectious virus after fusion with susceptible cells is not correlated with the number of viral equivalents per cell. However, the number of viral equivalents found in a transformed hamster cell line (60 for the H50 cell line) is higher than the mean value for mouse-transformed cells. This finding is to be related to the report of Tai and O'Brien (1969) who reported in the case of another SV40-transformed hamster cell line propagated in the animal, the equivalent of 64 viral genomes per cell. The number of cell lines studied is not sufficient to allow us to say whether a high number of viral DNA equivalents is characteristic of transformed or tumor hamster cells or whether the case of both cell lines is a particular one.

e. *Determination of the Physical Characteristics of the Integrated Viral DNA.* Westphal and Dulbecco (1968), determining the number of viral DNA equivalents in a series of polyoma and SV40-transformed cell lines, showed that all the DNA hybridizable with synthetic polyoma or SV40 DNA was found in the nucleus of the cell and not in the cytoplasm. The number of viral DNA equivalents varied with the different cell lines. Further studies by Sambrook *et al.* (1968) investigated the physical state of SV40 DNA in the SV3T3 cell line which contains twenty SV40 DNA equivalents per cell, and showed that transformed cells do not contain supercoiled forms of viral DNA, i.e., component I of SV40 DNA, nor do they contain free viral DNA of the same size or a similar configuration to that present in virions. The viral DNA is integrated in the transformed cell since hybridizable material is found in DNA of extracted chromosomes; SV40 DNA is therefore associated with cell chromosomes during metaphase. Hybridizable material is found in high molecular weight DNA. In an alkaline sucrose gradient, cellular DNA is well separated from forms I and II of viral DNA. The high molecular weight DNA isolated from the cells hybridized with SV40 RNA to the same extent as DNA extracted from nuclei of transformed cells. Comparing Py3T3 (control cell line) and SV3T3 for their ability to hybridize with SV40 DNA,

the increase in hybridized counts (between SV40 3T3 and Py3T3) corresponded to 20 viral DNA equivalents per cell, either with DNA extracted from the nuclei or with high molecular weight DNA extracted
from the cell. The two possible states for the integrated SV40 DNA are
thus either free form II molecules of a size larger than normal viral
DNA (arising from viral DNA by tandem duplication) or a form covalently linked to cellular DNA or to another structural component of the
nucleus. So, in SV3T3 cells, viral DNA is integrated in cell DNA by
alkali-stable covalent linkage, either as one large molecule at a single
insertion site, or as individual molecules at many insertion sites.

The number of viral equivalents in SV40-transformed cell lines is
higher than the one found in polyoma-transformed cell lines. But one cell
line, SV3T3-56, a clone of 3T3 cells transformed by nitrous acid-treated
virus, exhibits only seven viral DNA equivalents per cell, suggesting that
the expression of a viral gene may be required for the presence (by integration or duplication after insertion) of a large number of DNA
equivalents per cell.

f. *Determination of the Site of Integration of the Viral DNA*. Different approaches have been made by Weiss *et al.* (1968), Weiss (1970), and
by Marin and Littlefield (1968), and Marin and Macpherson (1969) to
try to determine the specific integration site of the DNA of the transforming virus. Weiss *et al.* (1968) fused SV40-transformed human cells with
normal mouse cells and obtained hybrid cells which spontaneously and
preferentially lost human chromosomes when subcultured. They tested
the different cell lines obtained, the hybrid line and the derived cell lines,
with variable proportions of human and mouse chromosomes, for the
presence of T-antigen. The starting SV40-transformed human cells contained T-antigen as well as the starting hybrid cell line. In the cell lines
with variable numbers of human chromosomes, the presence of T-antigen
could be correlated with the presence of the human chromosomes. Cell
lines having lost all the human chromosomes no longer contained T-
antigen; the ones with a few human chromosomes contained a mixture of
positive and negative cells. These results suggested that the viral DNA
was associated with the chromosomes of the transformed cell rather than
present as free particles either cytoplasmic or nuclear. Another possibility
was that the hybrid cells would have lost some cellular genes necessary
for the expression of the viral genome; this was ruled out since hybrid
cells negative for T-antigen synthesized T-antigen again after infection
with SV40. In related experiments, Marin and Macpherson (1969)
studied different properties of two revertant clones isolated as chromosomal segregants from a hybrid clone (obtained by fusion of two BHK21
subclones) transformed by polyoma virus. The characteristics of these

clones were as follows: they did not contain the complement-fixing antigen specific for polyoma virus and the transplantation antigen seemed to be reduced or even lost. However, both clones could be transformed again by polyoma virus, suggesting that the reversion is due to the loss of viral genes of the transformed cell and not to the loss of cellular genes necessary for the expression of the transformed phenotype. Reversion would then be due to the loss of polyoma genes, genes which control the transformed phenotype and which are associated with one or more chromosomes. The viral genome seems to be quite stably integrated in the chromosomes of the transformed cells: if the viral genes were periodically dissociated from their support chromosomes, and reintegrated randomly in another one, hybrid cells having lost all the human chromosomes and still positive for T-antigen could be expected to arise from the cell population, since the free viral genome could be integrated in mouse chromosomes. This was never observed even after 150 cell generations (Weiss *et al.*, 1968). Further studies by Marin and Littlefield (1968) and by Weiss (1970) looked for a relationship between the presence of the virus and some characteristics of the transformed cell. Marin and Littlefield used two BHK21 sublines. One had lost the enzyme inosinic acid pyrophosphorylase (IPP) and was resistant to 6-thioguanine; the other had lost the thymidine kinase (TK) and was resistant to 5-BUDR. These two cell lines were fused; the hybrid cell line obtained was IPP$^+$ and TK$^+$, and it was also sensitive to both analogs. This hybrid was then transformed by polyoma virus and an IPP$^-$ line was isolated by growing the hybrid in a medium containing 6-thioguanine. The cells of this line had a chromosome number lower than that of the starting hybrid: they probably acquired resistance to thioguanine by loss of the chromosome carrying the IPP gene. The growth habits of these revertant clones were different from those of the parent cell line. Furthermore, some of these clones had a normal phenotype; they had also lost the T-antigen. These results suggest that the polyoma DNA, integrated in a chromosome, had been lost while the cell acquired the resistance to 6-thioguanine. This fact tends to indicate that in this case viral DNA is located on a unique chromosome. Weiss (1970) looked for an eventual linkage between T-antigen and thymidine kinase by studying the relationship between the disappearance of T-antigen and the disappearance of the human chromosome specifying the enzyme thymidine kinase. Hybrid cell lines were obtained by fusion of a 3T3 cell line resistant to 5-BUDR and having lost the TK with either of the two different human cell lines transformed by SV40 and resistant to 8-azaguanine. They thus cannot use hypoxanthine + aminopterin + thymidine. The hybrid cell lines obtained were, on the contrary, able to develop in this HAT medium, since enzymic deficiencies of both parents were complemented. Furthermore, suitable culture medium allowed the selection of two kinds of hybrids: hybrids selected for TK by culture in the HAT medium, and hybrids selected against TK by culture in a medium containing 5-BUDR. The observation that hybrid cells having lost the T-antigen were still able to develop in the HAT medium—and this has been observed for the hybrids obtained with the two different human cell lines used—shows that the parental SV40-transformed cell lines contained at least one TK specified by a chromosome which did not contain the SV40 genome. Furthermore, the hybrids cultured in the presence of 5-BUDR and which were at the beginning positive for T-antigen, remained positive: the human chromosome which carries the information for TK does not, therefore, contain a unique integration site for SV40. It seems unlikely that a unique human chromosome carries the specific integration site for the SV40 genome. These results seem to indicate that different chromosomes carry the SV40 genomes in the two human parent cell lines transformed by SV40 and used in the fusion experiments.

g. *Necessity of a Continuous Persistence of the Expression of the Viral Genome for the Maintenance of the Transformed State in the Case of RSV-Transformed Cells.* In the case of polyoma virus, Fried (1965a,b) had demonstrated that the function, called the *Ts-a* function, was necessary for the initiation of the transformation in BHK21 cells but not for the maintenance of the transformed state since cells transformed at the permissive temperature and then shifted at the nonpermissive temperature always showed the characteristics of transformed cells. A certain number of temperature-sensitive mutants of polyoma virus have been isolated, but none of them are defective in the ability to stimulate DNA synthesis in confluent cells, to produce abortive transformation, and to maintain the transformed state. Goldé (1970) has shown that irradiation of certain strains of avian sarcoma virus results in the formation of viruses which retain the ability to grow but are no longer able to transform. This indicates that part of the viral genome which is required for transformation is not required for growth; it is different from that observed with the *Ts-a* mutant of polyoma virus whose temperature-sensitive function was needed both for transformation and replication (Fried, 1970; Vogt, 1970). G. S. Martin (1970) isolated, after treatment with the mutagen N-methyl-N'-nitro-N-nitrosoguanidine, a temperature-sensitive mutant of RSV with the following properties: this mutant develops as well at the nonpermissive temperature as at the permissive temperature; only transforming ability is affected at the nonpermissive temperature. The wild-type virus grows as well at 41°C. as at 36°C. Since the mutant is unable to produce foci at 41°C., it may thus be distinguished from the wild type which forms clones at 36°C. as well as at

41°C. These results indicate that part of the viral genome of this mutant is required for transformation but not for growth.

II. Nuclear Modifications

Cell transformation being above all an inheritable characteristic, one would expect to find the earliest and most apparent modifications at the level of the nucleus. In fact, apart from nonspecific morphological alterations, it has been possible to detect two forms of nuclear changes: first, modifications of the chromosomal structure and second, antigenic modifications with the appearance of a new antigen. Finally, we shall see the proof of the continuous activity of the integrated viral genome by the synthesis of a virus-specific RNA in the transformed cell.

A. KARYOLOGICAL STUDIES

As far as the viral DNA is integrated in the chromosomal material of the host cell, specific chromosomal modifications could be expected to occur. In fact, it seems that the type of modification is different in DNA virus transformation from that in RNA virus transformation. We shall study successively DNA viruses, RNA viruses, and RNA plus DNA viruses double transformation.

1. *Transformation by DNA Viruses*

a. *SV40 and Human Diploid Fibroblast-like Cells.* Embryonic or adult human fibroblast-like cells are suitable material for studying karyological modifications after infection by SV40. In fact, these cells have a stable karyotype in culture and undergo few spontaneous transformations. The most convenient period for infecting the cells is the later period of declining growth rate because at this time the latent period between infection and transformation is the shortest (Todaro *et al.*, 1963; Jensen *et al.*, 1963). The period of infection and adsorption of the virus does not show any chromosomal modification (Moorhead and Weinstein, 1966). During the whole abortive cycle in kinetic study these authors observed no anomalies of the karyotype. Chromosomal anomalies appeared only 2 days after the initiation of transformation. Extensive chromosomal and chromatid breakage, polyploidy, abnormal unstable chromosomes such as dicentric chromosomes, were the most frequent signs of transformation. S. R. Wolman *et al.* (1964) found dicentric chromosomes 5 days after infection. Possible disturbances of the spindle were indicated by the increase in tetraploidy observed 2 days after loss of inhibition of division. However, endoreduplication among the tetraploid cells may mean that a disturbance of DNA synthesis rather than of spindle formation was the more important consequence of the presence of the virus.

In conclusion, the important point of the SV40 and human cell interaction is that the chromosomal anomalies appear only when the cell is
definitively transformed and do not occur during the abortive cycle of the
virus.

b. *SV40 and Hamster Kidney Cells.* Chromosomal analyses of adult
hamster kidney cells were done by Prunieras and Jacquemont (1965). No
specific difference could be evidenced between normal cells, SV40 infected,
or SV40-transformed cells.

c. *Polyoma Virus and BHK21 Cells.* The karyotype of the normal
hamster was established by Lehman *et al.* (1963). Macpherson (1963)
observed few deviations of this karyotype in the BHK21/C13 line. He
studied also the C13 TC6 cell line which is a polyoma virus-transformed
subline of the C13 cell line. Most of the cells retained the normal karyotype of the C13 cells. However, he noted a progressive increase in the
proportion of tetraploid cells in the subcultures of this line. This effect
and the progressive appearance of abnormal chromosomes indicated that
an increased tendency toward mitotic errors accompanied this type of
transformation. Marin and Basilico (1967) studied the variability of
BHK21 cells' susceptibility to undergo transformation by polyoma virus
and thought that increased susceptibility was related to the doubling of
the genome of the cell before division; a difference in ploidy could account
for the genetic variation. For this reason, these authors studied a hybrid
line of Littlefield—the Hy3 cell line. The Hy3 cell line and the Hy3-5
studied by Marin and Macpherson (1969) were obtained by fusion of
two BHK21 variants, B1 and T6, which carry drug-resistance markers.
Its modal chromosome number was approximately the sum of the modal
values of the B1 and T6 cells. The transformation rate of the Hy3 cell
line was compared to that of the parental lines, B1 and T6. The difference
observed was too small to suggest a "two-hit" phenomenon which might
be expected if each of the parental chromosome complements had to be
transformed independently.

d. *Human and Simian Adenoviruses and BHK Cells.* Cooper and
Stich (1967) tried to determine whether the chromosome damaging
capacity is a common property of adenoviruses, whether the types of
induced chromosomal and mitotic anomalies are virus-specific, and
whether oncogenic and nononcogenic adenoviruses differ in their capacity
to induce chromosome aberrations. Cultured Syrian hamster cells were
used as host cells, as most of the adenoviruses can initiate but not complete a full replication cycle in these cells. The input multiplicity of the
virus can be related with the viral dose. Infection of BHK21 cells with
human adenoviruses types 2, 4, 7, 12, or 18 or with Simian adenoviruses
SV7 or SV15 induced chromosome aberrations, including chromatid break-

age, fragmentation, overcontraction, erosion, and mitotic anomalies. The incidence of metaphase plates with chromosome aberrations and the intensity of damage per cell depended upon the input multiplicity of each virus tested. However, there was no correlation between the types of damage induced and the oncogenic potential of the virus.

In conclusion, in the Syrian hamster-DNA virus system, we saw that the transformed cells can show chromosomal modifications either in the number (increase of the ploidy) or in the structure, i.e., chromosome fragmentations, chromatid breakage, rearrangement. In fact, no specific evidence of the virus at the chromosomal level has ever been shown.

2. RNA Viruses

a. *Rous Sarcoma Virus (RSV) and Chinese Hamster Cells.* The effect of RSV on the chromosomes of a Chinese hamster cell line was studied by Kato (1967). This system was chosen because of the very good cytological characteristics of the Chinese hamster chromosomes, including low chromosome number (22), unusually good morphological differentiation, and the facility of identification of sex chromosomes and most of the autosomes. Consequently, chromosome breakages, both spontaneous and induced by RSV, have been studied in a clonal tissue culture cell line of Chinese hamster fibroblasts designated CL1 by Kato (1967). Two RSV strains were utilized: the Schmidt-Ruppin strain (RSV-SR) and the Mill Hill strain (RSV-MH). The cells were fixed after 12, 24, and 48 hours of culture. The average doubling time of the CL1 population was 24 hours. Cells infected with RSV exhibited a higher incidence of chromosome breakage than noninfected cells. A modified system of subdivision of the idiogram was devised by Kato and used to localize the breaks. There was no appreciable difference between RSV-SR and RSV-MH-treated cells. There were different types of breaks; open breaks without reunion of broken ends were the most frequent. Multiple breaks were observed to range from a number of breaks in one or a few chromosomes to extreme shattering of all the chromosomes of a cell; these were examples of the pulverization phenomenon. The anaphases of virus-treated cells revealed a variety of mitotic disturbances, pseudochiasmata, bridges, and multipolarity of the spindle. In conclusion, the present results agree with previous observations on the efficiency of RSV-SR to induce chromosome breaks, and also on the general characteristics of the induced breaks.

The nonrandom distribution of chromosome breaks over chromosomes and chromosome regions was very striking in the Chinese hamster. Many hypotheses have been proposed to explain why chromosome breaks tend to accumulate in heterochromatic regions. Hsu and Somers (1961) suggested that BUDR, which is incorporated into DNA in place of thymidine, would be especially active in damaging chromosome regions rich in adenine-thymine pairs. Nichols (1966) correlated chromosome breakage with inhibition of DNA synthesis in specific chromosome regions that might be late replicating segments. He suggested as a possible mechanism either a direct action of the virus on the chromosomes or an indirect action through the cytoplasm, possibly by competitive exhaustion of nucleic acid precursors.

b. *Rous Sarcoma Virus and Human Cells.* The accumulation of breaks in specific chromosome regions has also been observed in human chromosomes, although their localization is less distinct than in the Chinese hamster cells. Boué *et al.* (1968) studied chromosome evolution in human cells transformed by RSV-SR. More than 50% of the breaks could be observed in chromosomes while the cells were growing *in vitro* after virus infection. The first stable lesion was a ring chromosome that was present in 65% of the cells. They could thus follow the evolution of chromosome number modifications. First, they could see trisomies as C + C, C + D, C + F (autosomes). However, only cells showing two chromosomes of group C in addition were viable. In conclusion, the RNA virus system seems different from the DNA virus system from a chromosomal point of view. The chromosomal modifications seem more specific and closely related to the viral transformation in the RNA system.

3. *DNA and RNA Viruses*

In our laboratory (Berebbi and Bonneau, 1971), we studied the karyological variations related to susceptibility to transformation by polyoma virus and RSV in the hamster cell line BHK21/C13. A comparison between polyoma-transformed and RSV-transformed clones revealed the following characteristics: Polyoma virus did not seem to modify the chromosome modal number of hamster cells which remained pseudodiploid (44 ± 2) as was shown by Defendi and Lehman (1965) who noted that only one cell line developed chromosome anomalies and became subtetraploid. We did not find any specific chromosome abnormalities in the polyoma-transformed clones. In accordance with these authors, we found no chromosomal anomalies specific for the transformation of BHK21/C13 cells by polyoma virus. On the contrary, the RB12 clone derived from the same BHK21 line but transformed by RSV (Bryan strain) was hypotetraploid. On the other hand, Kato (1967) using the Schmidt-Ruppin and the Mill Hill strains induced breakage in specific regions of Chinese hamster chromosomes. We observed chromosome breakage in the RB12 clone, but these breaks were nonspecific and appeared at random so that we cannot say that a tendency to tetraploidy was associated with the RSV Bryan strain. It is possible that the clonal cell line BHK21/C13 transformed by RSV Bryan strain was tetraploid in the beginning. Marin and Basilico (1967) studied heterogeneous clones transformed by polyoma virus which were diploid or tetraploid. It is not yet possible to correlate modal chromosome number and transformation. Moreover, all clones doubly transformed by both RSV and polyoma virus seem to maintain diploid or pseudo-diploid chromosomal modes with the exception of one substrain (RP 38) which is widely aneuploid. It does not seem that the introduction of two viral genomes into the cells induces fresh anomalies in their chromosome number. No particular structural abnormalities were found in transformed clones either by polyoma virus or by RSV or by both viruses. However, only one subline doubly transformed with UV-irradiated polyoma and RSV viruses (RB12 PyUV) was hypotetraploid with a mode of 70–72 chromosomes, and presented an abnormally long chromosome in all the metaphases studied. It is not possible to say whether this occurred at the time of supertransformation by polyoma virus or if it preexisted in the RB12 population.

After this brief review of the studies of chromosomal modifications in correlation with viral transformation, it can be concluded first, that DNA virus transformation did not cause specific chromosomal modification, second, that some Rous sarcoma virus strains may induce characteristic breaks on specific chromosome regions, and third, that super transformation by DNA virus on originally RNA-transformed cells does not bring about further chromosomal modifications.

B. Antigenic Modifications

The most important and specific modification of the nucleus that can be detected is the appearance of a new antigen. Huebner et al. (1963) have demonstrated its existence for SV40. The first method used was complement fixation; the antibodies were present in tumor-bearing hamsters. The antigen was evidenced in ground tumors or transformed cells. Habel (1965) demonstrated the same antigenicity in the polyoma system. The titers of antigens and of antibodies were lower than in the SV40 system. The immunofluorescence method allowed localization in the nucleus of this complement-fixing antigen. In SV40-transformed cells (Pope and Rowe, 1964) the antibodies were shown to be the same by immunofluorescence and by the complement fixation technique. The cells must be fixed by a solvent specific for lipids. This increases the permeability of the membranes, which allows a better penetration of antibodies. In polyoma virus, it was more difficult to obtain an immunofluorescent reaction and the results have been obtained only recently (Takemoto et al., 1966; Defendi and Taguchi, 1966; Meyer et al.,

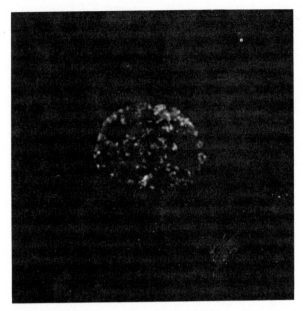

Fig. 1. T-antigen induced by polyoma virus in BHK21 cells at the twenty-fourth hour after infection, and revealed by the Coons method. The antigen appears as small dots all over the nucleus. The nucleolus remains unstained. ×2000.

1967b). The nuclear fluorescent antigen is seen as small dots scattered over the whole nucleus except the nucleoli (Fig. 1). No difference is observed in the aspects of antigens induced by different viruses.

1. Ultrastructural Localization of the T Antigen with Enzyme-Labeled Antibodies

The use of antibodies labeled either with ferritin or with different enzymes (peroxidase or phosphatase) has given a better localization of the nuclear antigens of the cells transformed by oncogenic viruses. Levinthal et al. (1967), studying adenovirus-infected and transformed cells, demonstrated that the ferritin particles were bound and concentrated at the following sites: (a) at the level of the filaments which appear early in the course of infection, (b) as intranuclear staining having a medium density to electrons, (c) as sediments of fibrogranular material, (d) as dense and homogeneous material which can be digested by pronase, (e) as material adjacent to the chromatin, and (f) connected to viral particles.

A similar study was undertaken with SV40-infected or transformed hamster cells (Levinthal et al., 1967). In transformed cells these authors demonstrated the existence of an accumulation of ferritin-labeled material in the nucleus corresponding probably to early antigens, and viral particles at all the stages of maturation surrounded by ferritin and located in the cytoplasm.

Ferritin is a large molecule and so enters the cells relatively poorly. Peroxidase is a smaller molecule and can enter more easily. The conjugation of the enzyme with antibodies denatures the latter to a small extent. Peroxidase marking was used by Wicker and Avrameas (1969) for the localization of the viral and tumor antigens of SV40, adenovirus 12, and rat K virus-infected or transformed cells. This technique allowed a direct comparison between light and electron microscopy. The T-antigen is seen as a cloudy network all over the nucleus except the nucleolus. Our findings were similar in polyoma virus-transformed hamster cells, BHK21 cells infected with polyoma virus, and polyoma virus-transformed mouse cells (Fig. 2). In all the experiments, the T-antigen was intranuclear, sometimes perinuclear, always leaving the nucleolus free as well as some parts of the chromatin. We never observed any viral structure.

2. Kinetics and UV Deletion of T-Antigen

The T-antigen was first described as a tumor antigen. Antibodies against this antigen were thought to be formed only in tumor-bearing animals. On the contrary, the presence of T-antigen was soon detected in the very early stage of the infectious cycle of cells *in vitro*. The name of T-antigen was also confusing and it was preferable to use Defendi's terminology: ICFA (induced complement-fixing antigen). Despite this fact, it was possible that a difference existed between the tumor antigen of tumor cells and the nuclear antigen revealed in the infectious cycle, especially in the case of adenoviruses. We shall prefer to use the terminology of tumor antigens and T-antigens.

Takemoto *et al.* (1966) described the kinetics of appearance of T-antigen in permissive cells for polyoma virus. In the same system, we studied the kinetics of synthesis of this protein. We used ^{3}H-leucine or mixed ^{14}C-amino acids. T-antigen was prepared from nuclear material (Chauveau *et al.*, 1956) and separated by polyacrylamide gel electrophoresis. This antigen was identified by radioimmunological titration in agar according to Ouchterlony. The method consists of two steps: labeled antigen and antibody reaction, then precipitation of this complex by antiglobulin serum. In this system, the synthesis of T-antigen began approximately 10 hours after infection, reached a maximum at the eighteenth hour, and decreased quickly after the twentieth hour (Fig. 3). This technique allowed the evaluation of the turnover of T-antigen: it

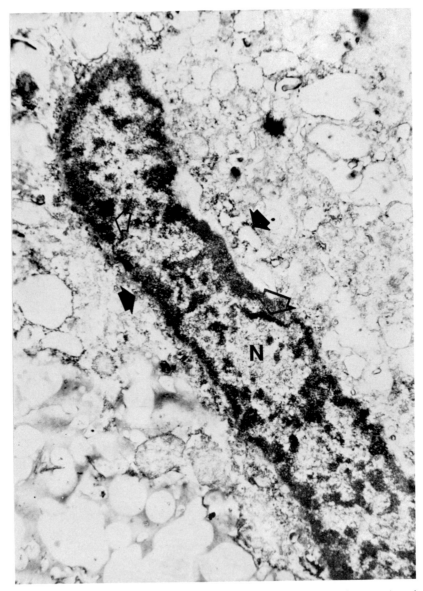

Fig. 2. Immunoelectron microscopy. T-antigen induced by polyoma virus in BHK21 cells at the twenty-fourth hour. Peroxidase-labeled antibodies are seen in the nucleus (N) in contact with chromatin (white arrow) and on the peri-nuclear membrane (black arrow). The cytoplasm remains unstained with few traces of marker nonspecifically adsorbed on membranes. ×15,000.

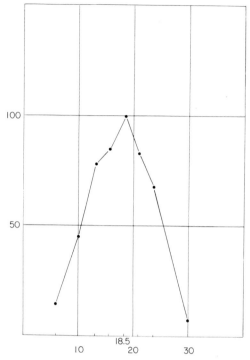

Fig. 3. Kinetics of synthesis of T-antigen in mouse embryo cells infected with polyoma virus (100 PFU/cell). The synthesis of T-antigen was followed by incorporation of ³H-leucine. T-antigen was prepared from nuclear material, separated by polyacrylamide gel electrophoresis, and identified by radioimmunological titration in agar according to Ouchterlony. In abscissa, hours after infection. In ordinate, the values of ³H-leucine incorporated are expressed as the percentages of the maximal incorporation.

was about 10% per hour and it is important to note that it did not increase in the decreasing phase of synthesis (Nicoli *et al.*, 1971). Similar studies are in progress in the transforming cycle.

From the time the T-antigen was discovered to be an early phenomenon, it was interesting to study its kinetics in a nonpermissive cell system (Meyer *et al.*, 1967b). By infecting BHK21 cells (Stoker and Macpherson, 1964) with polyoma virus, the number of cells with T-antigen increased very quickly (Fig. 4). The number of fluorescent cells was much greater than the number of cells undergoing transformation. After the twenty-fourth hour, the number of cells showing T-antigen decreased rapidly and after the forty-eighth hour only 6 or 7% of the cells showed this antigen. This was a demonstration of an abortive cycle of the virus in nonpermissive cells. This abortive cycle

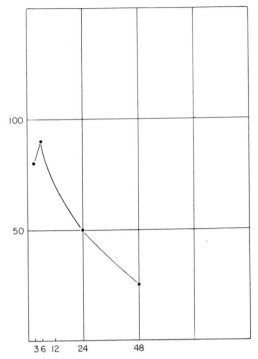

Fɪɢ. 4. Kinetics of appearance of T-antigen in BHK21 cells infected with polyoma virus (100 PFU/cell). As abscissa, hours after infection; as ordinate, percentage of cells with labeled nuclei.

has been confirmed (Stoker, 1968) from cell behavior in culture. In fact, it seems that all the cells were involved in the host cell and viral genome interaction, but most of the cells were "cured" of this infection. Probably only those cells where the viral genome could be integrated into the host genome showed the immunofluorescent antigen and underwent the subsequent steps of the transformation. Macpherson and Stoker (1962) have demonstrated that the ability to pass from the abortive cycle to the transforming cycle was not a property of the cell but seemed to be a random phenomenon. However, Basilico and Marin (1966) demonstrated that the possibility of the persistence of the viral genome in abortively infected cells was partially dependent on the phases of the growth cycle.

The same authors (Marin and Basilico, 1967) have demonstrated that polyploidy favored this passage, probably by the multiplication of reactive sites between chromosomes and virus.

The T-antigen was specific for the virus; it must then be coded by the viral genome. It was interesting to note the part of the viral genome involved in this coding. Research on SV40 (Carp and Gilden, 1965) and polyoma virus (Defendi *et al.*, 1967; Meyer *et al.*, 1969b) demonstrated that half of the viral genome necessary for replication was necessary for the coding of the T-antigen. To prove this fact, the virus was irradiated by UV or gamma radiation and a monolayer of nonpermissive cells was infected with the irradiated virus. The curves of deletion of the T-antigen were compared to those of the infectivity (Fig. 5). The ratio of the slopes of the different curves gave the part of the viral genome involved in the coding of the T-antigen. This technique also

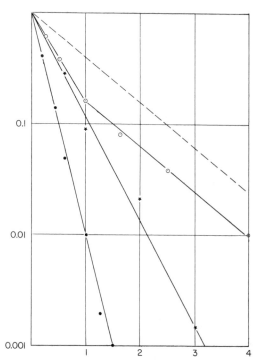

Fig. 5. Influence of UV-irradiation of polyoma virus on induction of T-antigen in BHK21 cells; comparison with inactivation of infectivity and transforming ability. UV doses ($\times 10^4$ ergs/mm.^{2}) are shown in abscissa. ●——●, virus infectivity as PFU. Infectivity of nonirradiated virus is 100%. ★——★, inactivation of T-antigen in BHK21 cells after UV-irradiation of polyoma virus; the percentage of cells with labeled nuclei is shown as a function of irradiation dose. Cells infected with nonirradiated virus are taken to show 100% fluorescence. ○——○, inactivation of transforming ability of UV-irradiated polyoma virus. Transforming ability is expressed in colony formation in soft agar. Transforming ability of nonirradiated virus is taken as 100%. —————, slope of the second part of the curve of inactivation of transforming ability.

allowed the comparison of the induction of T-antigen with the transforming ability of the virus studied. Basilico and Di Mayorca (1965), Benjamin (1965), Latarjet et al. (1967), and Defendi et al. (1967) had demonstrated that at least one-fifth of the viral genome was necessary to initiate the transformation. These results seemed contradictory. We have seen that the T-antigen is present in transformed cells but that the target of the function coding for transformation is 2.5 times smaller than the function coding for T-antigen. It is surprising that in a cell determined by only one-fifth of the viral genome, a function needing half of the viral genome necessary for infection can be expressed. The following argument may help to resolve this apparent contradiction. After the abortive infection, about 5% of the cells undergo transformation. However, if the same cell type is infected with polyoma virus, irradiated, for example, at 2×10^4 ergs/mm.^{2}, only 9% of these cells will show T-antigen. At the same time, the transforming ability is reduced to 1% of the whole cell population (Table VI). This 1% is now

TABLE VI
ABORTIVE AND PERMANENT TRANSFORMATION

Irradiation 10⁴ ergs/mm.²	T Ag. % cells	Colonies % cells	% T Ag. Colonies
0	90	5	5.5
1	30	2.25	7.5
2	9	1	11
3	2.7	0.42	15.5
4	0.84	0.2	24

11% of the cells which entered into the abortive cycle. It seems that by using irradiated polyoma virus, more cells of the abortive cycle underwent a definitive transformation. These results were confirmed by works in vivo (Defendi et al., 1967; Herberman and Ting, 1969) which demonstrated that irradiated polyoma virus had increased oncogenic ability. This could be due either to the fact that irradiation had selected oncogenic viruses or to specific radiation-induced oncogenic mutants.

3. Chemical Data on the Structure of T-Antigen

a. *Isolation of T-Antigen.* The fact that immunological techniques have been used to prove the existence of T-antigen indicates that techniques of protein isolation can be successful also. The following procedures have been used: T-antigen was prepared from different virus-transformed cultures. Tumor antigens were prepared from transplanted cells in compatible animals (Table VII). Adenovirus 12 and SV40 have been employed mostly as infecting agents. Two kinds of techniques may be used: one involves isolation of the nucleus and the other involves protein precipitation. To isolate nuclei, cell or tissue suspensions in saline solution were homogenized and centrifuged at 500g or more to give a nuclear pellet and a cytoplasmic supernatant. The nuclei were washed, resuspended, and disrupted by sonication. After centrifugation at more than 12,000g, the supernatant could be used for the purification of the T-antigen. Deoxycholate was used to separate the DNA (Delvillano et al., 1968; Tockstein et al., 1968a; Gilead and Ginsberg, 1968a). The precipitation technique could be used either alone or, as in most cases, following the isolation of the nuclear fraction. The most widely employed technique was ammonium sulfate precipitation (Fugmann and Sigel, 1967; Jainchill et al., 1969); at half saturation (Tativian et al., 1967; Gilden et al., 1968); at 32% saturation (Kit et al., 1966); and at 20–45% saturation (Lazarus et al., 1967). Other techniques have been used, such as calcium phosphate precipitation or pH 5 acetic acid precipitation (Kit et al., 1967a), magnesium chloride 0.1 M (Gilead and Ginsberg, 1968b), tris-chloride, cadmium chloride precipitation (Lazarus et al., 1967), and acetone precipitation (Jainchill et al., 1969; Gilead and Ginsberg, 1968a). However, they have not been proved to be more effective than the ammonium sulfate method.

All the present methods of purification require a large quantity of proteins (5 mg. or more). T-antigen did not exist in sufficient quantities to be used, thus tumor antigen had to be used in its place. All the methods used in the past have been insufficient for the total purification of T-antigen. Total purification would be obtained by combination of the following techniques, but the amount of proteins available was not sufficient. (a) Ultracentrifugation at 105,000g (Fugmann and Sigel, 1967). (b) Sucrose linear density gradients (Potter et al., 1969, 1970; Tativian et al., 1967; Tockstein et al., 1968b; Delvillano et al., 1968; Gilden et al., 1965; Gilden, 1968; Hollinshead et al., 1968). (c) Sephadex gel filtration from G-75 to G-200 (Fugmann and Sigel, 1967; Kit, 1966; Kit et al., 1967a; Gilden, 1968; Hollinshead et al., 1968). (d) DEAE-cellulose chromatography using either K_3PO_4, pH 7.3 and NaCl gradient (Tockstein et al., 1968a) or tris 0.05 M, pH 8, containing DDT 0.001 M and NaCl gradient (Lazarus et al., 1967; Fugmann and Sigel, 1967). (e) Hydroxylapatite chromatography (Tockstein et al., 1968b; Gilead and Ginsberg, 1968; Riggs et al., 1969). This method provides a 200–400-fold purification of T-antigen. The unique property which facilitates their lack of retention by hydroxylapatite columns is unknown. (f) Starch block electrophoresis (Riggs et al., 1969): all the recovered CF activity

TABLE VII
SOME CHARACTERISTICS OF SV40 AND ADENOVIRUS-T-ANTIGENS

References	Source of antigen	Method of identification	No. of species	M.W. daltons $\times 10^3$	S
Potter et al. (1970)	Adenovirus 12 CBA mice, Hamster cell lines: HEK, H Ep. 2	Rate-zonal centrifugation	2	70–80 40–50	
Tativian et al. (1967)	Adenovirus 12 Intraperitoneal hamster tumor KB cells	Sucrose gradient centrifugation	1	150	7.5
Tockstein et al. (1968b)	Adenovirus 12 KB cells	Rate-zonal centrifugation	4	84 52 40 24	5.1 3.9 3.7 2.2
Gilead and Ginsberg (1968b)	Adenovirus 12 KB cells Hamster cell line	Rate-zonal centrifugation	1		2.2–2.6
Jainchill et al. (1969)	Adenovirus 31. Solid hamster tumors	Rate-zonal centrifugation	1		2.93
Gilden (1968)	Adenovirus 12 KB cells	Sephadex. Rate-zonal centrifugation Membrane filtration	2	40–50 200	
Fugmann and Sigel (1967)	Adenovirus 12 Newborn Syrian hamster	Sephadex G-200	1	160	
Hollinshead et al. (1968)	Adenovirus 12 KB cells	Sephadex	2	67–68 23–27	
Hollinshead (1969)	Adenovirus 12 KB cells	Sephadex Rate-zonal centrifugation	1	25	
Potter et al. (1969)	SV40 trans- planted hamster tumor	Rate-zonal centrifugation	2	65–75 110–120	
Kit (1966)	SV40 GMK	Sephadex G-100	1	110–150	
Kit et al. (1967a)	SV40 Mouse kidney cells Hamster tumors	Sephadex G-200	1	200	

TABLE VII (*Continued*)

References	Source of antigen	Method of identification	No. of species	M.W. daltons × 10³	S
Gilden *et al.* (1965)	SV40 Human fibroblasts	Sucrose gradient centrifugation	1	600	
Delvillano *et al.* (1968)	SV40 Human fibroblasts	Rate-zonal centrifugation	1	60–70	

was present in one peak leading to a 10-fold increase in specific activity by a one-step procedure. A new technique, polyacrylamide gel electrophoresis, had never been used for purification of T-antigen although it has been used as a control (Tockstein *et al.*, 1968a; Gilden *et al.*, 1968; Jainchill *et al.*, 1969). This technique demonstrated more proteins than shown by serological tests. The same is also true for all the techniques mentioned above.

b. *Physicochemical Properties of the T-Antigen* (Table VII). Molecular weight has been estimated by rate-zonal centrifugation and Sephadex filtration techniques. The number and sizes of T-antigens reported in the literature present a confusing picture at the present time. They can be divided into five groups according to their molecular weights. (a) More than 200,000 daltons. Gilden *et al.* (1965) found a M.W. of 600,000 daltons for an antigenic species from SV40-infected human fibroblasts, but this species was probably not pure as it was bound to RNA. This could also apply to the antigen species having a M.W. of 200,000 daltons found by Kit *et al.* (1967a) and by Gilden (1968). (b) 150,000 daltons. Using the Sephadex method, a unique antigen species with a M.W. of 110,000–150,000 daltons was described by Kit (1966) and a unique species with a M.W. of 160,000 daltons by Fugmann and Sigel (1967). Using rate-zonal centrifugation, a unique species with a M.W. of 150,000 daltons was found by Tativian *et al.* (1967) and the largest species found by Potter *et al.* (1969) had a M.W. of 110,000–120,000 daltons. (c) 70,000–90,000 daltons. All experiments used rate-zonal centrifugation. The unique species found by Delvillano *et al.* (1968) and the smaller species found by Potter *et al.* (1969) have been shown to have this M.W. using T-antigen species from SV40. Using adenovirus 12 T-antigen, Potter *et al.* (1970) and Hollinshead *et al.* (1968) showed that the larger antigen had a similar molecular weight. These data were comparable to those of Tockstein *et al.* (1968b) who found this same molecular weight for the largest of four species. (d) 40,000–50,000 daltons. The smaller of the antigens found by Potter *et al.* (1970) having a M.W. of 40,000–50,000 daltons was comparable to the single species reported by Gilden *et al.* (1968). Tockstein *et al.* (1968b) reported two distinct T-antigen species in this position. (e) 20,000–25,000 daltons. An antigen species of estimated M.W. 20,000–25,000 daltons was reported as the only T-antigen species by Gilead and Ginsberg (1968a) and by Jainchill *et al.* (1969), as the smaller species by Hollinshead *et al.* (1968; Hollinshead, 1969), and as the smallest of the four species by Tockstein *et al.* (1968b). The data in groups 4 and 5 are limited to adenovirus only.

These studies do not necessarily conflict, as the interpretation of molecular weight from sedimentation coefficients assumes that molecules have the same shape and the same partial specific volume. The separation of multiple species of these antigens by rate-zonal centrifugation may indicate differences in molecular form rather than differences in molecular weight. It is also difficult to assume that all these antigen species are not an aggregate of the smallest species because only sodium deoxycholate was used as a dispersing agent.

Other physicochemical properties of the T-antigens induced by different viruses have been investigated. The SV40 T-antigen is a soluble protein (M.W.: 600,000 daltons) associated with nuclear RNA from which it may be dissociated by RNase (Gilden *et al.*, 1965). RNase treatment also caused a change in the distribution of SV40 T-antigen in rate zonal centrifugation (Delvillano *et al.*, 1968). The T-antigen and tumor antigens induced by adenoviruses could have physical differences (Gilden, 1968). The absorption spectrum of T-antigen had a maximum at 278 nm and a minimum at 250 nm; this is characteristic of proteins (Gilead and Ginsberg, 1968a). The antigenic activity of purified T-antigen was reduced at least 85% by digestion by trypsin for 1 hour at 37°C. (Gilead and Ginsberg, 1968a). The activity was not destroyed at a protein concentration of 2 mg./ml. by exposure to RNase 50 μg., trypsin 50 μg., chymopapaïn 0.2 mg., or papaïn 0.1 mg./ml. for 4 hours at 20°C (Jainchill *et al.*, 1969). The T-antigens were stable between pH 5.7 and 8.8 (Gilead and Ginsberg, 1968b), and near pH 4.5 (Jainchill *et al.*, 1969). These antigens may be acidic proteins (Tockstein *et al.*, 1968a). The T-antigens are temperature-sensitive at 56°C. (Gilead and Ginsberg, 1968b). Half of the CF activity was destroyed by heating to 56°C. for 5 minutes but the remaining activity was stable for 1 hour at 56°C. (Jainchill *et al.*, 1969). The T-antigen also appeared to be associated with or to contain a phospholipid, the removal of four-fifths of which rendered the T-antigen heat labile (Hollinshead, 1969).

The T-antigen contained 20% lipids (Hollinshead, 1969). It is lipophilic, and is associated with and probably aggregates on the cell membranes (Gilead and Ginsberg, 1968b). The solid tumor antigen is predominantly cytoplasmic (Jainchill et al., 1969). Three bands appeared to contain different proteins by nitrogen and group analysis: band 1, alanine and leucine; band 2, alanine and isoleucine; and band 3, alanine (Hollinshead, 1969).

c. *Enzymic Properties.* In the case of SV40, the T-antigen and the thymidine kinase differed in thermal stability and in adsorption on calcium phosphate gel. Both were insoluble in 32% ammonium sulfate (Kit, 1966). The T-antigen was tightly adsorbed by calcium phosphate gel, precipitated by acetic acid at pH 5 and by ammonium sulfate at about 20–32% saturation. These properties differed from deoxycytidylate deaminase, thymidylate kinase, thymidine kinase, and dihydrofolic reductase. DNA polymerase activity resembled the T-antigen in adsorption on calcium phosphate, in precipitation by ammonium sulfate, and at pH 5 by acetic acid. However, the polymerase activity could be partly separated from the T-antigen by Sephadex gel chromatography (Kit et al., 1967a).

In the case of adenovirus 12, the T-antigens were not pure in polyacrylamide gel electrophoresis and did not have any enzymic properties as did thymidine kinase, DNA polymerase, RNA polymerase, DNase, and RNase (Tockstein et al., 1968b).

4. Internuclear Transfer of T-Antigen

Fogel and Defendi (1967) had shown that in myotubes infected either with polyoma virus or with SV40, neither T-antigen nor viral antigen can be revealed by immunofluorescence. On the contrary, when infection was made at the time the myotubes were not fully formed, they could observe both the induction of cellular DNA synthesis as revealed by autoradiography, some viral DNA synthesis, and also the synthesis of the T-antigen. Up to 40% hamster muscle cells were positive after infection by polyoma virus, 25% rat cells in the case of rat cells; only 0.6% cells were positive when human muscle cells were infected with SV40. A very interesting problem would be to specify the mechanism by which the infecting virus induces a synchronous change in groups of nuclei in a myotube. The most probable explanation is that the information for the synthesis of virus-specific products is brought by one of the cells which fused to make the myotube and that this information was transferred to the other nuclei either by a chain induction or by a common derepression. Further studies of Fogel and Defendi (1968) dealt with the transfer of the SV40 T-antigen from virus-free

SV40-transformed human cells to the nuclei of rat myotubes upon coculture of both types of cells. Results showed that the SV40 T-antigen could be transferred from the virus-free SV40-transformed cells to myotubes of different species and to rat cells in particular. However, this transfer is a very rare event. The reason may be that the incorporation of a transformed human cell in a fusing myotube may be required; such a transfer does not occur by simple cell proximity or cocultivation.

Several explanations for this phenomenon can be proposed: (a) The T-antigen is synthesized in the cytoplasm of the donor cell and is then transferred to the nuclei of the myotube. However, T-antigen has never been detected in the cytoplasm. (b) The T-antigen migrates from one nucleus to another. (c) The T-antigen is induced by subviral particles which are transferred from one nucleus to the other nuclei. These experiments show that a specific cell product, such as T-antigen, may be transferred between heterospecific cells. Steplewski *et al.* (1968) further investigated the mechanism of the internuclear transmission of the SV40 T-antigen in heterokaryocytes. The investigation of the action of the SV40 by means of fusion between SV40-transformed cells and susceptible monkey cells showed that T-antigen was transmitted to the nucleus of nontransformed cells. The fusion may result in the production of infectious virus.

Different metabolic inhibitors were tested for their effect on the transmission of the T-antigen: FUDR, cycloheximide, and actinomycin D. The synthesis of T-antigen must indeed be directed by a portion of the viral genome; this transmission may occur following one of these modalities: (a) The transmission of T-antigen may be mediated by the transfer of the viral genome from the donor cell to the recipient cells. This model needs the synthesis of both messenger RNA and protein. (b) The transmission may be a passive transfer of already synthesized antigen. (c) Messenger RNA may be transferred from the donor cell to the recipient cell where T-antigen is then synthesized. (d) T-antigen is synthesized in the cytoplasm of the heterokaryocyte and is then incorporated in the recipient nuclei. Addition of FUDR to the culture medium does not affect the internuclear transfer of T-antigen. DNA replication is therefore not needed for internuclear transfer of T-antigen. The addition of cycloheximide (which inhibits protein synthesis) blocks the transmission of T-antigen; *de novo* protein synthesis would then seem to be required for the transmission. The addition of actinomycin D blocks the transmission of T-antigen whatever the species of origin of the transformed cell lines. These different results indicate first, that the replication of the gene directing the synthesis of T-antigen is not necessary for the transmission; second, that a passive transfer of already synthesized antigen from one nucleus to another does not occur since the presence of cycloheximide had not blocked such a transfer and third, that there is an actual block of the internuclear transmission of T-antigen by actinomycin D. The site of the synthesis of T-antigen will be matter for conjecture as long as it is not known whether such a protein can be synthesized in the nucleus. In fact, it is most probably synthesized in the cytoplasm where it may be under a "nonantigenic form," which would not allow its recognition.

C. Expression of the Viral Genome in Transformed Cells

We have already seen that in transformed cells, a fraction of the total messenger RNA, capable of specifically hybridizing with the DNA of the transforming virus, could be demonstrated. Since it is not known for the majority of the transformed cells whether the cell contains a complete or defective viral genome, it is rather difficult to estimate the amount of RNA produced (or even the amount of integrated DNA) except when the complete viral genome can be rescued after fusion with permissive indicator cells. In the case of polyoma virus-transformed 3T3 or BHK21/C13 cells, Benjamin (1966) showed that a certain fraction of the viral genome was transcribed into RNA, the amount of RNA produced per cell being equal to one to five half-polyoma DNA equivalents. Fujinaga and Green (1966), looking for virus-specific RNA in polyribosomes of adenovirus-transformed cells, found that up to 1 to 5% of the polysomal RNA was virus-specific. Numerous studies were then undertaken in many laboratories to try to determine the amount of virus-specific RNA produced in SV40-transformed cells and its relations to virus-specific RNA produced in infected cells.

During infection of permissive cells, viral-specific RNA is produced in two steps: immediately after infection, a small quantity of an early RNA appears. After the synthesis of cellular and viral DNA has ceased, late RNA is produced in amounts 30 to 40 times that of early RNA. Thus it is relatively easy to isolate late RNA for competition hybridization experiments, but it is rather difficult to succeed in isolating enough early RNA for such experiments. Different authors (Aloni et al., 1968; Oda and Dulbecco, 1968; Sauer and Kidwai, 1968; M. A. Martin and Axelrod, 1969; M. A. Martin, 1969) tried to characterize the viral-specific RNA produced and looked for its relationship with RNA of infected corresponding cells.

Therefore, in all the SV40-transformed cell lines studied, the DNA-RNA hybridization reveals the presence of virus-specific RNA, this RNA transcribing variable parts of the viral genome. The degree of homology of this RNA with the late RNA of infected cells is more or less important. It is, however, rather difficult to determine its degree of homology with early RNA of infected cells which is produced only in small quantities. The proportion of RNA transcribed seems to vary with the type of transformed cells (Table VIII). Sauer and Kidwai (1968) showed that in originally permissive SV40-transformed cells, the RNA produced shows a degree of homology with the late RNA of transformed cells which is twice the degree of homology of the RNA of SV40-transformed mouse cells (nonpermissive cells). In mouse cells, a

TABLE VIII
VIRUS-SPECIFIC RNA PRODUCED IN VARIOUS SV40-TRANSFORMED CELLS

References	Cells	Amount of virus-specific RNA produced	Properties of the RNA synthesized
Aloni et al. (1968)	SV3T3-10 clone 1 (Green and Todaro)	Similar to the amount of early RNA detected in virus-yielding cells	Competition hybridization experiments with late RNA of infected cells: $\frac{1}{3}$ of the viral genome is transcribed. Base composition is different from that of both early and late RNA of virus-yielding cells (BSC-1)
Oda and Dulbecco (1968)	SV3T3 (Green)	Similar to the amount of early RNA	RNA transcribed is different from early RNA: expression of viral DNA sequences not expressed in early lytic infection. Sequences transcribed correspond to almost $\frac{1}{3}$ of the late RNA of infected cells.
Sauer and Kidwai (1968)	3T3 transformed by SV40 (nonpermissive cells)		The fraction of DNA transcribed into RNA shows 40% homology with late RNA of infected cells. RNA of transformed cells seems to inhibit almost completely the binding of early RNA.
Sauer and Kidwai (1968)	GMK cells transformed by SV40 (originally permissive transformed cells)		The fraction of DNA transcribed into RNA shows 80% homology with late SV40 RNA of productively infected cells.
M. A. Martin and Axelrod (1969)	5 different SV40-transformed mouse cell lines	15–50% of the viral genome	

special property of the host cell might be responsible for the restricted transcription, compared to what is observed in transformed GMK cells. It is noteworthy that the RNA produced shows such an homology with the late RNA of infected cells: the functions of viral origin observed in the transformed cells are early functions, synthesis of T-antigen, induction of cell DNA synthesis, and induction of cell surface modifications. It remains to determine whether or not the virus-specific RNA produced in transformed cells exhibits an homology with the early RNA of infected cells.

It is essential for the maintenance of transformation that the expression of the viral genome be regulated, but one may ask how this regulation is made. Pettijohn and Kamiya (1967) showed that the purified DNA-dependent RNA polymerase of *E. coli* attaches specifically to some sites of the polyoma DNA molecule in ionic strength conditions allowing enzymic activity. The number of sites, corresponding to a "specific saturation" of the DNA, is equal to 4 to 7 molecules of RNA polymerase per molecule of polyoma DNA. Pettijohn and Kamiya postulated that, in addition, the affinity of the different fixation sites may not be identical. Such differences may represent an important mechanism for the regulation of the relative rates of transcription of the different DNA cistrons.

The analogy existing between lysogeny and cell transformation by oncogenic viruses leads different authors to postulate the existence of a repressor, analogous to that evidenced in *E. coli* cells lysogenized by the lambda bacteriophage (Ptashne, 1967a). This repressor, which is the product of the C1 gene of the phage, attaches to the two operator sites of the integrated chromosome of the phage, these two operators controlling the two sets of genes which are read in opposite senses (Ptashne, 1967b). It can be questioned whether such a repressor and such a repression mechanism exist in nonpermissive transformed cells. Different authors had different experimental approaches. The results obtained were also different, the alternative being that there is no repressor in SV40-transformed cells (Jensen and Koprowski, 1969) or that there is a repressor in the cells infected or transformed by SV40 (Cassingena *et al.*, 1969) or by polyoma virus (Cramer, 1969; Zamfiresco, 1970).

Jensen and Koprowski (1969) thought that no repressor exists. The following experiments were done: fusion between transformed cells and other SV40-transformed cell lines which were originally permissive for the virus. The nonpermissive transformed cells were the SV3T3 cell line and various transformed hamster cells. Transformed human cells, which were resistant to the superinfection by the virus, or green monkey kidney cells (AGMK) were the cell types used as permissive cells. The GMK E-VA clone and derived subclones which were resistant to the superinfection by SV40 but could be reinfected by SV40 DNA were especially used. Cocultivation or fusion experiments between nonpermissive transformed cells and originally permissive transformed cells showed that infectious virus is rarely obtained by cocultivation while almost all the heterokaryons obtained by fusion with β-propionolactone-inactivated Sendai virus produced virus.

These results argue against the presence in SV40-transformed cells of a compound inhibiting the replication of SV40. A repressor can be evidenced in SV40 or polyoma virus-transformed cells (Cassingena and Tournier, 1968; Zamfiresco, 1970). Cassingena and Tournier showed a repressor, in SV40-transformed cells, which is a protein molecule and reduces SV40 multiplication in monkey cells. There is an optimal concentration of the repressor to obtain an effect. Furthermore, it is necessary to add to the culture medium a basic polymer (such as poly-L-lysine) which increases the cellular permeability. The action of the repressor is evidenced by a technique of the "decrease of the plaques": the results are expressed as the percentage of reduction of the number of plaques in the test versus the number of plaques in the control which received no addition of the cellular extract containing the repressor. SV40-transformed cells give a mean inhibition rate of 30%. With a similar technique, Zamfiresco (1970) demonstrated that a specific repressor can be evidenced in polyoma-transformed hamster or rat cell extracts. This repressor is a protein; it is sensitive to trypsin and to high temperature, resistant to DNase or RNase treatment, and would be coded for by the virus. Cassingena et al. (1969) and Cramer (1969) respectively demonstrated an inhibitor in SV40 abortively or productively infected cells and in polyoma abortively infected cells. The inhibitor synthesized in the case of BHK21 cells infected with polyoma virus was also found in BHK21 clones transformed by polyoma virus, in a clone of BHK21 doubly transformed by polyoma virus and Rous virus (Montagnier et al., 1969), and in spontaneously transformed cells. Hybrid mouse-hamster cells were also tested for the presence of such an inhibitor. They do not contain such an inhibitor, which would show that there is no dominant information in hamster cells. Further experiments are needed to know if there is really an inhibitor in virus-transformed cells or in cells which undergo an abortive infection and, if this is the case, to elucidate its mode of action. Does it act, like the lambda repressor, directly at the DNA level and so inhibit the transcription of viral DNA in the transformed cells? Transformation would thus only be a matter of DNA transcription.

In conclusion, it can be considered that the essential event at the nuclear level is the persistence of the viral genome with its integration into the cell's chromosomal stock. The result of this supplementary genetic information is the synthesis of new proteins directed by viral-specific RNA. Regulation of the entire cellular machinery is disturbed without (and that is where we find the originality of the transformation) causing cell death. In this context, morphological modifications of the nucleus are only secondary.

III. Cell Surface Modifications

A. INTRODUCTION

It seems to be well established that the transformed cell has a modified plasma surface. The initial evidence was immunological as shown by Habel (1961) and Sjögren et al. (1961) in the polyoma system; there is a manifestation of a new antigen, the homograft rejection antigen. Adaptation to agar, changes of electrophoretic mobility correlated to modifications of the superficial charges, ability to grow in suspension, and, most recently, the evidence of a new antigen by immunofluorescence, are the most recent tests of the modifications of the cell surface. These events appear to be important not only in the evolution of the transformed cell, but also because some of them could be the basis of the transformation itself.

The homograft rejection antigen has been reviewed by Deichman (1969). We are only concerned with comparison of this antigen with the other surface modifications. We will describe successively the morphological modifications seen by light and electron microscopy, chemical modifications, and antigenic modifications revealed by different techniques.

B. BRIEF REVIEW OF THE MEMBRANE STRUCTURE AND
   ITS RELATION WITH THE NEIGHBORHOOD

1. Structure

Adhesiveness on glass or plastic surface, intercellular adhesiveness, contact inhibition of movement, and contact inhibition of division are the typical features of normal cells growing in vitro. We know, after Wallach's studies (1969), that all these phenomena may be explained by particular membrane activities. In fact, to justify this explanation, we must consider cell surface membrane as the borderline between extracellular and intracellular medium. The first model for membranes was proposed by Danielli and Davson in 1936. They believed that the membrane consisted of a double layer of lipid molecules joined by their hydrophobic tails and sandwiched between two protein layers, these proteins being the internal and external borderings. The electron microscopic counterpart of the lamellar structure was the unit membrane of J. Robertson (1959). In recent years, however, an increasing amount of evidence points to a different structure called granular, globular, hexagonal, or repeating unit pattern. In fact, the first model could not explain all the exchange properties of the cell. It also seems that the surface proteins are not holoproteins but glyco and/or lipoproteins. Recent results also show that parts of the membrane possess a regional specialization. The different structures for the membrane and the different models proposed have been usefully analyzed in recent reviews on this problem (Elbers, 1964; Curtis, 1967; Stoeckenius and Engelman, 1969; M. Wolman, 1970; Danielli, 1968).

It is important to give a definition of cell surface membrane: cell surface membrane is constituted of structural coordinations consisting, on the one hand, of a differentiated particular cytoplasmic zone, toward the intracellular medium, and on the other hand, of a mosaic formed by elements elaborated by the cell near the extracellular medium, and of extracellular elements modified by the presence of the membrane. The particular behavior of tumor cells and generally of transformed cells could be explained by modifications of the cell surface membrane. We will try to elucidate this point. Among many papers describing the behavior of transformed cells *in vitro*, we shall describe some well-defined experiments which seem to be particularly related to our subject.

2. *Mechanical Requirements for Cell Growth*

For growing and propagating in culture, normal cells need a solid support: this is the phenomenon of anchorage dependence. *In vitro*, this support is the glass or the plastic of the bottle used. In a semiliquid medium containing methylcellulose, normal cells do not grow if there are no glass fibrils in the medium on which the cells can fix themselves and elaborate colonies (Stoker, 1968). These fibrils, measuring about 0.5 mm in length, are able to take the place of a solid support. On the contrary, silica fragments shorter than the size of cells cannot fill the place of solid support. However, some virus-transformed cells or some tumor cells do not require solid support and propagate themselves in a semi-liquid medium (Sanders and Burford, 1964). This method of culture in suspension has been used by Montagnier and Macpherson (1964). These authors demonstrated that only polyoma-transformed BHK21 cells grew in suspension in a medium containing 0.35% agar, whereas normal BHK cells did not grow. *In vitro*, semiliquid medium containing agar, from a mechanical point of view, is closely related to pericellular

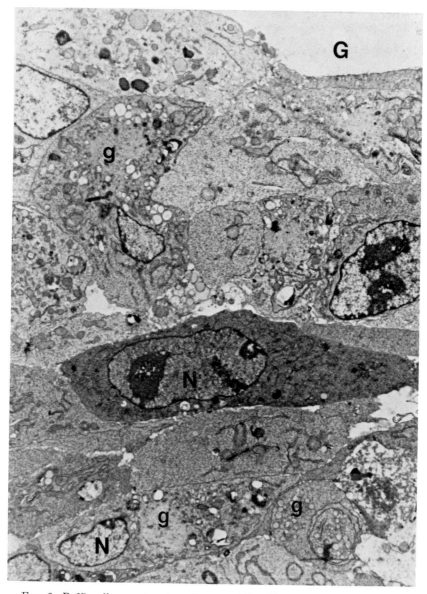

Fig. 6. Py27 cells growing in soft agar (G). The cells are round and well differentiated. Golgi apparatus is prominent (g). ×6000.

environment *in vivo*. Thus we can approximate that *in vitro*, this model resembles the model that was observed *in vivo* (Figs. 6 and 7).

3. *Cellular Environment and Intercellular Communications*

When two normal cells come in contact in culture, they remain motionless; this is contact inhibition of movement. They also stop dividing; this is contact inhibition of replication. Transformed cells in culture lose contact inhibition and show a characteristic appearance with three-dimensional growth. In order to observe contact inhibition, movement phenomena and replication, mixed cultures of both transformed and normal cells were required. Borek and Sachs (1966), studying normal cells and the same cells transformed either spontaneously or by different chemical carcinogens, or by a DNA virus, had concluded that a normal cell contact-inhibits and is contact-inhibited by normal cells and transformed cells. Similar experiments between normal cells and transformed cells demonstrated that transformation is the result of a change in the regulating mechanism and that the transformed cell was only contact-inhibited by cells of another type, either normal cells or cells transformed by an agent different from its own transforming agent. Stoker *et al.* (1966) and Stoker (1967) studying BHK21 cells transformed by polyoma virus and normal fibroblasts reported that the growth of transformed cells was inhibited by normal cells of the same type or by transformed cells of another origin.

Contact inhibition of movement and division are specific phenomena. Wallach (1969) refers to Stoker for the interpretation of these facts: "contact inhibition requires both a transmitter and a receptor mechanism and . . . the neoplastic cell can receive a specific message leading to contact inhibition but cannot send this message to a cell of its own kind." The normal cells are supposed to exchange information, the result of which is contact inhibition of movement and division when cells approach one another. The nature of these intercellular exchanges is unknown. Bellanger and Harel (1969) thought it could be possible that a diffusible factor exists that is responsible for inhibition of protein synthesis in the cells. This inhibitor is a small thermostable and dialyzable molecule.

Todaro *et al.* (1965) working on 3T3 cells in contact inhibition observed that after addition of calf serum, it was possible to verify an increase of RNA synthesis followed by protein synthesis and by some DNA synthesis. Holley and Kiernan (1968) demonstrated in the case of 3T3 cells that the final cellular density obtained after the stop of division was directly proportional to the quantity of serum added to the medium. The serum would therefore contain one or several factors needed for the division of 3T3 cells, called "serum factor(s)." It is to

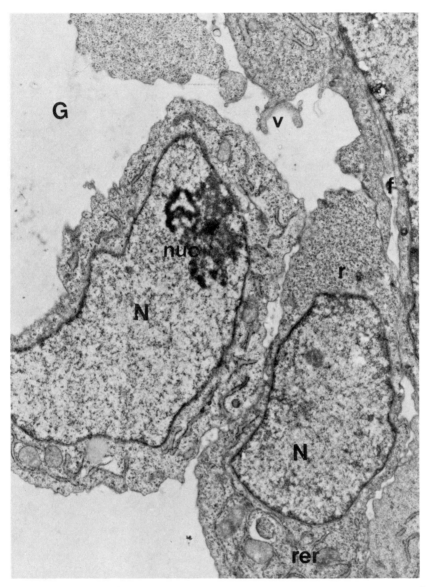

FIG. 7. Py27 growing in soft agar. These cells represent the growing part of a microcolony. These cells show "rosette"-like ribosomes (r) and rough endoplasmic reticulum (rer). Between the cells there are fibrillar materials (f) or microvilli (v). The nucleolus is prominent (nuc). ×18,000.

be noticed that virus-transformed 3T3 cells have a greatly reduced
requirement for these serum factors.

C. Aspects of Membrane Modifications According to Different Techniques

1. *Optical Microscopy*

Our model for normal cell culture is the hamster embryo secondary
culture which can be considered as reference cells. However, for practical
reasons we utilized mainly fresh subcultures of the BHK21/C13 strain
which can be considered as nearly normal (Stoker and Macpherson,
1964). Further studies (Montagnier, 1970) showed that this cell line
has probably jumped Montagnier's first stage. An inverted microscope
allows growth of cells on glass to be followed: the cells stay in ordered
direction and do not form foci or microcolonies; the cellular layer
gradually becomes homogeneous. In old cultures only, cells intersect
themselves and thus grow in several layers. This can be seen perfectly
in cross section in the electron microscope (Figs. 8 and 9).

Microcinematographic examinations of this cell type enabled Abercrombie and Ambrose (1958) to study the details of their movements.
Normal cells have a phase of progression productive of microvilli; the
opposite pole is constituted by stretching of the cytoplasm. When two
normal cells come in contact there is a change in polarity of the villi;
the direction of movement of the two cells also changes, the parts being
separated in contact. Cells multiply and when the culture reaches con-
fluence, the points of contact between the cells become more and more
numerous. Contacts persist, cellular movements stop, and divisions also
cease. In BHK21/C13 cells, cessation of division does not occur and
the cells run over onto neighboring cells. Cellular limits on fixed cells
can be seen better when the Harris-Shorr staining method is used:
culture is homogeneous and the elongated fibroblastic-type cells lie in
parallel on the glass support. All cells present contacts and have a pro-
pensity to move one upon another if the culture is not stopped. The
chromatin is dusty and regularly scattered. Nucleoli, which are easily
seen in this technique, are of equal volumes and are not very heavily
stained; only one nucleolus is apparent. Giant or numerous nucleoli
joined to heavily stained nucleoli indicate the aging of these cells. Heavy
cytolysis does not occur. Dulbecco (1969) demonstrated that cells transformed by oncogenic viruses have a very different behavior: they do not
undergo contact inhibition and there is no change of direction of migration after the contact, and the overlapping on several surfaces occurs
before completion of the monolayer. Some microcolonies, like perceptible
foci, can be seen by an inverted microscope and look like cellular foci

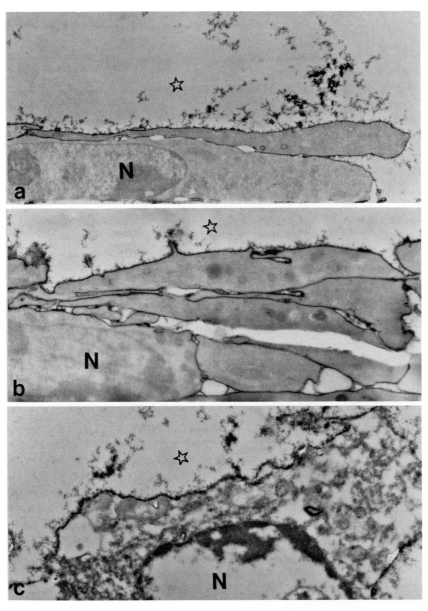

Fig. 8. Kinetics of growth of the BHK21/C13 on glass. Sections are perpendicular to the growing surface. Ruthenium red was mixed with glutaraldehyde solution. (a) First day of culture: monolayer or bilayer of BHK cells; there are no microvilli on the surface. ×7000. (b) Third day: four or five layers of cells are overlapping. We note the U or Y-like endings of the cells. ×10,000. (c) Eighth day: the lytic process occurs; the nucleus is pycnotic. The RR-stained membrane is however, well preserved. ×10,000.

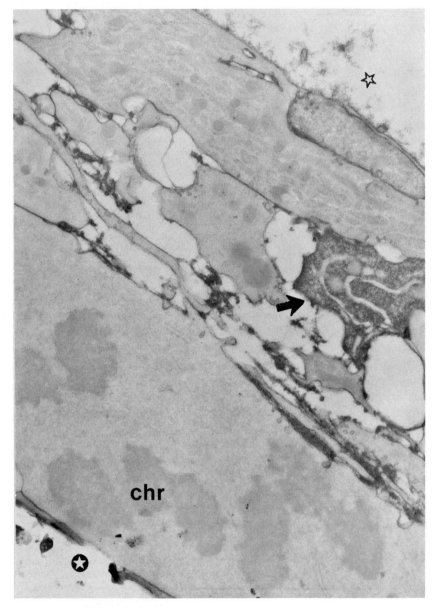

Fɪɢ. 9. Kinetics of growth of the BHK21/C13 on glass. The RR stain was mixed with glutaraldehyde. Eighth day: the lytic process is indicated by the black arrow and mitoses occur (chr) near the glass surface. ×13,500.

in cytology. Central cells of these foci are necrotic and peripheral cells seem to slip off anywhere. In these foci, the nucleoli are irregular and hypertrophied, chromatin is condensed, more basophilic, and the cytoplasm is poorly developed and cellular limits, consequently, much more distinct. In conclusion, all the aspects shown in the different models studied permit us to clearly state three phases of a culture: contact inhibition of culture exhibited by hamster embryo cells, semicontact inhibition exhibited by confluent BHK21/C13 cells, and lack of contact inhibition exhibited by polyoma-transformed BHK21/C13 cells.

It is possible (Pollack *et al.*, 1968) that contact inhibition of division and its determinism have the same regulatory factor as cell growth *in vivo*. The degree of contact inhibition in culture could be correlated to the ability of tumor formation: decreased contact inhibition *in vitro* would correspond to a lower tumor-inducing ability *in vivo*. This hypothesis is contradictory to Rabinowitz and Sachs' results (1969): epithelioid variants of polyoma-transformed BHK21 cells issued from fibroblastic-transformed cells show a decrease of plating efficiency and some properties characteristic of normal cells (autocontact inhibition and contact inhibition with parental cells). On the contrary, they have an increased tumorigenicity. This discrepancy between tumorigenicity and *in vitro* cellular properties could be caused by a modification of the cell surface in these variants. The apparent conflict in the results is possibly dependent upon the choice of models. Criteria for transformation, cancerous state, and tumorigenicity remain to be established and at this time no general rule can be made.

2. *Electron Microscopy*

The electron microscope allows us to see distinctly the cell-limiting unit membrane and some variations of its structure, variations which reflect specific activity at this level. Some sophisticated techniques have helped the study of the three-dimensional growth of cells in culture. Duhal and Césarini (1967) and Martinez-Palomo and Brailovsky (1968) described improved techniques to clarify this point.

We studied the BHK21/C13 system extensively by a sequential analysis of the evolution of this clone from time zero (corresponding to the plating of the cell) to the fourteenth day of culture. A parallel study of the transformation of this clone by polyoma virus was undertaken. We analyzed at the same time different clones of cells transformed by the same virus strain and/or related virus strains. We also used ultrastructural histochemistry in order to study the modifications of the cell surface.

a. *Criteria for Membrane Activities.* The following criteria have been taken for testing the membrane modifications: (a) membrane profile (straight, large-waved, short-waved); (b) membrane expansions (large microvilli, short microvilli, ball-like structures); (c) stopping-lateral contacts (Y-like, simple overlapping); (d) micropinocytosis at the upper and the under sides of the cell, forming either lines or clumps; (e) fibrillar material and microtubules; (f) nature of intercellular contacts (large space between two cells, tight junction, desmosomes).

b. *Histochemical Criteria.* We used mainly two techniques to evidence membrane glycoproteins. First, the affinity of ruthenium red (RR) for hyaluronic acid and chondroitin sulfuric acid as noted by Morgan (1968) who quoted Luft (1966). Sialic acid is not labeled by RR stain. RR seems to be dense under the electron microscope and thus appears black on the micrographs. Second, ultrathin sections of material embedded in glycol-methacrylate (GMA) (Leduc and Bernhard, 1967) were stained by Rambourg solution (Rambourg, 1967). This technique is similar to a PAS reaction for electron microscopy when carried out at pH 1.0. With GMA we can digest the thin sections by neuraminidase which specifically extracts its substrate.

With RR, we studied some particular points (thickness, electron density, smokelike projections, accumulation at the upper side of the cell) at the level of cellular contacts.

c. *Kinetics of BHK21/C13 Growth.* Twenty-four hours after seeding, most cells have stuck to the glass and have begun to spread. Cells are elongated, with rare short expansions; the cellular extremities are in contact. Micropinocytosis is limited. There is no formation of a dense material accumulation (which we shall henceforth call "plugs") and the surface offers a regular layer labeled by RR (thickness about 15 to 18 nm.). Thick smokelike projections escape from this layer; intercellular contacts are produced in parallel lines (Fig. 8). On the third day, two or three cell layers, regularly scattered on the surface, can be seen. Cell surface presents large waves and slender extensions of their extremities. Pinocytosis is greater, contacts of extremities are either U-shaped or Y-shaped. Plugs of material labeled with RR are more and more numerous.

On the eighth day, five or six layers are superposed, with very important micropinocytosis, longer microvilli, and a great number of intercellular plugs. RR contrasted filaments extend from cell to cell. Two phenomena, perhaps in conjunction, appear: deep mitosis and auto-lysomes (Fig. 9).

On the fourteenth day, the culture dissociates by foci in some regions and the cells reveal signs of slow destruction: vacuolated nuclei, disappearance of mitochondria, granulation of cytoplasm, but the mem-

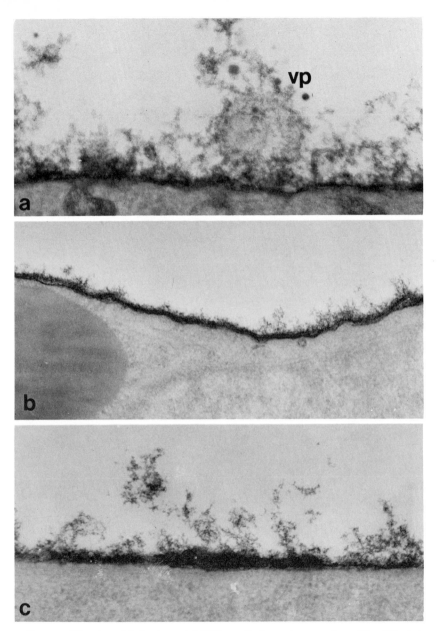

Fɪɢ. 10. Kinetics of infection of BHK21 cells by polyoma virus. The RR stain was mixed with glutaraldehyde. (a) Three hours after infection, numerous virus particles (vp) are seen in close contact with glycoproteins coating the cell surface membrane. The dense RR layer is 15 nm. thick. ×90,000. (b) Six hours after infection, no more virus particles are seen. The RR layer is 15 nm. thick. ×50,000. (c) Forty-eight hours after infection, some cells exhibit a very thick and dense layer of RR-stained material, about 22 nm. thick. ×50,000.

brane paradoxically is in a state of preservation and RR layer is thicker. This state is the prelude to the complete breakdown of the cell.

d. *Evolution of BHK21/C13 Cells Infected by Polyoma Virus.* In culture, 3 hours after infection, cellular aspects are practically the same as normal aspects of noncontaminated cells. Pinocytosis increases; some viral elements can be seen at the level of the smokelike projections, and in the vesicles situated immediately under the membrane. After 6 hours of culture, some cells show impairment symptoms, increasing and breaking of the glycocalix, and mitotic activity. At the eighteenth hour after infection (the second day of culture) four or five cellular layers are found with very loose intercellular spaces. We noticed at this stage a strange phenomenon: the deepest cells stayed in monolayer although the uppermost cells seemed to be without any connection with this deep layer. This superficial population appeared to develop by itself and exhibited very long, cloudy expansions. When no RR positive plugs existed, the cells overlapped. The synthesis of free material closed between cells is very extensive. On the other hand, a focus of cells after 48 hours of culture (24 hours of infection) has a normal arrangement. Forty-eight hours after infection superficial cells are coated by RR and smokelike projections (Fig. 10).

After 8 days of culture, cells relax their multiplication: the stops in U and Y are seen, long villosities disappear and mucus plugs gather and mitotic activity persists. Thickness of RR layer at the level of these foci reaches 20 to 25 nm. (Fig. 11).

e. *Parallelism between Some Different Polyoma Virus-Transformed Cell Strains.* We first studied the Py27 strain, a BHK21 cell line which has been transformed by a small plaque variant of polyoma virus. This clonal cell line is highly tumorigenic and the cells carry T-antigen. At the twenty-fourth hour of culture, cells pile up (Fig. 12) and show numerous U-like stops. The layer labeled by RR is 20 to 23 nm. thick; it winds its ways between the cells. There are only a few plugs. The cytoplasm of these cells contains more fibrils than in the case of the BHK21; it is also much more differentiated. At the fourth day of culture there is a great activity of the surface and numerous microvilli appear. RR stains the surface regularly. The membrane is rather wavy and some signs of lysis appear. The RR layer, however, is conserved. Under the same conditions of culture and techniques we compared some clones of BHK cells transformed either by the small plaque Toronto strain of polyoma virus or by a large plaque polyoma virus supplied by Tournier. In the previous paragraph we reported the kinetics of development of BHK21 cells infected by a small plaque variant of polyoma virus. Before reporting the results on these different transformed cell

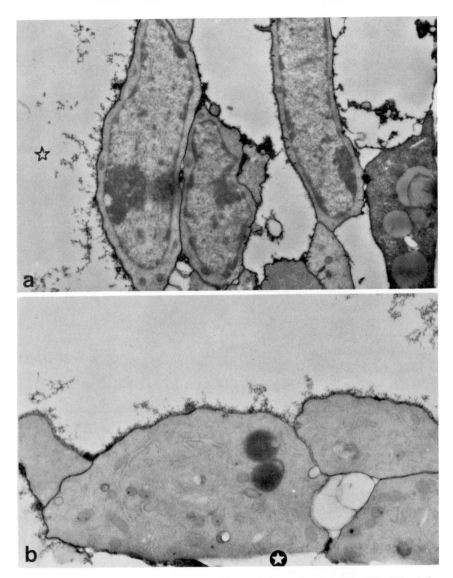

Fig. 11. Kinetics of infection of BHK21 cells by polyoma virus. The RR stain
was mixed with glutaraldehyde. (a) Three days after infection, a group of normal
cells showing numerous disruptions appears. The RR layer is about 15 nm. thick.
×14,000. (b) Eighth day: a group of transformed cells near the glass surface is
seen. The RR layer is 22 nm. thick. There is no U-like stop. ×12,500.

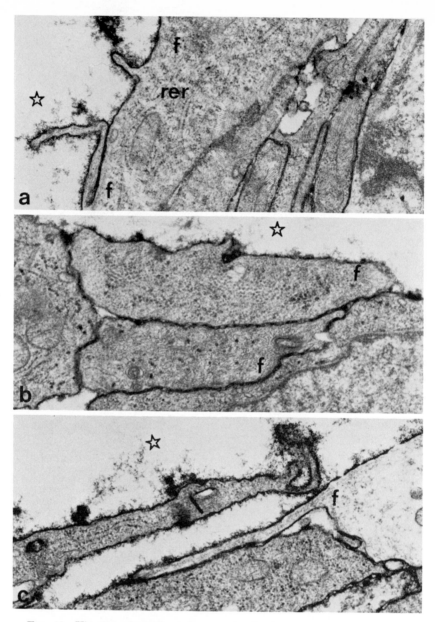

Fig. 12. Kinetics of Py27 strain growth. Sections are perpendicular to the growing surface. RR was mixed with glutaraldehyde solution. (a) First day of culture: there are three cell layers and numerous microvilli at the free cell surface. The cells are well differentiated with microfilaments (f) and rough endoplasmic reticulum (rer). ×30,000. (b) Third day of culture: in some areas of the culture, cells are stopping with Y-like stops. RR enters between the cells. ×30,000. (c) Third day of culture: in other areas of the culture, cells overlap each other; the RR layer is smoky. ×30,000.

lines, we want to note that RR applied to hamster embryo cells under the same conditions gives a RR-labeled layer of about 12 ± 2 nm. These results are very similar to those of the different authors mentioned in the discussion.

In the case of cell strains transformed by small plaque variants of polyoma virus, the layer labeled by RR is about 20 ± 3 nm. thick (Fig. 13). This has been found in the case of five cell lines. When BHK21 was transformed by a large plaque polyoma virus, the RR-labeled layer was about 12 ± 2 nm. thick. We finally studied BHK21/C13 cells of different origins which had been kept in liquid nitrogen for different periods of time. The layer labeled by RR was generally 15 ± 3 nm. thick.

    f. *Discussion of the Results and Critical Study of the Value of RR.* The membrane of the BHK21/C13 cells did not show numerous modifications during culture growth. The activity of micropinocytosis and the presence of cytoplasmic fibers showed more or less cyclic variations: they seemed to decrease while the culture was aging. On the contrary, in all the transformed strains, microfibrils were abundant, which paral-

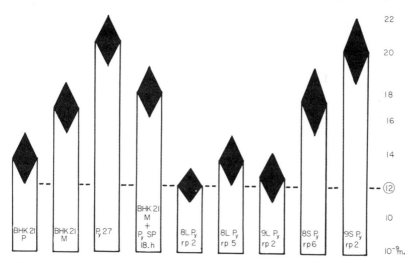

FIG. 13. Comparison of the thickness of the RR stain-taking layer in the case of some polyoma virus-transformed cells strains, BHK21 cells, and hamster embryo cells. The large diagonal of the rhombus indicates the maximal and minimal limit values; the horizontal line represents the values of the RR-labeled layer in the case of hamster embryo cells, which are the reference cells. The thickness of the labeled layer is increased in the case of BHK21 cells; in the case of the LP polyoma virus-transformed cell strains, the thickness of the labeled layer does not increase as compared to BHK21 cells. On the contrary, in the case of SP polyoma virus-transformed cell strains, the thickness of this labeled layer is increased.

leled increased glycolytic activity. Microfibrils might play a role in locomotion of the cells and their greater number in transformed cells increased cell mobility and ATP consumption. Sophisticated work of Follett and Goldman (1970) on BHK21/C13 cells using replica technique observed with a transmission and a scanning electron microscope pointed out that microvilli were in connection with microfilaments and that they played an important role mainly in mitosis. More recently, Ambrose et al. (1970) demonstrated particular subsurface structures in normal and malignant cells.

The microvilli persisted in the material we studied during all phases of the cycle of transformed cells. In the cells undergoing transformation by polyoma virus and also in many cell lines stably transformed, we observed the presence of ball-like enlargements. A section of these enlargements often possessed a periodic structure recalling the pseudo-myelin figures assumed by phospholipids. This resembles what was observed on the surface of ascitic tumor cells. Ambrose (1967) was inclined to think that these phospholipids could belong to the cell surface and could be in an exposed form. Montagnier (1970), from a different point of view, showed that phospholipids can be unmasked during transformation and that their electronegative charge was able to fix RR in great amounts, consequently increasing in some cases the thickness of the RR-labeled layer.

We previously pointed out that RR probably combined with polymerized hyaluronic acid and with chondroitin sulfuric acid. On the contrary, it was not fixed by sialic acid. RR also had an affinity for polymerized acidic mucopolysaccharides, which can be proven by the disappearance of the RR-labeled layer after action of hyaluronidase. This layer was resistant to the action either of trypsin or neuraminidase. RR showed, therefore, a great affinity for acidic mucopolysaccharides (AMPS) containing hyaluronic acid. These data support the experiments reported by Bonneau and Césarini (1968) on normal and polyoma virus-transformed BHK21 cells, either with RR or with the technique reported by Rambourg (1967). This is a true PAS-staining for electron microscopy. In vivo, Rambourg's stain showed at the surface of tumor cells an irregular line of heavily stained material. The same technique in vitro revealed a more regular surface material. There was no correlation between the thickness of the RR-labeled layer and the Rambourg-stained layer. Neuraminidase digestion of the ultrathin sections before action of the Rambourg stain revealed a clear area between the membrane unit and the densely stained material. The Rambourg stain revealed all the glycoproteins, some of which were removed by neuraminidase treatment.

Defendi and Gasic (1963) pointed out that the amount of muco-polysaccharides of the cell surface of polyoma virus-transformed cells was quantitatively increased since Hale's reaction was more intensive, but disappeared completely after neuraminidase action. It disappeared only partially after treatment with hyaluronidase. Alternatively, pepsin treatment increased the intensity of the reaction. Martinez-Palomo et al. (1969) demonstrated that the thickness of the RR-labeled layer increased to 23 nm. in SV40-transformed cells. In the case of adenovirus 12-transformed cells, the thickness of the labeled layer was 33 nm. Further studies of Vorbrodt and Koprowski (1969) showed that in SV40-trans-formed cells, the contrasted layer might have a thickness similar to that of normal cells (13 nm.) and might even be diminished in the case of some spontaneous or SV40-induced hamster tumors. On the other hand, experimental studies by Morgan (1968) demonstrated that in the case of an RNA-containing oncogenic virus (RSV), the RR-labeled layer was of unequal thickness in the case of cells transformed by different virus strains. We noted no difference between BHK21 cells and BHK21 cells transformed either by the Bryan or the Schmidt-Ruppin strains of RSV (Césarini, 1969). On the contrary, overtransformation of these cells by polyoma virus, done by Montagnier et al. (1969), showed an increase to 20 nm. of the RR-labeled layer (Torpier and Montagnier, 1969).

Thus it appears that the thickness of the RR-labeled layer (in reality, the quantity of electronegative material with the exception of sialic acid) is highly variable and that oncogenic viruses have different properties according to the strains. RR affinity cannot parallel the in-crease of surface electronegativity revealed by electrophoresis of these cells (Forrester et al., 1962, 1964) and abolished by neuraminidase treatment.

It becomes urgent to study in a very well-fixed cell system model the relationship between surface electronegativity, sialic acid content, and glycoprotein nature of the normal and transformed cell lines.

D. MEMBRANE MODIFICATIONS REVEALED BY CHEMICAL OR IMMUNOCHEMICAL METHODS

1. Chemical Methods

Different observations indicated that the membrane of transformed or tumor cells was different from that of the corresponding normal cell, in antigenic properties and modified electrophoretic mobility (Forrester et al., 1962, 1964). However, these observations at the cell level only evidenced differences in the behavior of the cells. On the contrary, biochemical analysis is able to reveal the differences at the molecular level. This analysis is rather difficult since cell surface membrane must be isolated in a rather pure form; it is necessary to avoid denaturation. The external part of the membrane is mostly composed of different carbohydrates and glycolipids. Different studies suggest that the specificity of the cell surface is determined not only by the quantity and the quality of glycolipids but also by their spatial organization at the cell surface, which is clear from the works of Burger (1969) and Inbar and Sachs (1969). Changes in glycoproteins or glycolipids may occur during transformation by viruses. Characterization of the glycolipids of both normal and polyoma-transformed BHK21 cells was made by Hakomori and Murakami (1968). The glycolipids were extracted from whole cells and their amounts measured by suitable procedures. The main glycolipid found in hamster cells was N-acetylneuraminyl lactosylceramide; a second fraction found was another glycolipid, lactosylceramide. The quantities of hematoside and lactosylceramide present in a cell showed a reciprocal relationship depending on whether the cells were derived from BHK21 or from the transformed cell lines. The hematoside content was the highest in the normal fibroblast line but the polyoma-transformed line contained only one-fifth the quantity found in the normal fibroblast. Furthermore, the quantities of lactosylceramide showed the inverse relationship: the level in normal BHK was only one-tenth that found in the virus-transformed cell line. Thus the main glycolipid of BHK was an hematoside type of glycolipid which contained N-acetylneuraminic acid. It appeared that the content of this hematoside was greatly diminished in polyoma virus-transformed cells. On the contrary, a minor glycolipid of normal cells, lactosylceramide, was greatly increased in transformed cells. It is noteworthy that lactosylceramide is a precursor of the hematoside. Furthermore, a correlation seems to exist between the hematoside content and the degree of contact inhibition of the cell line tested: the more contact-inhibited cell line contained more complete glycolipids and less incomplete hematoside.

The differences in the electrophoretic behavior of normal and virus-transformed cells (Forrester et al., 1962, 1964) was attributed to an increase in sialic acid content in the case of the transformed cell and especially in the case of cells transformed by polyoma virus. However, Ohta et al. (1968) reported that the sialic acid content of the virus (polyoma or adenovirus)-transformed cells was consistently lower than that of the corresponding normal cells, BHK21 or 3T3. Since the enzymes of sialic acid metabolism are not affected in any one of their parameters in the case of the transformed cells, they concluded that there was no positive correlation between sialic acid content and the degree of contact inhibition. Correlated observations of Mora *et al.* (1969) on the content of ganglioside homologs in normal 3T3 and SV40-transformed 3T3 showed that a decrease was observed in the higher ganglioside homologs, disialoceramide-tetrahexoside and monosialo-ceramidetetrahexoside in the transformed cell line. It should be noted that such a change could be correlated with increased saturation density in tissue culture and also with the rejection in immunologically competent syngenic hosts.

Different labeling experiments have been made to determine the relative contents of various sugar components. Several of these experiments looked for the glucosamine, galactosamine, and sialic acid contents of both normal and SV40-transformed mouse fibroblasts 3T3 (Wu *et al.*, 1968, 1969; Meezan *et al.*, 1969). Normal and transformed cells were grown in the presence of either ^{14}C or ^{3}H-glucosamine, then harvested and mixed in the following combinations: ^{14}C — 3T3 + ^{3}H — SV40 3T3 and ^{3}H — 3T3 + ^{14}C — SV40 3T3. After mixing, the subcellular fractions were separated according to Wallach's method. The ^{3}H/^{14}C ratios were determined in the total homogenate and in the particulate fractions, corresponding roughly to plasma cell membrane. The analysis of the relative compositions of glycoproteins and glycolipids of the membrane in both cell lines showed that sialic acid and galactosamine contents decreased and that there was a relative increase in the percentage of glucosamine in the SV40 3T3 cell line. Such differences were observed in the particulate fractions but not in the sugar nucleotide pool of the cell. This change was therefore not due to a lack of the necessary precursors. A comparative study of spontaneously transformed 3T3 cells also revealed an increase in the content of the neutral and amino sugars. The overall composition of glycoproteins of the membrane fractions of SV40 3T3 cells was relatively low in N-acetylneuraminic acid and galactosamine and high in glucosamine as compared with the composition of the 3T3 fraction. More recently, Onodera and Sheinin (1970) also investigated a macromolecular glucosamine-containing component of the surface of 3T3 cells. Comparative study of this component, which can be removed by trypsin treatment without damaging the plasma membrane, revealed that it was different in normal 3T3 and in the same SV40-transformed cells. Analysis of surface component released by trypsin treatment of 3T3 cells revealed the presence of at least five fractions, whereas a similar treatment of SV40-transformed 3T3 cells revealed the presence of only three fractions. All these results showed qualitative or quantitative differences in sugar components of the membrane. This parallels the findings of Bosmann (1969) of an increased glycolytic activity in transformed fibroblasts. Polyoma or SV40-transformed 3T3 cells were tested together with normal 3T3 cells for the enzymic activity of a number of glycosidases such as N-acetyl-β-D-glucosaminidase, α-D-glucosidase, α-D-galactosidase. The enzymic activities, either on a cell or protein basis, were always found to be increased in the transformed cells as compared to the normal cells.

2. *Immunochemical Methods*

Since direct approach to the modifications of the plasma membrane after transformation is rather difficult, some indirect methods have been used which allow the detection of these modifications. Aub *et al.* (1963) showed that an impurity of a "wheat germ lipase" preparation agglutinated specifically some tumor cells. Burger and Goldberg (1967) purified this minor component of the preparation, which was revealed to be a glycoprotein of M.W. 26,000. The different characteristic values of the protein and particularly the relation between the axis (equal to 4 or 5) are consistent with the model of an elongated protein which could carry two recognition sites, one at each end, which would allow it to act as a bridge in the agglutination process. The molecule contains 4.5% sugar.

In different studies (Pollack and Burger, 1969; Burger and Goldberg, 1967; Burger, 1969) the characteristics of this agglutination were sought. Only the transformed cells (tested in parallel with the normal cells from which they derive) were agglutinated by this agglutinin. The surface "determinant" of the transformed cell responsible for agglutination has been identified by agglutination inhibition, assuming that this agglutination reaction is an interaction of the antigen-antibody type. Different sugars have been tested as haptenic inhibitors. These experiments showed that N-acetylglucosamine was the one with inhibitory properties; the agglutination, however, is also inhibited by chitobiose, the disaccharide of N-acetylglucosamine. This agglutination reaction is reversible since after addition of N-acetylglucosamine to agglutinated cells, the agglutination reaction is reversed and homogeneous cell suspensions are obtained. The treatment with trypsin (or another proteolytic enzyme such as chymotrypsin, papain, or ficin) converts the cells from a nonagglutinable state to an agglutinable state. This also occurs in different nonagglutinable cell lines such as BHK-D and 3T3. In optimal conditions and after trypsin treatment, the agglutinability of normal cells is identical to that of the virus-transformed nontreated cells (Table IX).

Subsequently, the number of receptor sites for agglutinin and the affinity for agglutinin seemed to be identical for the virus-transformed cells and the normal cells from which they were derived and which have been treated by trypsin. Burger (1969) suggested three hypotheses in order to explain this difference in agglutinability between normal cells and virus-transformed cells. Either a *de novo* synthesis (which must be

TABLE IX

THE CHARACTERISTICS OF AGGLUTINATION BY THE WHEAT GERM AGGLUTININ

Cells tested	Agglutina-bility	Treatment by different enzymes	Agglutina-bility[a]	References
Normal cells: BHK	0			Burger and
Transformed cells: polyoma-BHK	+	Neuraminidase	0	Goldberg (1967)
Normal cells: BHK or 3T3	0	Trypsin	+	Burger (1969)
		Chymotrypsin	+	
		Ficin, papain	+	
		DNase or RNase	0	
		Collagenase	0	
		Glycosidases	0	
Transformed cells: polyoma trans-formed BHK21 or 3T3 cells	+ (varying with the cell type)	Trypsin	+	

[a] After treatment with the different enzymes.

excluded since normal BHK cells can be agglutinated at a very high agglutinin concentration) or an increase in the formation of sites (which must also be excluded since, after trypsin treatment, normal cells acquire the same agglutinability as transformed cells). Subsequently, transformation must comprise an architectural rearrangement of the cellular surface. This rearrangement can eventually lead to the altered surface properties of the transformed cells, by analogy with the trypsin treatment.

Similar experiments have been made with concanavalin A (con. A), a protein which specifically attaches different sugars, particularly α-methyl-D-glucopyranoside (α-MG) (Inbar and Sachs, 1969). This protein contains a nickel atom. The labeling of the protein with ^{63}Ni allows the determination of the number of fixation sites. Con. A is extracted from Jack bean meal and has a M.W. of 60,000. Different cell lines have been tested for their ability to bind con. A: nontransformed cells like 3T3, Syrian hamster embryo cells, and the same cell lines transformed by polyoma virus or by treatment with dimethylnitrosamine. The results showed that the amount of con. A fixed by transformed cells was higher than the amount fixed by normal cells even in the presence of α-MG. Supposing that the cells are spherical, and knowing their number and their volume, it was easy to calculate the number of fixation sites for con. A per cell. The results indicated that normal 3T3 cells have 5 to 10 $\times$ 10^3 sites and that hamster cells have 4 to 8 $\times$ 10^3 sites. The same cells transformed by polyoma virus have 23 to 58 $\times$ 10³ sites per square micron of cellular surface.

It was interesting to determine if the minor number of sites at the surface of normal cells could be increased by treatment with a proteolytic enzyme as in the case of wheat germ agglutinin. Normal hamster cells treated by trypsin have been tested for their ability to bind con. A and the number of fixation sites per square micron of cellular surface was determined. The number of sites varies from 4 to 8 $\times$ 10³ for untreated cells to 23 to 46 $\times$ 10³ for the cells treated with trypsin. Thus trypsin treatment of normal cells resulted in the exposition of formerly "cryptic" sites. Furthermore, the number of unmasked sites was similar to the number of sites evidenced in the case of transformed cells.

In a similar manner, it has been shown that "variants" (Inbar *et al.*, 1969) (obtained from polyoma virus-transformed cells grown in the animal and then subcultured *in vitro,* and which exhibited a reversion of the *in vitro* properties of transformed cells but always retained the ability to synthesize T-antigen) exhibited a total or partial loss of agglutinability by con. A. As in the case of normal cells, this agglutinability can be restored by trypsin treatment. Considering, therefore, the surface properties revealed by agglutinability by con. A, transformed cells can revert to the structure of normal cells. The synthesis of T-antigen, probably due to the DNA integrated in the cell, is not sufficient to prevent this reversion; thus the presence of T-antigen is not a guarantee of the transformed character of a cell.

The sites revealed either by con. A or by the wheat germ agglutinin, are apparently different since each of these proteins has an affinity for different sugars. They present, however, common characteristics: (a) transformed cells only are agglutinated—or bind the protein and this occurs in both cases: the sites revealed by both methods are unmasked simultaneously; (b) trypsin treatment (or treatment by any other proteolytic enzyme) reveals in the case of nonagglutinated cells or cells which do not bind con. A, a number of fixation sites which are equal to the number of sites revealed by agglutination or equal to 85% of the sites unmasked in transformed cells in the case of agglutination by con. A; (c) the mechanism of unmasking of these sites which exist on the normal cell in a cryptic state will be discussed further.

E. Antigenic Modifications

1. *Introduction*

The morphological modifications of the cell membrane which we have just described correspond to antigenic modifications of the cell surface.

Two groups of techniques were used to explore these antigenic modifications: (a) *In vivo,* the tumor homograft rejection after preparation of the animal by a well-adapted protection was used. Since 1961, this method has made it possible to reveal the existence of a specific antigen of the inducing virus: the "transplantation-specific tumor antigen" (TSTA). The history and biology of this particularly interesting antigen have been described by Deichman in this review (1969) and we shall no longer refer to it except for comparisons with the antigens revealed *in vitro.* (b) Numerous *in vitro* techniques were used which can be divided into two groups: first, methods using lymphocytes which reveal the cell-mediated immune reactions and second, methods using antisera of protected animals such as cytotoxicity, mixed hemadsorption, or immunofluorescence on living cells. The results of these different methods are not absolutely identical except, perhaps, for the mixed hemadsorption and the immunofluorescent tests which clearly explore the same phenomenon. We shall take as an example the description of the immunofluorescent test. We shall then compare these results to those obtained by the other methods.

2. Cell Surface Antigen in Immunofluorescence

This technique is based on the method first described by G. Möller (1961). He was able to show mouse isoantigens by immunofluorescence on living cells. Klein and Klein (1964) applied this technique to tumor homograft rejection antigens in the Moloney system. Tevethia *et al.* (1965) demonstrated cell surface antigen in the SV40 system; Irlin (1967), Lhérisson *et al.* (1967), and Malmgren *et al.* (1968) pointed it out in the polyoma system. The principle of this method is the following: living cells are incubated with antisera of animals protected against tumor graft. After washing, immunofluorescence is revealed by labeled antigammaglobulins. The critical point of this technique is that the cell membrane must not be damaged when the cells are detached from the glass, either by trypsinization or by scraping. When the cell surface is damaged, labeled antibodies can enter the cell and color the whole cell by a cytoplasmic fluorescence. When the technique is correct, the presence of surface antigen is seen as a crown of pearls bordering the cell (Fig. 14). By varying the focus, we acknowledge that the whole membrane is strewn with these pearls and that the crown look is equivalent to a section. This antigen is specific for the inducing virus. We shall see in the discussion that this specificity is partially discussed at this time chiefly in relationship to a Forssman-type antigen. Nevertheless, we found no cross-reaction either within antisera obtained from animals protected by polyoma virus, SV40, or RSV and tumor cells or cells transformed by the

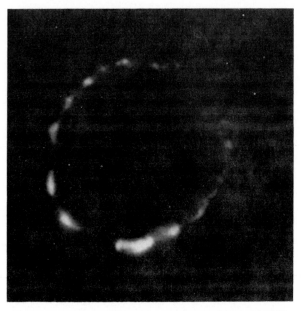

F_IG. 14. Cell surface antigen induced by polyoma virus on BHK21 cells at the nineteenth hour after infection, and revealed by the indirect method. Cell surface antigen looks like a crown of small pearls on the cell surface membrane. ✕ near 2000.

same viruses. On the other hand, doubly transformed cells (Montagnier *et al.*, 1969) showed positive reaction with sera of animals protected against Rous and polyoma tumors. One could suppose that the appearance of this antigen was in relation to the transformation of the cell. It was also interesting to study the kinetics of its appearance after infection of nonpermissive cells. This antigen appears very early on BHK21 cells infected at high input multiplicity with polyoma virus (Meyer *et al.*, 1969a). Some cells bear this antigen from the third hour after infection. The maximum average of cells bearing this antigen is found between the eighteenth and twentieth hour after infection (Fig. 15). Then the rate of labeled cells decreases quickly, and after 2 or 3 days it is about 6 or 7%, remaining constant until the twelfth day. We were surprised by these results because we believed the membrane antigen would appear much later and that it would be contemporary with the morphological transformation. In fact, we see that this antigen is one proof of an abortive cycle of polyoma virus in BHK21 cells. To try to prove that the viral genome is involved in coding for surface antigen, we analyzed the part of the viral genome involved in this coding (Meyer and Birg, 1970). The experimental system chosen was polyoma virus and the BHK21 cell line.

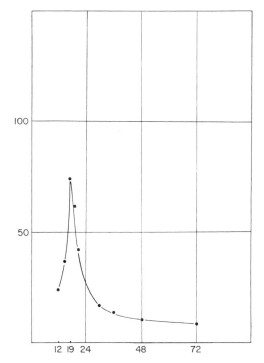

Fig. 15. Kinetics of appearance of cell surface antigen in BHK21 cells infected with polyoma virus (100 PFU/cell). As abscissa, hours after infection and as ordinate, percentage of cells with cell surface antigen.

The virus had been irradiated with increasing doses of UV light ranging from 3000 to 10,000 ergs/mm.[2] The rates of cells bearing the cell surface immunofluorescence antigen were counted and plotted against the UV doses (Fig. 16). The slope of the exponential curve obtained was measured and compared with the loss of infectivity under the same conditions. It could be concluded that half of the viral genome necessary for replication was involved in specification of the surface antigen, the coding of this antigen being direct or indirect by a derepression mechanism. We recall that similar results have been found for the coding of T-antigen (Meyer *et al.*, 1968).

3. Cell Surface Antigen in Immunoelectron Microscopy

By replacing the fluorochrome used in fluorescence microscopy by a marker detectable by the electron microscope (such as ferritin or peroxidase-labeled antibodies) we hoped to detect the virus-induced surface antigens. With the aid of both high resolution and magnification

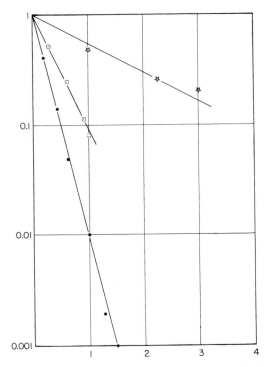

Fig. 16. Influence of UV-irradiation of polyoma virus on infectivity and on induction of cell surface and homograft rejection antigens. UV-irradiation doses
($\times 10^4$ ergs mm.$^{-2}$) are shown in abscissa. ●——●, virus infectivity as PFU.
Infectivity of nonirradiated virus is 100%. □——□, inactivation of cell surface
antigen in BHK21 cells after infection with UV-irradiated polyoma virus. The
percentage of fluorescent cells is shown as a function of the irradiation dose. Cells
infected with nonirradiated virus are taken to show 100% fluorescence. ✪——✪,
inactivation of homograft rejection antigen. Activity is expressed as the mean
reciprocal of the time of tumor appearance in immunized animals: the control
at 100% represents protected animals without tumors following administration of
nonirradiated polyoma virus. For details of statistical data, see Meyer *et al.*
(1969b).

afforded by the electron microscope, we hoped to find the exact localization of these surface antigens. Virus-induced antigens have never been
sought by such a technique. However, Aoki *et al.* (1969) studied mouse
histocompatibility loci with ferritin or virus as markers while Bretton
and Lespinats (1969) studied a transplantable mouse plasmocytoma with
peroxidase as a marker. We tried to demonstrate the cell surface antigen
in polyoma-induced transformation using peroxidase-labeled rabbit anti-
hamster α-globulins in a sandwich procedure (Baxendall *et al.*, 1962).
Labeled antibodies were prepared according to Avrameas (1969). For the

detection of surface antigen, we used either the procedure of Leduc *et al.* (1969) for SV40, omitting the step of freezing-thawing or we used the method of Bretton and Lespinats (1969).

We have tested established cell lines transformed *in vitro* by polyoma virus and transplantable tumor strains induced *in vivo* in hamsters (primary culture). We studied the kinetics of events in BHK21 cells infected by polyoma virus in parallel with immunofluorescence. In this case, samples were taken every 3 hours for the first 2 days and, thereafter, day by day for 2 weeks. The same controls as in immunofluorescence were used for all experiments. A particular control is very important and must be used when peroxidase is used as a marker. It is necessary to test peroxidase activity of the cells, and especially its activity in tumor cells. The surface antigen in immunofluorescence resembles a fine ring structure with small pearls. The examined cells are whole and superposition of planes may be confusing. When cells treated for electron microscopy are examined with the optical microscope (Fig. 17), a very dense line is seen at the periphery of the cell. There are also some small dark spots in the cytoplasm. The stained structures correspond to the localization of peroxidase activity. In electron microscopy the thin sections prevent mistakes induced by superposition. On a section, per-

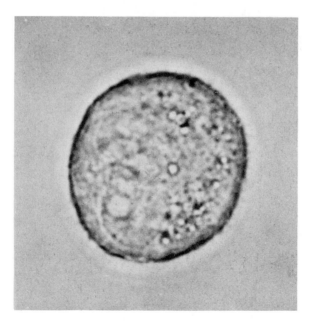

Fig. 17. Optical immunochemical techniques: the peroxidase takes the place of fluorochrome. An appearance very similar to that of Fig. 11. × near 2000.

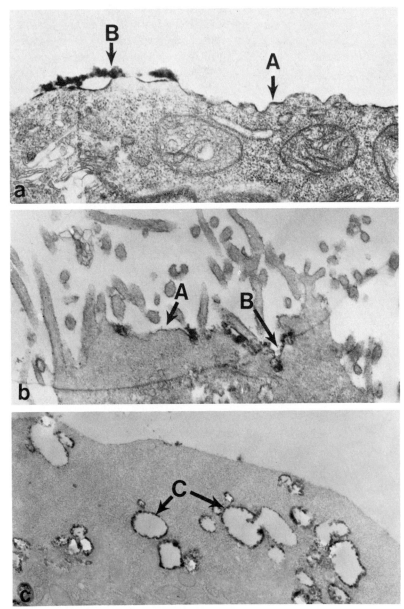

Fɪɢ. 18. Immunoelectron microscopy: membrane antigen induced by polyoma virus on BHK21 cells revealed by the indirect method. (a) Type A reaction (very thin dense layer) and type B reaction are seen at the cell surface. These reactions are specific. (BHK21 cells infected with polyoma virus at the nineteenth hour). ×27,000. (b) Types A and B reactions on an established cultured tumor cell line (CT54). ×27,000. (c) Example of nonspecific reaction observed on BHK21/C13. This is called the type C reaction. ×18,000.

oxidase activity can be classified according to four different aspects (Césarini *et al.*, 1970) : (a) a nonspecific adsorption of the conjugated antibody on the cell surface. For physical reasons, the γ-globulin complex is adsorbed at the cell surface and cannot be entirely removed by washing. This fact is clearly seen on cells growing on glass. The free surface is regularly stained but the anchoring side is irregularly stained; (b) at the level of the cell surface membrane we can see a very thin layer of dense material. This material is irregular, in small plaques on the outer leaflet of the membrane, which is perfectly preserved under this layer. On the other hand, some accumulation of dense material is observed on the surface of transformed cells. We call this reaction type A reaction [Fig. 18(a)] ; (c) when suspended cells present numerous microvilli, some dense material is seen between them. This phenomenon is observed in the case of *in vivo*-induced tumors. We call this reaction type B reaction [Fig. 18(b)]. In this case, we also see type A reaction. We believe that both type A and B reactions are specific reactions. They may be the electron microscopic translation of immunofluorescent aspects; (d) in some transformed strains and in BHK21/C13 we see a peroxidase activity in micropinocytotic vesicles in correlation with cell surface and endoplasmic reticulum [Figs. 18(c) and 19(b)]. This activity is observed in a layer of about 2 to 4 μ thick under the cell surface [Fig. 19(a)]. We can interpret this aspect as the result of absorption of labeled γ-globulins by living cells. This reaction is not specific and may correspond to the small pearls sometimes seen by immunofluorescence. In some cases 15% of the cells in control groups present this phenomenon. This reaction is called type C reaction. The Klein index takes care of the positive cells in the controls and we think that the cells with type C reaction are counted as positive cells.

In summary, immunoelectron microscopy results with peroxidase-labeled γ-globulins agree with those obtained by immunofluorescence although the method is not as accurate as hoped. The interpretation of micrographs may be very difficult. This fact may be due either to technical artifacts or to nonspecific adsorption of labeled globulins at the cell surface.

4. *Comparison of the Different Techniques used in Testing Surface Antigen*

Our description has been based on the results of immunofluorescence (IF) upon living cells and on results in homograft rejection; however, other techniques permit the observance of surface antigen(s). Mixed hemadsorption may be used by using serum antibodies (Metzgar and Oleinick, 1968; Espmark and Fagraeus, 1962). The results are, in fact, the same as in IF. This method is perhaps more sensitive than IF, but

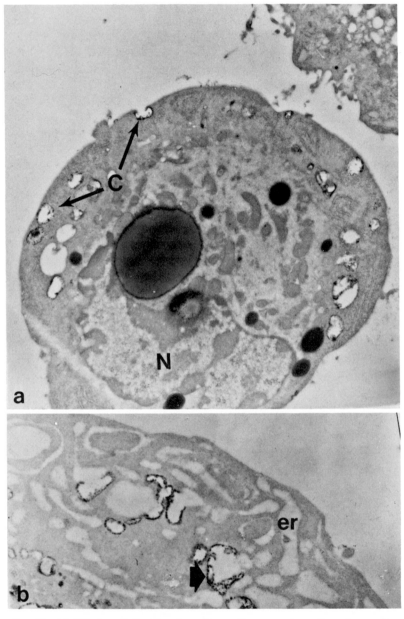

Fig. 19. (a) Whole cell showing type C reaction near the cell surface and connected with outer space. All the organelles are well preserved. ×6000. (b) Particular
aspects of the labeling of endoplasmic reticulum (er) by peroxidase-labeled globulins: the dense marker is located in vesicles (black arrow) in direct correlation
with endoplasmic reticulum. ×18,000.

from our point of view, is less reproducible and more subjective. Another serum-mediated technique involves the use of complement: the cytotoxicity test (E. Möller and Möller, 1962) and particularly the improved method of I. Hellström and Sjögren (1965) of colony inhibition (CI). The results obtained are very similar to those obtained in IF. Tevethia *et al.* (1970) demonstrated the identity of the antigens revealed by CI and surface IF. On the other hand, the antibodies responsible for the reaction in these two tests do not seem to be identical, the complement-needing antibodies which are 7 S IgA 2 immunoglobulins and the non-complement-needing antibodies which are 7 S IgA 1 immunoglobulins.

Agar immunoprecipitation shows all cellular antigens at the same time as some surface antigens. According to De Vaux Saint-Cyr *et al.* (1969), some other antigens revealed are identical with the surface antigens demonstrable by immunofluorescence. The inhibition of macrophage migration is also related to circulating antibodies, but this method involves also a cellular component. The cell-mediated reaction can be evidenced *in vitro* by CI with sensitized lymphocytes (I. Hellström, 1967); this test is closely related to the *in vivo* homograft rejection test and probably reflects the same phenomenon.

5. Relation between Cellular Antigens and Virus-Specific Antigens in Transformed Cells

The origin of the antigenic modifications of the cell surface after transformation is not unequivocally clear at present. The question is whether these modifications are new proteins coded for directly by the virus, whether there is a conversion of the carbohydrates of the peripheral layer of the cell membrane (as has been seen in the action of some lysogenic phages), or whether there is a derepression of some cellular genes and the subsequent appearance of antigens preexisting in the membrane. This last hypothesis could explain the appearance of the carcinoembryonic antigens. This type of "cell-directed" modification could also explain the appearance of common antigens of a Forssman type. Many authors (Fogel, 1963; O'Neill, 1968; H. T. Robertson and Black, 1969) described this type of antigen after viral transformation.

In the case of SV40, it is possible that the Forssman antigen is identical with the immunofluorescent surface antigen (De Vaux Saint-Cyr, 1971). We tested our tumor and transformed cells for the presence of the Forssman type antigen. All the polyoma-induced tumors were found to be Forssman positive. The BHK21/C13 cell line was Forssman negative but after transformation by polyoma virus in most cases became Forssman positive. The appearance of this Forssman antigen in kinetic experiments was not found in the abortive cycle of the virus on BHK cells but only in cloned, transformed lines. This is the first proof that this antigen is different from the immunofluorescent virus-induced surface antigen. On the other hand, our sera, which revealed the specific immunofluorescent antigen, could not be absorbed with boiled sheep red cells.

These results suggest that after transformation in polyoma-transformed BHK21 cells, at least two types of antigens appear: first, an early type antigen, present in the abortive cycle, virus-specific, and coded for directly or indirectly by half the part of the viral genome necessary for replication; and second, a late type antigen only present in transformed cells and not present in the abortive cycle of the virus. This late type antigen depends on the type of the cells which are transformed and not on the type of transforming virus. In fact, SV40 or RSV-transformed BHK21 cells are also Forssman positive. Other experiments are in progress in order to determine the relation of the early and late antigens with TSTA.

6. Comparison between TSTA and Antigens Revealed by Immunofluorescence

We have described two possible immunoreactions directed against cell surface antigens: humoral and cell-mediated. The question arose whether these different responses were induced either by the same antigen or by two types of antigens. Studying the different functions coded for by the polyoma genome, and their loss after UV-irradiation of the virus, we were also interested in the part of the viral genome involved in coding for the TSTA (Meyer et al., 1969b). The experiments needed for studying this function were more sophisticated than the ones needed for the in vitro expressed functions; the statistical data had to be carefully checked. In a first step, we had to determine the 50% protecting virus dose against a well-known polyoma-induced tumor (Bonneau et al., 1967). This tumor was a hamster transplantable fibrosarcoma (CT54). The tumor dose 50% (DT50) was stable and the latency period of development of the tumor was regular. We also determined the mean dose of virus necessary to protect the animal against 10 DT50 (Meyer et al., 1967a). After irradiation of the virus by different UV doses, we observed the appearance of tumors, their latency period, and their doubling time. The statistical analysis (Meyer et al., 1968) allowed the construction of an exponential curve. When reported on a semilogarithmic scale, the slope of this curve is proportional to the resistance of this function to UV-irradiation. This function appeared particularly resistant to UV-irradiation. Applying the target hypothesis, it seems that the target of this function is five times smaller than the function of replication; in other words, the part of the viral genome involved in the coding of this antigen is one-fifth of the part necessary for replication (Fig. 16). Alstein *et al.* (1966) found similar results for TSTA of SV40. We recall that the part of the viral genome necessary for the coding of the immuno-fluorescent cell surface antigen is one half of the part of the viral genome necessary for replication. Consequently, it was possible that these two functions were different and that the two antigens revealed by these two different techniques of different sensitivities were themselves different.

In order to test this hypothesis we tested a polyoma virus mutant defective for one of these antigens. Tevethia *et al.* (1968) had demon-strated a lack of relationship between these two antigens using, in the case of SV40, a mutant defective for TSTA. We never found a mutant defective in immunofluorescent antigen inducing the TSTA, but Hare (1967) described a large plaque mutant of polyoma virus defective for TSTA. We verified this point and tested the induction of the immuno-fluorescent antigen; we found positive results. According to these results, these antigens could be considered as different, but the evidence is not definitive. In fact, the two techniques for revealing these antigens have a very different sensitivity, the *in vitro* method being much more sensitive than the *in vivo* method. The definitive proof will be reported only if someone is able to isolate a mutant inducing TSTA and not the immuno-fluorescent antigen. However, the experiments of K. E. Hellström and Hellström (1969) are in favor of the unity of these antigens. The virus-transformed cells were tested in colony inhibition with lymphocytes of peritumoral lymph nodes. The CI could be blocked by recovering the target cells with antitumor antisera of the same origin but without adding complement. If this blocking effect is not due to a steric hindrance, the unity of these antigens could be proved. Nevertheless, this technique of blocking allows a critical analysis of the antigenic "mosaic" of the cell surface and many studies are in progress using this method. We recall that this blocking effect might be an explanation of the enhancement phenomenon and of the outspread of the tumor in immunocompetent animals.

F. Conclusion

In conclusion, modifications of the transformed cell membrane are detected by a series of different techniques. The problem is to know whether these methods apply to only one phenomenon or if each method reveals a different change. From an immunological point of view we have already seen that two different changes can be detected, at least in the BHK21 cell model: one is viral-specific and the other is dependent upon the earlier cell state. The problem of the difference between the antigens revealed by tissue reaction and serum reaction does not seem to be definitively resolved.

In tumor cells, increase of migration speed in electrophoresis reveals an increase of the cell surface electronegative charge. This is a very general phenomenon involving different normal and transformed cell systems. Using different techniques, we have tried to specify the nature of the constituents responsible for this electronegativity. Sialic acid does not seem to play an important role; biochemical analyses of cell fractions have shown its level to be lowered in transformed cells. On the other hand, sialic acid does not fix ruthenium red and its selective digestion by neuraminidase permits its localization near the membrane unit. It is far from representing the totality of the heavy layer revealed by Rambourg's staining. Chondroitin sulfate and hyaluronic acids, both constituents of glycoproteins, could play the role of fixing agents for ruthenium red. Action of trypsin unmasks a certain number of membrane constituents at the surface of normal cells, cells which then seem to possess some characteristics similar to those of transformed cells, for example, agglutinating ability. According to Montagnier's hypothesis (1970), changes induced by polyoma virus, Rous virus, or even unknown factors, bring about the appearance of many negative sites at the surface, sites which are normally hidden by more superficial proteins and glycoproteins. Antigenicity of the Forssman type that can be seen on certain transformed cells seems to appear in connection with this antigenic uncovering of cell membrane sites which are normally hidden or repressed.

Some glycolipids support a part of the newly acquired antigenicity of the transformed cells. Whether these glycolipids are incomplete or hidden, their appearance in transformed cells must be under the dependence of regulatory mechanisms disturbed by the oncogenic virus.

IV. General Conclusions

After the account of these facts, we want to review our knowledge of cellular transformation by oncogenic viruses.

The first established fact is the integration of genetic information of viral origin into the stock of cellular genetic information. We do not know the exact site of this integration, but it is well established that it takes place at the chromosome level. We do not know if this integration occurs at random or at specific chromosomal sites. Furthermore, it is unknown whether the numerous DNA equivalents are integrated as one large molecule at a single insertion site or as individual molecules at many insertion sites.

It has been shown that the important point of the transformation is that the virus does not undergo the complete vegetative cycle. The question is whether this incapacity to multiply is of viral origin or of cellular origin. We have shown two contradictory hypotheses: one calls upon an inhibitor of cellular origin in the nonpermissive cells; the other is in favor of a viral inability, and would prove the viral deficiency in this type of cells. We used "inhibitor" in the broad sense of the word. There exists perhaps in the transformed cell, as in the lysogenized cell, a repressor inhibiting the autonomous multiplication of the virus. Alternatively, transformation is perhaps the result of a restrained transcription of the information of viral origin with regard to infection. This could be realized by sigma factors of the nonpermissive cells.

Once the integration is carried out, the interesting phenomena are the consequences of the expression of the genetic information of viral origin at the level of the cell. For a long time, initiation of cellular DNA synthesis has been considered as one of the essential actions of the viral genome in the transformed cell. Certain authors have even thought that this multiplication of cellular DNA was the particular event leading to the transformation. However, Fried (1970) demonstrated with the help of temperature-sensitive mutants of polyoma virus that these two phenomena were independent. Another expression of viral genetic information is the synthesis of T-antigen, but its significance and its role are still unknown. On the other hand, one fact we have learned is that the initiation of the modifications specific for transformation is not sufficient for maintaining this transformed state in the case of chicken cells transformed by RSV (G. S. Martin, 1970). In this case, the function necessary for transformation must be continually expressed. However, this function is not necessary for infection or replication. A third set of established facts is the modification of the cell membrane by the virus. Here also we have seen that this modification is not sufficient to definitively transform the cell, at least for antigenic modifications revealed by serological techniques. The problem cannot be solved for antigenic modifications revealed by cell-mediated techniques.

With our present knowledge, how can we understand viral action in the transformation? Two hypotheses, not necessarily contradictory, can be used to explain this essential point: the action is either centrifugal or centripetal. In the centrifugal hypothesis, irregularity is above all nuclear in nature; virus-induced initiation of cell DNA synthesis causes uncontrolled and wild mitoses. Any other virus-induced central action can be imagined: inactivation of a mitotic control function and/or activation of cell growth control. However, no experimental proof has yet confirmed this supposition, and besides, initiation of DNA synthesis does not lead to complete mitotic division. The centripetal hypothesis suggests that the regulation of cell division is dependent upon surface membrane information which may be perturbed by the virus-induced modifications of the cell surface. By analogy with bacteria, it seems that centripetal information is essential in determining cell division. We have seen that contact inhibition, which is unquestionably one of the regulatory factors in cell division of the normal cell, is deeply disturbed in the transformed cell. This disturbance could be due to an increase in negative charges at the cell surface. Whether it is due to an increase in material directly responsible for the negative charges or to an unmasking of certain pre-existing sites responsible for these charges, electronegativity can act in two different ways: repulsion of cells beyond the limit of 30 Å which are necessary for cell to cell information, or modification and neutralization of structures which carried information. We cannot completely eliminate the hypothesis that negative charges neutralize the cell's normal receptors. The defects in intracellular information can depend upon modifications of the state of the membrane constituents (for example, glycoproteins) and particularly upon the physical state of the water linked to these membranes (Pethica and Cambrai, 1970). On the other hand, we know very little about the linkage mechanism between membrane information and its repercussions at the nuclear level. The choice between the two hypotheses of regulatory mechanism of cell growth cannot be made with the present data and requires further studies.

When transformed, the cell behaves as an autonomous unit which is independent and isolated from its environment as is a prokaryote cell. The only mechanisms which would slow down disorganized multiplication of the transformed cell are, at this stage, either nutritional factors or, in the case of transplantation, immunological factors. For the latter, the part taken by the cell membrane is at least as important as the part taken by it in growth regulation. We have seen that its new antigenicity can give, on the one hand, rejection phenomena by attracting the host's cell-mediated defenses and, on the other hand, enhancement phenomena by causing production of particular antibodies.

The study of viral genome fractions involved in each of the observed modifications could guide our understanding of the mechanism of transformation. Table X summarizes these results. It is remarkable to note that the different functions to which are attributed one-fifth of the viral genome are not sufficient to maintain transformation, except for the "transforming fraction." This proves our ignorance on this specific matter. A second fact that can be deduced from this table is that finally a change in one hundred millionth of the total genetic information of the cell is sufficient to disturb an equilibrium, however stable. One can imagine how difficult it is to localize this one hundred millionth part of the genetic information of the cell and a fortiori, to explain its point of impact.

TABLE X
PART OF VIRAL GENOME INVOLVED IN DIFFERENT VIRAL FUNCTIONS

Functions	Part (%)
Infectivity assumed as	100
Induction of T-antigen	50
Induction of S-antigen	50
Initiation of cell DNA	20
TSTA	20
Transformation (colonies)	20

ACKNOWLEDGMENTS

I would like to thank Pr. Bonneau for helpful discussions, Dr. J. P. Césarini for invaluable contribution to the electron microscopy report; Miss M. Berebbi for karyological data; Dr. J. Nicoli, Dr. J. P. Kleisbauer, Dr. D. Vague, Miss M. R. Martin, Miss M. A. Nosny for helpful advice; J. Ingrand, M. Leibowitz and M. Tarayre for excellent technical assistance and for secretarial help. I thank Miss F. Birg for having collected the references and importantly contributing to the preparation of the manuscript.

REFERENCES[1]

Abel, P., and Crawford, L. W. (1963). *Virology* 19, 470–474.
Abercrombie, M., and Ambrose, E. J. (1958). *Exp. Cell Res.* 15, 332–345.
Aloni, Y., Winocour, E., and Sachs, L. (1968). *J. Mol. Biol.* 31, 415–429.
Alstein, A. D., Deichman, G. I., and Dodonova, N. N. (1966). *Virology* 30, 747–750.
Ambrose, E. J. (1967). *In* "Mechanisms of Invasion in Cancer" (P. Denoix, ed.), Vol. 6, pp. 130–139. Springer, Berlin.
Ambrose, E. J., Batzdorf, U., Osborn, J. S., and Stuart, P. R. (1970). *Nature (London)* 227, 397–398.
Aoki, T., Hämmerling, U., de Harven, E., Boyse, E. A., and Old, L. J. (1969). *J. Exp. Med.* 130, 979–1002.
Aub, J. C., Tieslau, C., and Lankester, A. (1963). *Proc. Nat. Acad. Sci. U. S.* 50, 613–619.
Avrameas, S. (1969). *Immunochemistry* 6, 43–52.
Axelrod, D., Bolton, E. T., and Habel, K. (1964). *Science* 146, 1466–1468.
Basilico, C., and Di Mayorca, G. (1965). *Proc. Nat. Acad. Sci. U. S.* 54, 125–127.
Basilico, C., and Marin, G. (1966). *Virology* 28, 429–437.
Basilico, C., Matsuya, Y., and Green, H. (1969). *J. Virol.* 3, 140–145.
Baxendall, J., Perlmann, P., and Afzelius, B. A. (1962). *J. Cell Biol.* 14, 144–151.
Bellanger, F., and Harel, L. (1969). *C. R. Acad. Sci., Ser. D* 113–116.
Benjamin, T. L. (1965). *Proc. Nat. Acad Sci. U. S.* 54, 121–124.
Benjamin, T. L. (1966). *J. Mol. Biol.* 16, 359–373.
Berebbi, M., and Bonneau, H. (1971). *Rev. Eur. Etudes Clin. Biol.* (in press).
Black, P. H. (1968). *Annu. Rev. Microbiol.* 22, 391–426.
Black, P. H., Rowe, W. P., and Cooper, H. L. (1963). *Proc Nat. Acad. Sci. U. S.* 50, 847–854.

[1] Literature survey completed on October 1, 1970.

Blackstein, M. E., Stanners, C. P., and Farmilo, A. J. (1969). *J. Mol. Biol.* **42**, 301–315.

Bonneau, H., and Césarini, J. P. (1968). *Electron Microsc. 1968, Proc. Eur. Reg. Conf., 4th, 1967, Rama, Italy,* Vol. 2, pp. 577–578.

Bonneau, H., Meyer, G., Lhérisson, A. M., and Césarini, J. P. (1967). *Proc. 1st Transplant. Congr. 1967, Paris,* **1**, 499–501.

Borek, C., and Sachs, L. (1966). *Proc. Nat. Acad. Sci. U. S.* **56**, 1705–1711.

Bosmann, H. B. (1969). *Exp. Cell Res.* **54**, 217–221.

Boué, A., Montagnier, L., and Vigier, P. (1968). *C. R. Acad. Sci., Ser. D* **266**, 178–181.

Bourgaux, P., Bourgaux-Ramoisy, D., and Stoker, M. G. P. (1965). *Virology* **25**, 364–371.

Bretton, R., and Lespinats, G. (1969). *C. R. Acad. Sci., Ser. D* **268**, 3223–3225.

Burger, M. M. (1969). *Proc. Nat. Acad. Sci. U. S.* **62**, 994–1001.

Burger, M. M., and Goldberg, A. R. (1967). *Proc. Nat. Acad. Sci. U. S.* **57**, 359–366.

Burns, W. H., and Black, P. H. (1969). *Int. J. Cancer* **4**, 204–211.

Carp, R. I., and Gilden, R. V. (1965). *Virology* **27**, 639–641.

Cassingena, R., and Tournier, P. (1968). *C. R. Acad. Sci., Ser. D* **266**, 644–646.

Cassingena, R., Tournier, P., May, E., Estrade, S., and Bourali, M. F. (1969). *C. R. Acad. Sci., Ser. D* **268**, 2834–2837.

Césarini, J. P. (1969). Unpublished data.

Césarini, J. P., Lhérisson, A. M., Meyer, G., and Bonneau, H. (1966). *C. R. Soc. Biol.* **160**, 2155–2163.

Césarini, J. P., Meyer, G., Birg, F., and Bonneau, H. (1970). *Proc. Int. Congr. Electron Microsc., 10th, 1970, Grenoble* Vol. 3, pp. 941–942.

Chauveau, J., Moulé, Y., and Rouiller, C. (1956). *Exp. Cell Res.* **11**, 317–327.

Cooper, J. E. K., and Stich, H. F. (1967). *Virology* **33**, 533–541.

Cramer, R. (1969). *C. R. Acad. Sci., Ser. D.* **268**, 3142–3145.

Cramer, R., Demerseman, P., and Atanasiu, P. (1967). *C. R. Acad. Sci., Ser. D* **265**, 378–381.

Crawford, L. V. (1962). *Virology* **8**, 177–181.

Crawford, L. V. (1964). *Virology* **22**, 149–152.

Crawford, L. V., and Black, P. H. (1964). *Virology* **24**, 388–392.

Crawford, L. V., Dulbecco, R., Fried, M., Montagnier, L., and Stoker, M. G. P. (1964). *Proc. Nat. Acad. Sci. U. S.* **52**, 148–152.

Curtis, A. S. G. (1967). "The Cell Surface: Its Molecular Role in Morphogenesis," p. 405. Academic Press, New York.

Cuzin, F., Vogt, M., Dieckmann, M., and Berg, P. (1970). *J. Mol. Biol.* **47**, 317–333.

Danielli, J. F. (1968). *In* "Molecular Associations in Biology" (B. Pullman, ed.), pp. 929–952. Academic Press, New York.

Danielli, J. F., and Davson, H. (1936). *Biochem. J.* **30**, 316–319.

Defendi, V. (1966). *Progr. Exp. Tumor Res.* **8**, 125–188.

Defendi, V., and Gasic, G. (1963). *J. Cell. Comp. Physiol.* **62**, 23–31.

Defendi, V., and Lehman, J. M. (1965). *J. Cell. Comp. Physiol.* **66**, 351–409.

Defendi, V., and Taguchi, F. (1966). *Ann. Med. Exp. Biol. Fenn.* **44**, 232–241.

Defendi, V., Jensen, F., and Sauer, G. (1967). *In* "The Molecular Biology of Viruses" (S. J. Colter and W. Paranchych, eds.), pp. 645–663. Academic Press, New York.

Deichman, G. I. (1969). *Advan. Cancer Res.* **12**, 101–136.

Delvillano, B., Carp, R. I., Manson, J. L., and Defendi, V. (1968). *Transplantation* **6**, 632–634.

De Vaux-Saint-Cyr, C. (1967). *C. R. Acad. Sci., Ser. D* **265**, 1015–1017.

De Vaux-Saint-Cyr, C. (1971). Personal communication.

De Vaux-Saint-Cyr, C., Herbet, A., Sobczak, E., Wicker, R., and Grabar, P. (1969). *Int. J. Cancer* **4**, 616–625.

Di Mayorca, G., Eddy, B. E., Steward, S. E., Hunter, W. S., Friend, C., and Bendish, H. (1959). *Proc. Nat. Acad. Sci. U. S.* **45**, 1805–1808.

Di Mayorca, G., Callender, J., Marin, G., and Giordano, R. (1969). *Virology* **38**, 126–133.

Dubbs, D. R., and Kit, S. (1969). *J. Virol.* **3**, 536–538.

Duhal, J. P., and Césarini, J. P. (1967). *J. Microsc. (Paris)* **6**, 50a.

Dulbecco, R. (1963). *Science* **142**, 932–936.

Dulbecco, R. (1969). *Science* **166**, 962–968.

Dulbecco, R., and Vogt, M. (1963). *Proc. Nat. Acad. Sci. U. S.* **50**, 236–243.

Dulbecco, R., Hartwell, L. H., and Vogt, M. (1965). *Proc. Nat. Acad. Sci. U. S.* **53**, 403–410.

Eckhart, W. (1969a). *Virology* **38**, 120–125.

Eckhart, W. (1969b). *Nature (London)* **224**, 1069–1071.

Elbers, P. F. (1964). *Recent Progr. Surface Sci.* **2**, 443–503.

Enders, J. F. (1965). *Harvey Lect.* **59**, 113–153.

Espmark, J. A., and Fagraeus, A. (1962). *Acta Pathol. Microbiol. Scand., Suppl.* **154**, 258–262.

Fogel, M. (1963). *Acta Unio Int. Contra Cancrum* **19**, 175–180.

Fogel, M., and Defendi, V. (1967). *Proc. Nat. Acad. Sci. U. S.* **58**, 967–973.

Fogel, M., and Defendi, V. (1968). *Virology* **34**, 370–373.

Fogel, M., and Sachs, L. (1969). *Virology* **37**, 327–334.

Fogel, M., and Sachs, L. (1970). *Virology* **40**, 174–177.

Follett, E. A. C., and Goldman, R. D. (1970). *Exp. Cell Res.* **59**, 124–136.

Forrester, J. A., Ambrose, E. J., and Macpherson, I. A. (1962). *Nature (London)* **196**, 1068–1070.

Forrester, J. A., Ambrose, E. J., and Stoker, M. G. P. (1964). *Nature (London)* **201**, 945–946.

Fried, M. (1965a). *Proc. Nat. Acad. Sci. U. S.* **53**, 486–491.

Fried, M. (1965b). *Virology* **25**, 669–671.

Fried, M. (1970). *Virology* **40**, 605–617.

Fugmann, R. A., and Sigel, M. M. (1967). *J. Virol.* **1**, 678–683.

Fujinaga, K., and Green, M. (1966). *Proc. Nat. Acad. Sci. U. S.* **55**, 1567–1574.

Fujinaga, K., Mak, S., and Green, M. (1968). *Proc. Nat. Acad. Sci. U. S.* **60**, 959–966.

Gerber, P. (1964). *Science* **145**, 833.

Gerber, P. (1966). *Virology* **28**, 501–509.

Gershon, D., and Sachs, L. (1963). *Nature (London)* **198**, 912–913.

Gershon, D., Hausen, P., Sachs, L., and Winocour, E. (1965). *Proc. Nat. Acad. Sci. U. S.* **54**, 1584–1592.

Gilden, R. V. (1968). *Transplantation* **6**, 645–647.

Gilden, R. V., Carp, R. I., Taguchi, F., and Defendi, V. (1965). *Proc. Nat. Acad. Sci. U. S.* **53**, 684–692.

Gilden, R. V., Kern, J., Freeman, A. E., Martin, C. E., MacAllister, R., and Turner, H. C. (1968). *Nature (London)* **219**, 517–518.

Gilead, Z., and Ginsberg, H. S. (1968a). *J. Virol.* **3**, 7–14.

Gilead, Z., and Ginsberg, H. S. (1968b). *J. Virol.* **2**, 15–20.

Gillespie, D., and Spiegelman, S. (1965). *J. Mol. Biol.* **12**, 829–842.

Goldé, A. (1970). *Virology* **40**, 1022–1029.

Habel, K. (1961). *Proc. Soc. Exp. Biol. Med.* **106**, 722–725.

Habel, K. (1963). *Annu. Rev. Microbiol.* **17**, 167–178.

Habel, K. (1965). *Virology* **25**, 51–61.

Hakomori, S., and Murakami, W. T. (1968). *Proc. Nat. Acad. Sci. U. S.* **59**, 254–261.

Hanafusa, H. (1969). *Advan. Cancer Res.* **12**, 137–165.

Hare, J. D. (1967). *Virology* **31**, 625–632.

Hare, J. D. (1970). *Virology* **40**, 978–988.

Hellström, I. (1967). *Int. J. Cancer* **2**, 65–68.

Hellström, I., and Sjögren, H. O. (1965). *Exp. Cell Res.* **40**, 212–215.

Hellström, K. E., and Hellström, I. (1969). *Advan. Cancer Res.* **12**, 167–223.

Herberman, R. B., and Ting, R. G. (1969). *Proc. Soc. Exp. Biol. Med.* **131**, 461–465.

Holley, R. W., and Kiernan, J. A. (1968). *Proc. Nat. Acad. Sci. U. S.* **60**, 300–304.

Hollinshead, A. C. (1969). *J. Gen. Virol.* **4**, 433–435.

Hollinshead, A. C., Alford, T. C., Oroszlan, S., Turner, H. C., and Huebner, R. J. (1968). *Proc. Nat. Acad. Sci. U. S.* **59**, 385–392.

Hsu, T. C., and Somers, C. E. (1961). *Proc. Nat. Acad. Sci. U. S.* **47**, 396–403.

Hudson, J., Goldstein, D., and Weil, R. (1970). *Proc. Nat. Acad. Sci. U. S.* **65**, 226–233.

Huebner, R. J., Rowe, W. P., Turner, H. C., and Lane, W. T. (1963). *Proc. Nat. Acad. Sci. U. S.* **50**, 379–389.

Inbar, M., and Sachs, L. (1969). *Nature (London)* **223**, 710–712.

Inbar, M., Rabinowitz, Z., and Sachs, L. (1969). *Int. J. Cancer* **4**, 690–696.

Irlin, I. S. (1967). *Virology* **32**, 725–728.

Jainchill, J. L., Candler, E. L., and Anderson, N. G. (1969). *Proc. Soc. Exp. Biol. Med.* **130**, 770–775.

Jensen, F., and Koprowski, H. (1969). *Virology* **37**, 687–689.

Jensen, F., Koprowski, H., and Ponten, J. A. (1963). *Proc. Nat. Acad. Sci. U. S.* **50**, 343–348.

Kato, R. (1967). *Hereditas* **58**, 221–247.

Kit, S. (1966). *In* "Subviral Carcinogenesis" (Y. Ito, ed.), pp. 116–143. Editorial Comm. First Intern. Symp. Tumor Viruses, Nagoya.

Kit, S. (1968). *Advan. Cancer Res.* **11**, 73–221.

Kit, S., Dubbs, D. R., Frearson, M., and Melnick, J. L. (1966). *Virology* **29**, 69–83.

Kit, S., Melnick, J. L., Anken, M., Dubbs, D., De Torres, R. A., and Kitahara, T. (1967a). *J. Virol.* **1**, 684–692.

Kit, S., Piekarsky, L. J., and Dubbs, D. R. (1967b). *J. Gen. Virol.* **1**, 163–175.

Klein, G., and Klein, E. (1964). *I. Nat. Cancer Inst.* **32**, 547–568.

Knowles, B. B., Jensen, F. C., Steplewski, Z., and Koprowski, H. (1968). *Proc. Nat. Acad. Sci. U. S.* **61**, 42–45.

Koprowski, H., Jensen, F. C., and Steplewski, Z. (1967). *Proc. Nat. Acad. Sci. U. S.* **58**, 127–133.

Latarjet, R., Cramer, R., and Montagnier, L. (1967). *Virology* **33**, 104–111.

Lazarus, H. M., Sporn, M. B., Smith, J. M., and Henderson, W. R. (1967). *J. Virol.* **1**, 1093–1097.

Leduc, E. H., and Bernhard, W. (1967). *J. Ultrastruct. Res.* **19**, 196–199.

Leduc, E. H., Wicker, R., Avrameas, S., and Bernhard, W. (1969). *J. Gen. Virol.* **4**, 609–614.

Lehman, J. M., Macpherson, I. A., and Moorhead, P. S. (1963). *J. Nat. Cancer*

Inst. **31,** 639–650.

Levinthal, J. D., Cerottini, J. C., Ahmad-Zadeh, C., and Wicker, R. (1967). *Int. J. Cancer* **2,** 85–102.

Lhérisson, A. M., Meyer, G., and Bonneau, H. (1967). *Bull. Cancer* **54,** 419–422.

Luft, J. H. (1966). *Electron Microsc., Proc. Int. Congr., 6th, 1966* Vol. 2, pp. 65–66.

Macpherson, I. A. (1963). *J. Nat. Cancer Inst.* **30,** 795–815.

Macpherson, I. A., and Stoker, M. G. P. (1962). *Virology* **16,** 147–151.

Malmgren, R. A., Takemoto, K. K., and Carney, P. G. (1968). *J. Nat. Cancer Inst.* **40,** 263–268.

Marin, G., and Basilico, C. (1967). *Nature (London)* **216,** 62–63.

Marin, G., and Littlefield, J. W. (1968). *J. Virol.* **2,** 69–77.

Marin, G., and Macpherson, I. A. (1969). *J. Virol.* **3,** 146–149.

Martin, G. S. (1970). *Nature (London)* **227,** 1021–1023.

Martin, M. A. (1969). *J. Virol.* **3,** 119–125.

Martin, M. A., and Axelrod, D. (1969). *Proc. Nat. Acad. Sci. U. S.* **64,** 1203–1210.

Martinez-Palomo, A., and Brailovsky, C. (1968). *Virology* **34,** 379–382.

Martinez-Palomo, A., Brailovsky, C., and Bernhard, W. (1969). *Cancer Res.* **29,** 925–937.

Meezan, E., Wu, H. C., Black, P. H., and Robbins, P. W. (1969). *Biochemistry* **8,** 2518–2524.

Metzgar, R. S., and Oleinick, S. R. (1968). *Cancer Res.* **28,** 1366–1371.

Meyer, G., and Birg, F. (1970). *J. Gen. Virol.* **9,** 127–131.

Meyer, G., Fondarai, J., and Lhérisson, A. M. (1967a). *C. R. Soc. Biol.* **161,** 2215–2218.

Meyer, G., Lhérisson, A. M., and Bonneau, H. (1967b). *Bull. Cancer* **54,** 79–86.

Meyer, G., Lhérisson, A. M., Fondarai, J., and Bonneau, H. (1968). *C. R. Soc. Biol.* **162,** 1535–1538.

Meyer, G., Birg, F., and Bonneau, H. (1969a). *C. R. Acad. Sci., Ser. D.* **268,** 2848–2849.

Meyer, G., Lhérisson, A. M., and Bonneau, H. (1969b). *Int. J. Cancer* **4,** 520–532.

Michel, R. M., Hirt, B., and Weil, R. (1967). *Proc. Nat. Acad. Sci. U. S.* **58,** 1381–1388.

Möller, E., and Möller, G. (1962). *J. Exp. Med.* **115,** 527–553.

Möller, G. (1961). *J. Exp. Med.* **114,** 415–434.

Montagnier, L. (1970). *Int. Symp. Tumor Viruses, 2nd,* pp. 19–32.

Montagnier, L., and MacPherson, I. A. (1964). *C. R. Acad. Sci., Ser. D.* **258,** 4171–4173.

Montagnier, L., Meyer, G., and Vigier, P. (1969). *C. R. Acad. Sci., Ser. D* **268,** 2986–2989.

Moorhead, S., and Weinstein, D. (1966). *In* "Recent Results in Cancer Research" (W. H. Kirsten, ed.), pp. 104–111. Springer, Berlin.

Mora, P. T., Brady, R. O., Bradley, R. H., and MacFarland, V. W. (1969). *Proc. Nat. Acad. Sci. U. S.* **63,** 1290–1296.

Morgan, H. R. (1968). *J. Virol.* **2,** 1133–1146.

Nichols, W. W. (1966). *Hereditas* **55,** 1–27.

Nicoli, J., Meyer, G., and Martin, M. R. (1971). *J. Gen. Virol.* (in press).

Oda, K., and Dulbecco, R. (1968). *Proc. Nat. Acad. Sci. U. S.* **60,** 525–532.

Ohta, N., Pardee, A. B., MacAuslan, B. R., and Burger, M. M. (1968). *Biochim. Biophys. Acta* **158,** 98–102.

Okada, Y. (1962). *Exp. Cell Res.* **26**, 98–107.

O'Neill, C. H. (1968). *J. Cell Sci.* **3**, 405–422.

Onodera, K., and Sheinin, R. (1970). *J. Cell Sci.* **7**, 319–336.

Payne, F. E., and De Vries, L. (1967). *Science* **158**, 533–534.

Pethica, B. A., and Cambrai, M. (1970). *Recherche* **1**, 433–440.

Pettijohn, D., and Kamiya, T. (1967). *J. Mol. Biol.* **29**, 275–295.

Pollack, R., and Burger, M. M. (1969). *Proc. Nat. Acad. Sci. U. S.* **62**, 1074–1076.

Pollack, R., Green, H., and Todaro, G. J. (1968). *Proc. Nat. Acad. Sci. U. S.* **60**, 126–133.

Pope, J., and Rowe, W. (1964). *J. Exp. Med.* **120**, 121–127.

Potter, C. W., MacLaughlin, B., and Oxford, J. S. (1969). *J. Virol.* **4**, 574–579.

Potter, C. W., Oxford, J. S., and MacLaughlin, B. (1970). *J. Gen. Virol.* **6**, 105–116.

Prunieras, M., and Jaquemont, X. (1965). *Ann. Inst. Pasteur, Paris* **109**, 185–203.

Ptashne, M. (1967a). *Proc. Nat. Acad. Sci. U. S.* **57**, 306–313.

Ptashne, M. (1967b). *Nature (London)* **214**, 232–234.

Rabinowitz, Z., and Sachs, L. (1969). *Virology* **38**, 336–342.

Rambourg, A. (1967). *C. R. Acad. Sci., Ser. D* **265**, 1426–1428.

Rapp, F., and Melnick, J. L. (1966). *Progr. Med. Virol.* **8**, 349–399.

Reich, P. R., Black, P. H., and Weissman, S. M. (1966). *Proc. Nat. Acad. Sci. U. S.* **56**, 78–85.

Riggs, J. L., Teitz, Y., Cremer, N. E., and Lennette, E. H. (1969). *Proc. Soc. Exp. Biol. Med.* **132**, 527–532.

Robertson, H. T., and Black, P. H. (1969). *Proc. Soc. Exp. Biol. Med.* **130**, 363–370.

Robertson, J. (1959). *Biochem. Soc. Symp.* **16**, 3–10.

Rokutanda, M., Rokutanda, H., Green, M., Fujinaga, K., Kumar-Ray, R., and Gurgo, C. (1970). *Nature (London)* **227**, 1026–1028.

Sabin, A. B., and Koch, M. A. (1963). *Proc. Nat. Acad. Sci. U. S.* **50**, 407–417.

Sambrook, J., Westphal, H., Srinivasan, P. R., and Dulbecco, R. (1968). *Proc. Nat. Acad. Sci. U. S.* **60**, 1288–1295.

Sanders, F. K., and Burford, B. O. (1964). *Nature (London)* **201**, 786–787.

Sauer, G., and Defendi, V. (1966). *Proc. Nat. Acad. Sci. U. S.* **56**, 452–457.

Sauer, G., and Kidwai, J. R. (1968). *Proc. Nat. Acad. Sci. U. S.* **61**, 1256–1263.

Sheinin, R. (1966a). *Virology* **28**, 47–55.

Sheinin, R. (1966b). *Virology* **29**, 167–170.

Sjögren, H. O., Hellström, I., and Klein, G. (1961). *Cancer Res.* **113**, 329–337.

Spiegelman, S., Burny, A., Das, M. R., Keydar, J., Schlom, J., Travnicek, M., and Watson, K. (1970). *Nature (London)* **227**, 1029–1031.

Steplewski, Z., Knowles, B. B., and Koprowski, H. (1968). *Proc. Nat. Acad. Sci. U. S.* **59**, 769–776.

Stoeckenius, W., and Engelman, D. M. (1969). *J. Cell Biol.* **42**, 613–646.

Stoker, M. G. P. (1967). *J. Cell Sci.* **2**, 293–304.

Stoker, M. G. P. (1968). *Nature (London)* **218**, 234–238.

Stoker, M. G. P., and Macpherson, I. A. (1964). *Nature (London)* **203**, 1355–1357.

Stoker, M. G. P., Shearer, M., and O'Neill, C. H. (1966). *J. Cell Sci.* **1**, 297–310.

Stoker, M. G. P., O'Neill, C. H., Berryman, S., and Waxman, V. (1968). *Int. J. Cancer* **3**, 683–692.

Svoboda, J., Chyle, P., Simkovic, D., and Hilgert, I. (1963). *Folia Biol. (Prague)* **9**, 77–81.

Tai, H. T., and O'Brien, R. L. (1969). *Virology* **38**, 698–701.

Takemoto, K. K., Malmgren, R. A., and Habel, K. (1966). *Science* **153**, 1122–1123.

Tativian, A., Peries, J., Chuat, J., and Boiron, M. (1967). *Virology* **31**, 719–721.

Temin, H. M., and Mizutani, S. (1970). *Nature (London)* **226**, 1211–1213.

Tevethia, S. S., Katz, M., and Rapp, F. (1965). *Proc. Soc. Exp. Biol. Med.* **119**, 896–901.

Tevethia, S. S., Diamandopoulos, G. T., Rapp, F., and Enders, J. (1968). *J. Immunol.* **101**, 1192–1198.

Tevethia, S. S., Crouch, N. A., Melnick, J. L., and Rapp, F. (1970). *Int. J. Cancer* **5**, 176–184.

Thorne, H. V. (1968). *J. Mol. Biol.* **35**, 215–226.

Thorne, H. V., Evans, J., and Warden, D. (1968). *Nature (London)* **219**, 728–730.

Tockstein, G. V., Polasa, H., and Green, M. (1968a). *Transplantation* **6**, 637–638.

Tockstein, G. V., Polasa, H., Piña, M., and Green, M. (1968b). *Virology* **36**, 377–386.

Todaro, G. J., and Green, H. (1966). *Virology* **28**, 756–759.

Todaro, G. J., Wolman, S. R., and Green, H. (1963). *J. Cell. Comp. Physiol.* **62**, 257–265.

Todaro, G. J., Lazar, G. K., and Green, H. (1965). *J. Cell. Comp. Physiol.* **66**, 325–331.

Torpier, G., and Montagnier, L. (1969). *Ann. Inst. Pasteur Lille* **20**, 203–210.

Trilling, D. M., and Axelrod, D. (1970). *Science* **168**, 268–270.

Vinograd, J., Leibowitz, J., Radloff, R., Watson, R., and Laipis, P. 1965. *Proc. Nat. Acad. Sci. U. S.* **53**, 1104–1111.

Vogt, M. (1970). *J. Mol. Biol.* **47**, 307–317.

Vorbrodt, A., and Koprowski, H. (1969). *J. Nat. Cancer Inst.* **43**, 1241–1248.

Wallach, D. F. H. (1969). *N. Engl. J. Med.* **280**, 761–767.

Watkins, J. F., and Dulbecco, R. (1967). *Proc. Nat. Acad. Sci. U. S.* **58**, 1396–1403.

Weil, R., and Hancock, R. (1970). *Bull. Schweiz. Akad. Med. Wiss.* **25**, 35–46.

Weil, R., and Vinograd, J. (1963). *Proc. Nat. Acad. Sci. U. S.* **50**, 730–738.

Weil, R., Michel, R. M., and Ruschmann, G. K. (1965). *Proc. Nat. Acad. Sci. U. S.* **53**, 1468–1476.

Weiss, M. C. (1970). *Proc. Nat. Acad. Sci. U. S.* **66**, 79–86.

Weiss, M. C., Ephrussi, B., and Scaletta, L. J. (1968). *Proc. Nat. Acad. Sci. U. S.* **59**, 1132–1135.

Westphal, H., and Dulbecco, R. (1968). *Proc. Nat. Acad. Sci. U. S.* **59**, 1158–1165.

Wicker, R., and Avrameas, S. (1969). *J. Gen. Virol.* **4**, 465–472.

Winocour, E. (1965a). *Virology* **25**, 276–288.

Winocour, E. (1965b). *Virology* **27**, 520–527.

Winocour, E. (1967). *Virology* **31**, 15–28.

Winocour, E. (1968). *Virology* **34**, 571–582.

Wolman, M. (1970). *Recent Progr. Surface Sci.* **3**, 262–271.

Wolman, S. R., Hirschorn, K., and Todaro, G. J. (1964). *Cytogenetics (Basel)* **3**, 45–61.

Wu, H. C., Meezan, E., Black, P. H., and Robbins, P. W. (1968). *Fed. Proc., Fed. Amer. Soc. Exp. Biol.* **27**, 814.

Wu, H. C., Meezan, E., Black, P. H., and Robbins, P. W. (1969). *Biochemistry* **8**, 2509–2517.

Zamfiresco, M. (1970). *C. R. Acad. Sci., Ser. D* **270**, 2139–2141.

PASSIVE IMMUNOTHERAPY OF LEUKEMIA
AND OTHER CANCER

Roland Motta

Institut de Cancérologie et d'Immunogénétique, Hôpital Paul-Brousse,
94-Villejuif, France and Unité de Génétique, Université Paris VI,
Paris, France

I. Introduction

Aiding the natural defense of an organism in the rejection of a malignant disease by injecting circulating antibodies directed against the transformed cells is a simple idea which has led to numerous experiments and clinical trials. In fact, the first attempts date from the end of the nineteenth century and, as early as 1895, Hericourt and Richet tried to treat patients with dog and donkey antisera directed against the malignant cells.

We shall define "passive immunotherapy" as the transfer to an organism of antibodies produced by another organism belonging to the same or a different species. By contrast, "active immunotherapy" is an attempt to raise in the organism an active response against the neoplasm, and "adoptive immunotherapy" consists in the injection of living cells capable of taking the place of or strengthening the immunological defense of the host against the malignant cells. Despite numerous and various attempts, passive immunotherapy applied to malignant disease has not, until now, given hoped for results, and this form of therapy was soon regarded with great distrust.

Recently, a reverse tendency seems to have appeared, probably owing to improvement in our understanding of the immunological mechanism involved in defense against malignant cells. We may now hope to be able to combine, in a more judicious way, passive immunotherapy with other types of therapy. The results obtained, the difficulties encountered and the possible further development of this method will be described from an experimental point of view.

II. Experimental Basis

A. ROLE OF ANTIBODIES IN THE DEVELOPMENT OF MALIGNANT DISEASE

The presence in the primary host of circulating antibodies directed against tumor-associated antigens has been demonstrated in animals (Fefer *et al.*, 1968; Alexander *et al.*, 1966; Pilch and Riggins, 1966; G. Möller, 1964; Narcissov and Abelev, 1959) and in man (Graham and Graham, 1955; Bonatti *et al.*, 1964; Hellström *et al.*, 1968; Doré *et al.*, 1967; Lewis, 1967; Gold, 1967; Parigot *et al.*, 1958). In the very special case of Burkitt's lymphoma, the presence of considerable amounts of circulating antibodies (G. Klein *et al.*, 1968) having cytotoxic activity *in vitro* against the lymphoma cells (Fass and Herberman, 1970) may be related to the occurrence of spontaneous regression in the disease (Burkitt *et al.*, 1965). The various effects of circulating antibodies on mammalian cells have been extensively studied *in vitro* and *in vivo*. Nevertheless, their exact role in the immunological defense against tumors and leukemia is still under discussion. However, it is no longer in doubt that under some experimental conditions the passive administration of antibodies induces or accelerates the rejection of a neoplasm.

Several experimental systems have been used to study the possibilities of passive immunotherapy. In many studies tumor cells are grafted and differ from the host by histocompatibility antigens. We shall consider in this chapter only those instances where the malignant cells are syngenic with the host so that rejection phenomena are caused by the presence of leukemia- or tumor-associated antigens.

1. *Inhibition of Growth*

In tumor induced by the murine sarcoma viruses, Law *et al.* (1968) have shown that injection of antiserum directed against the virus can reduce the number of takes and the growth rate of the tumors. With the Moloney sarcoma, Fefer (1969, 1970) obtained, by injection of specific immune serum, a high percentage of regression, followed by the disappearance of tumors, which were palpable at the beginning of the treatment. The passive transfer of immune serum during the latent period gives protection against the carcinogenic induction due to the murine sarcoma virus (Harvey) (Bubenik *et al.*, 1969). In Friend leukemia, the direct injection into the newborn or the transfer by the milk of antibodies injected into the mother prevents the subsequent induction of leukemia by the Friend virus in the newborn (Wahren, 1968).

When syngenic malignant cells are grafted into a host, passive immunotherapy has been demonstrated to be effective. Old *et al.* (1967) treating a grafted leukemia originally induced by Gross virus in the $C_{57}Bl_6$ mice strain with rat antiserum specific for the G⁺ leukemias, obtained total protection. When the tumor or the leukemia is chemically induced, we only need to consider the action of antibodies against the cells. Delayed growth (Reif and Kim, 1969; G. Möller, 1964) regressions, or no takes (Alexander *et al.*, 1966) have been reported following immunotherapy of these tumors.

2. *Enhancement Phenomenon*

It is not possible to discuss the effect of antibodies on the growth of malignant cells without mentioning the enhancement phenomenon. It has been possible to demonstrate, in some instances, that the active production by the host of antibodies directed against the tumor-associated antigens could be related to an enhancement of tumor growth (Abdou and McKenna, 1969). In women suffering from placental choriocarcinoma, production by the patient of antibodies directed against the husband's antigens, showing a cytotoxic activity, have been correlated with an unfavorable prognosis (Amiel *et al.*, 1967). Similarly, passive injection of specific antibodies to malignant cells very often produces an enhancing effect. This phenomenon has been reported by many authors (Tokuda and McEntee, 1967; Chard *et al.*, 1967; Chard, 1968; Voisin, 1963; Voisin *et al.*, 1969; Bremberg *et al.*, 1967; Bubenik and Koldovsky, 1964; Bubenik *et al.*, 1965c; Bubenik and Turano, 1968; Ferrer and Mihich, 1968; Cruse *et al.*, 1965; Mildenhall and Nelson, 1968). As pointed out by Bachelor (1968), the mechanisms of the enhancement phenomenon have to be understood before we can hope to be able to employ passive immunotherapy in man. It is necessary to learn more about the factors which can orient the response to a passive injection of antibodies toward either an accelerated rejection of the neoplasm or an enhanced growth.

B. Different Factors Influencing the Results of Passive Immunotherapy

Those factors that have already been discussed in passive immunotherapy of animals (Caso, 1965; Bachelor, 1968; Old *et al.*, 1967; K. E. Hellström and, Möller, 1965; Alexander, 1968; Cinader, 1963) and in man (Nigro, 1967; Mardiney *et al.*, 1969; Kodovsky, 1966; Woodruff, 1964; Southam, 1961; Vidal, 1911; Baldwin, 1967; Mathé, 1965; Kaliss, 1966), have often been studied in nonsyngenic systems. However, the rejection mechanisms of isologous or heterologous grafts seem to be analogous, at least qualitatively, to those of the tumor rejection in autologous or isologous systems. We propose in some instances to extrapolate conclusions from one system to the other.

1. *Quantity of Injected Antibodies or the Ratio of Antibodies to Target Cells*

One of the most important factors influencing the results of passive immunotherapy is without doubt the quantity of injected antibodies or, more precisely, the ratio of the quantity of antibody to the number of target cells in the body. This point has been mentioned by several authors (Hutchin *et al.*, 1967; Boyse *et al.*, 1962). It was established that, in some target cells/antiserum systems, the injection of small quantities of antibodies produced an enhancing effect although greater quantities were inhibitory (Phillips and Stetson, 1962; Gorer and Kaliss, 1959; G. Möller, 1963a). In the treatment by passive immunotherapy, these facts argue for short and massive administration of antibodies rather than for a chronic administration which might have effects other than the one desired.

2. *Type of Injected Immunoglobulin*

A certain number of investigators have tried to correlate the properties of the various classes of immunoglobulins with the inhibitory or enhancing effects of antisera (Voisin *et al.*, 1969; Chard, 1968; Bubenik *et al.*, 1965a,b,c). In theory, the properties of corresponding classes of immunoglobulins may differ from one species to another, but some general rules seem to emerge. The majority of authors have observed that the 7 S complement-fixing antibodies have an inhibitory action while the noncomplement fixing 7 S antibodies seem to have an enhancing effect. In mice, 19 S antibodies which fix complement with great efficiency have been demonstrated generally to have no effect in either direction. However, it is possible that the studies made with hyperimmune sera have not answered the question because of the low quantities of 19 S antibodies present in such sera.

On the contrary, Bubenik *et al.* (1965c) found in mice "enhancing antisera" with an enhancing activity in 19 S as well as in 7 S antibodies, with the maximum in the 7 S. In mice inhibitory antiserum the inhibitory activity was found in 19 S and 7 S antibodies but with the maximum in the 19 S. Andersson *et al.*, (1967) studying the properties of mice immunoglobulins, showed a relationship between the greatest proportion of 19 S antibodies produced by the strain $C_{57}Bl_6$ and the high efficiency of this strain in graft rejection. He proposed that these 19 S antibodies could be responsible for a part of this rejection activity.

The relationship between the inhibiting activity and the capacity to fix complement is clearly demonstrated by the work of Chard et al. (1967; Chard, 1968) and Broder and Whitehouse (1968) who have shown that antibodies, cytotoxic in vitro and "inhibitory" in vivo become enhancing if, by digestion with papain or pepsin, the Fc fragment responsible for the complement fixation is split. In the same sense, it has been shown that the nephrotoxicity of an injected antiserum depended on complement participation, and antibodies deprived of the Fc fragment were not aggressive against the kidney (Baxter and Small, 1963).

Finally, a factor which is perhaps important in passive immunotherapy is the affinity of the injected antibodies for their antigenic determinant. Fauci et al. (1970) have shown that the antibody affinity was directly related to the efficiency of complement fixation.

3. Quantity of Complement and Properdin in the Organism

It is well established that complement plays an important role in the destruction of extraneous cells in an organism. This is as true for a graft of normal cells as for malignant cells. The importance of the four factors of complement C1, C2, C3, and C4 has been demonstrated in the neutralization of mouse virus (Linscott and Levinson, 1969; Daniels et al., 1970). It has been shown that in patients with cancer or leukemia the level of complement was significantly increased (McKenzie et al., 1967). More precisely, this level increased during the evolutionary phases of the disease and decreased during the remissions (Kolar et al., 1967). Although the reasons for this were not understood, one hypothesis proposed was that this increase is due to an aspect of the immunological reaction of the organism against the neoplasm. It is possible to think that passively injected antibodies need a considerable, rapidly available quantity of complement in the organism to exhibit detectable activity. Inversely, the level of properdin seems diminished in cancer patients (Southam and Pillemer, 1957; Rottino and Levy, 1957). A parallelism between the level of properdin in the serum and the capacity for graft rejection has been demonstrated in animals (Herbut and Kraemer, 1956) and in man (Southam and Pillemer, 1957).

It has been suggested that treatment able to increase the level of this factor in the serum, for example, injection of small quantities of zymozan or polysaccharide, could help the natural defenses of the organism to increase the efficiency of immunotherapy (Landy and Pillemer, 1956a,b; Pillemer and Ross, 1955). However, in cancer patients, administration of small quantities of polysaccharide has not produced the expected increase of properdin (Southam, 1958).

Passive injection of guinea pig serum causes rejection of the ascitic form of Murphy Sturm lymphoma in the rat, probably by supplying properdin (Ainis *et al.*, 1958; Jameson *et al.*, 1958). Winn (1960) has shown that the efficiency of passive immunotherapy of $6C_3HED$ lymphosarcoma in C_3H mice is increased by injection of guinea pig serum. Passive administration of rat properdin inhibits significantly the growth of rat Yoshida sarcoma (Pfordte and Ponsold, 1969). Guinea pig properdin is active against Ehrlich cells and $6C_3HED$ tumor *in vitro* and *in vivo* (Oravec and Cambelova, 1969). Passive injection of properdin to cancer patients has shown very rapid clearance, as it was used up very quickly by a factor peculiar to these patients (Southam, 1958). In the eventuality of an attempt to supply a cancer patient with the fractions of complement which appear necessary for the complete efficiency of passive immunotherapy, one must verify the compatibility of the complement fractions injected with those of the recipient. Tamura (1970) has drawn attention to incompatibility between the C2 human component with the C4 guinea pig component. Some antibodies found in the serum of patients with sarcomas and directed against the sarcoma-specific antigens can only fix human complement (Eilber and Morton, 1970).

4. *Number and Density of Antigenic Sites on the Target Cell Surface*

If it is to be hoped that injected antibodies can kill the greatest quantity of target cells present in the organism, it is necessary that the number of antibody fixation sites by cells be sufficient to give a high probability of cell death. In fact, it has been demonstrated that the sensitivity of cells to the antibody action is correlated with the quantity of complement able to be fixed on their surface (E. Möller and Möller, 1962; Winn, 1962). In general, the sensitivity of cells to antibody action *in vitro* and *in vivo* varies in a similar way. The importance of the parameters of density and numbers of antigenic sites for the agglutinating and lytic reactions has been studied in detail using the red blood cell system (Hoyer and Trabold, 1970; Pasanen and Mäkelä, 1969). It seems necessary that the antibody fixation sites be sufficiently near to one another for an efficient complement action.

However, it is likely that, in addition to variation in the number and disposition of the antigenic sites of transformed cells (E. Möller and Möller, 1962; Bases, 1963), other physicochemical modifications may interfere with the antibody action at the cell membrane level (Troup and Walford, 1965). The presence of large quantities of mucopolysaccharide on the surface of some malignant cells could be one of these factors. Finally, one factor capable of rendering malignant cells more resistant to the action of injected antibodies could be the coating by immunoglobulins produced either by the cell itself or by other cells of the body (Brody and Beizer, 1963).

5. Situation of Cells in the Organism

Although some correlation exists for a given cell type between the sensitivity to antibodies in vitro and in vivo, one often observes cells which are sensitive to antibodies in vitro but are resistant to those antibodies in vivo. In such cases, we have to consider the cell's accessibility to the injected antibodies. Witz et al. (1968) measured the ^{125}I-labeled antibody fixation level in different organs after injection in mice. The various organs show very different intensities of labeling. These variations seem to be due, not only to the various quantities of antigens in these organs, but equally to the differences in the accessibility of antigenic sites for the injected antibodies. This fact can be related to the observation that the ascitic or leukemic cells are more susceptible to antibodies than those of solid tumors (Gorer and Kaliss, 1959). Witz et al. (1969) have shown in Moloney lymphoma that injected antibodies specific for malignant cells were fixed in the spleens of mice bearing the tumors, even though the fixation on the tumor itself was negligible. Finally, humoral antibody action has been noticed to be more efficient against metastases than against the primary tumor (Kröger et al., 1966, 1967).

6. Interference or Cooperation with the Host Immune Reaction

The inhibitory effect for the immune response to a given antigen, of antibodies corresponding to this antigen is well known (Uhr and Baumann, 1961; Motta, 1970a; G. Möller, 1963b; Bernardini et al., 1970; Dixon et al., 1967). It is possible that passive injection of antibodies may decrease an eventual host reaction against the disease. However, it has been demonstrated that this inhibitory effect is particularly important when the antibodies come from the same species as the recipient; inversely, antigen-antibody complexes where the antibodies are heterologous in respect to the recipient may have an immunogenic power higher than those of the antigen alone. Under these conditions, it is hoped that the injection of heterologous antibodies can increase an active immune response. Furthermore, it has been demonstrated in mice that suppression of the active response occurred when 7 S antibody was injected, even though 19 S was capable of increasing the response (Henry and Jerne, 1968). The influence of antibodies on the augmentation of phagocytic activity is known (Argyris, 1969) and cooperation between humoral antibodies and macrophages in the destruction of tumor cells has been demonstrated *in vitro* (Bennett *et al.*, 1964) and *in vivo* (Yamada *et al.*, 1969).

Many workers have produced evidence of a synergistic action between antibodies and immune lymphoid cells (Hutchin *et al.*, 1967; Slettenmark and Klein, 1962; Mazurek and Duplan, 1963; Alexander *et al.*, 1966; Bachelor *et al.*, 1960). Consequently, we can hope for synergy between the injected antibodies and the host's cellular immune response. Conversely, it is possible that these antibodies protect the target cells against the host immune lymphoid cells' aggression. Opinion on this subject is divided. E. Klein and Sjögren (1960) and Brondz (1965) have shown that facilitating antibodies have not the capacity to protect target cells from immune lymphoid cells, *in vitro* and *in vivo*, even though I. Hellström *et al.* (1969), G. Möller (1963b), and E. Möller (1965) found results to the contrary. The great complexity of the relations between humoral and cellular immunity is most certainly the origin of these different results.

7. *Immunoselection of Immunoresistant Cells*

If passive immunotherapy were to exist for a long period, it is probable that the development of immunoresistant cell lines could take place. Fenyo *et al.* (1968) obtained cell lines from Moloney lymphoma bearing a lowered quantity of specific antigens on their surface by successive passage through preimmunized hosts. The immunoselective phenomenon is therefore an additional argument for a short and massive treatment in order to prevent the immunoselection of the less immunogenic cells.

8. *Specificity of Antibodies Against Malignant Cells*

Normal and malignant cells of an animal generally show a large degree of antigenic identity. Any allogenic or heterologous antisera directed against malignant cells will have a great proportion of their activity directed equally against the normal cells of the animal. The degree of specificity of antisera to a given type of malignant transformed cell in various systems in the animal (Asakuma and Reif, 1968; Woodruff and Smith, 1970) and in man (G. L. Miller and Wilson, 1968; Perper *et al.*, 1970) has been studied. If antiserum is not highly specific for the leukemic cells, it will have an immunodepressive action owing to its antilymphocytic action. Where the host has some capacity of reaction against the malignant cells, this immunosuppressive effect could nullify the advantage, owing to an eventual antileukemic action of the injected antibodies. The aggravating effect of antilymphocytic serum has been demonstrated by the appearance of malignant tumors induced by viral (Hirsch and Murphy, 1968; Hirsch, 1970; Law, 1970; Allison et al., 1967; Allison, 1970) or chemical carcinogens (Cerilli and Treat, 1969; Woods, 1969; Grant and Roe, 1969), their development (Fisher et al., 1969; Deodhar et al., 1968; Cerilli and Treat, 1969; Anigstein et al., 1966) and chiefly by their metastatic spread (Deodhar and Crile, 1969; Fisher et al., 1969; Gerson and Carter, 1970; Hellmann et al., 1968). It has even been suggested that prolonged treatment of man with antilymphocyte serum could provoke cancer by interfering with the normal immunological surveillance of the body (Editorial, 1969; McKhann, 1969). However, this effect is not absolutely general and in some systems the antilymphocytic serum injection can cause an inhibition of tumor growth (Bremberg et al., 1967; Woodruff and Smith, 1970). A suggested explanation is that antibody activity directed against antigens common to normal and cancer cells can participate in the destruction of cancer cells. Another explanation could be that the immunosuppressive effect prevents production of enhancing antibodies by the host.

The classical way to obtain specific immune serum for a given type of malignant cell is to absorb an antiserum directed against this type of cell by the corresponding normal cells. However, only a small fraction of antibody activity is kept in the serum by this process. In addition, for this process to work, a sufficient quantity of normal cells is required and this is not always the case. Attempts have been made to overcome these difficulties so as to obtain directly antiserum specific to the tumor-associated antigens. Various experimental protocols have been tried. Levi et al. (1966; Levi, 1963; Levi and Schechtman, 1963; Levi and Zerubavel, 1966) have shown that it is possible to make animals tolerant to normal cells at birth, then when they are adults to immunize them with tumor cells. The study of the in vitro (Levi et al., 1966; Holeckova et al., 1963; Sekla and Holeckova, 1962) and in vivo (Levi and Zerubavel, 1966; Sekla et al., 1967) effect of such antisera has shown the usefulness of this process to produce antiserum more specific for tumor-associated antigens.

Motta (1970a) with the same goal in mind, has obtained antiserum specific for the Friend leukemia-associated antigens by immunizing various species of animals by a mixture of Friend leukemic cells and antinormal cell antiserum. These antinormal cell antisera injected passively, largely prevent the animal from being immunized against normal antigens. The remaining response against leukemic antigen is then notably increased. Another reason to prefer antiserum specific for tumor antigens is the danger of damage of some organs like the kidney, which in some instances can be fatal (De La Pava *et al.*, 1962). The importance of such an attack is related to the quantity of antibody injected and the quantity of complement present in the body. The probability of efficiency of the treatment is related to the same parameters. This is a further argument for the use of antibodies highly specific for the target cells.

C. Possible Modifications of the Principle of Passive Immunotherapy

Generally, in passive immunotherapy experiments, it is considered that the injected antibodies will kill the target cells *in vivo* by the action of complement. But it is possible to use antibodies only as carriers for products such as radioactive isotopes, chemical drugs, toxins, or enzymes. In this case, the role of the antibody is only to concentrate the cytotoxic product at the target cell.

1. *Transfer of Radioactive Product by Antibodies*

Woodruff and Smith (1970) injected mice with heterologous antibodies tagged by ^{131}I and observed their concentration in tumors. Bale *et al.* (1960) obtained total regression of rat lymphosarcoma by treatment with ^{131}I-tagged antibodies. Ghose *et al.* (1967) have shown the efficiency of ^{131}I-tagged rabbit globulins against Ehrlich cells. Balb/c mice inoculated with 2.5×10^7 Ehrlich cells are completely protected by these antibodies. The selection of the isotope is important for antibody labeling. It is necessary to irradiate the target cells sufficiently to prevent their multiplication; consequently the specific radioactivity of tagged antibodies has to be as high as possible in order that even a small quantity of antibody on cells be efficient. Equally, it is interesting to use an isotope with short-range penetration radiation in order to have specific irradiation of target cells. At least it is necessary to choose a product with a half-life of the same order of duration as that of the treatment, in order to limit the effects of the radiation on the rest of the body.

2. *Transport of Chemical Drugs by Antibodies*

The elective transport and the concentration of a drug at the tumor level has been studied by Mathé *et al.* (1958; Mathé and Tran Ba Loc, 1959). Hamsters grafted with L1210 mice leukemia cells and then treated by a single injection of amethopterin coupled to hamster antibodies against L1210 cells have exibited a very significantly augmented survival time. Among the control groups was a group receiving antibodies and amethopterin alone. A therapeutic trial based on the same principle but using ACTH as carrier protein was made on two patients with adrenal cortical tumors, resulting in incomplete but significant regression of the tumors (Mathé and Tran Ba Loc, 1959).

3. *Transport of Toxins or Enzymes by Antibodies*

Moolten and Cooperband (1970) have shown that antibodies against mumps antigens conjugated to diphtheria toxin were capable of lysing selectively monkey kidney cells bearing new surface antigens induced by infection with mumps virus.

It is possible to attach various enzymes to antibodies (Avrameas and Uriel, 1966). It would be interesting to know the effect of a concentration of enzymes having a specific action against tumor cells. This action could be either directed toward the cell itself or to the surroundings of the target cell.

4. *Indirect Passive Immunotherapy*

It is rare to find enough specific antigenic sites on a malignant cell surface so that the antibodies can efficiently kill the cell. It is possible to try to increase this antigenicity artificially. Various processes have been proposed. Burke *et al.* (1966; Burke, 1969) have used L-phenylalanine mustard in intravenous injection in order to modify specifically the tumor antigens, followed by an injection of antibodies directed against the injected hapten (L-phenylalanine mustard). This system, despite its toxicity, has proved efficient in causing tumor cell destruction. It is equally possible to consider injected heterologous antibodies, specific for malignant cells, as "new antigens" of the target cells whereby an active immunological reaction of the host against the injected heterologous immunoglobulins will be provoked. It would be possible in a similar manner to make a second passive antibody transfer, but this time with an antiglobulin specific for the globulins injected during the first passive transfer.

A possibility has been shown *in vitro*, of increasing by means of an antiglobulin the cytotoxic activity of an antiserum directed against either normal cell antigens (Fass and Herberman, 1969; Motta, 1970b) or leukemic transplantation antigens (Motta, 1970b). It is clear that this indirect method for fixing a higher quantity of immunoglobulin at the target cell level can be combined with the various modifications that we have reviewed: transfer of radioactive product (Harder and McKhann, 1968), toxin, enzymes, or drugs.

D. Synergy between Passive Immunotherapy and
   Other Forms of Therapeutics

1. Passive Immunotherapy and Radiotherapy

We have discussed previously the tagging of antibodies with a radio-active product. Radiotherapy permits a considerable reduction in the number of cells of an organism without regard to the original number of cells in the organism. It is predictable that the successive utilization of radiotherapy and immunotherapy will give better results than immunotherapy alone. Jacquet and Steeg (1966) report a study on rat epithelioma where combined treatment with radiotherapy and serotherapy gave better results than individual treatments.

2. Passive Immunotherapy and Chemotherapy

As indicated previously for radiotherapy, chemotherapy has an action complementary to immunotherapy, as it does not depend on the number of target cells. Mihich (1969) obtained interesting results with L1210 leukemia in DBA_2 mice. This leukemia is well known to be poorly antigenic in DBA_2, its strain of origin. The combination of various drugs and passive or adoptive immunotherapy succeeded in protecting a high percentage of mice (85% protection after injection of 10^2 cells by animals when 10^1 cells normally kill all the controls). Similarly with the L1210 leukemia, D. G. Miller et al. (1968) obtained better results by the association of rabbit or goat anti-L1210 antiserum and cyclophosphamide or 6-mercaptopurine.

3. Passive Immunotherapy and Other Forms of Immunotherapy

Numerous authors have called attention to the fact that various forms of immunotherapy gave better results when associated in treatment. Injections of antibodies gave more important inhibition when they were associated with immunized cells (Hutchin et al., 1967; Slettenmark and Klein, 1962; Mazurek and Duplan, 1963; Alexander et al., 1966; Bachelor et al., 1960). There is no doubt that the various forms of immunotherapy can complement one another; active or adoptive immunotherapy can be followed by passive immunotherapy, for example.

4. Various Techniques Derived from Passive Immunotherapy

Some embryonic antigens have been demonstrated in various tumors in man (Krupey et al., 1967; Zilber and Ludogovskaya, 1967; Gold and Freedman, 1965; Gold, 1967; Freedman et al., 1969; Uriel et al., 1967; Burtin et al., 1970; Von Kleist and Burtin, 1969) and animals (Furusawa *et al.,* 1965). Antimice embryo antiserum has a cytotoxic activity against Ehrlich ascitic cells (Sedallian, 1966; Sedallian and Jacob, 1967). Some trials have used such antiserum in passive immunotherapy without much success (Sedallian, 1966; Sedallian and Jacob, 1967). Evidence has been presented that some neoplastic tissues had the property to fix fibrinogen either directly or by the intermediation of the inflammation caused by the tumor growth (Day *et al.,* 1959a,b). Back *et al.* (1966) have shown a marked and specific fixation of human fibrinogen and plasmin on Murphy-Sturm lymphosarcoma in the rat. Rabbit antifibrinogen and plasmin antibody are concentrated electively in these tumors. Bale *et al.* (1960) treating rat-bearing tumors by rabbit antirat fibrinogen antibodies and heavily labeled with ^{131}I, have obtained rapid and complete regressions of tumors. These antibodies were principally localized at the tumor level and delivered specific radiotherapy. Finally, antibodies directed specifically against Walker ascites tumor nuclear antigens have exibited an *in vitro* and *in vivo* activity (Zitman *et al.,* 1968). This observation is related perhaps to the presence of antinuclear antibodies in the sera of some cancer patients (Hamard *et al.,* 1964). The role of these antibodies, if they have one, is perhaps worthy of being studied.

III. Clinical Applications

As I have pointed out at the beginning of this review, the first attempts to apply passive immunotherapy in man are far from recent. Antibody injections have been used principally to reduce the number of malignant cells, hoping that the patient might subsequently have a better reaction to another therapy. The use of antilymphocytic serum directed against normal cells should be mentioned (Laszlo *et al.,* 1968; Grace *et al.,* 1957; Mathé *et al.,* 1967). More numerous attempts were made employing antiserum directed against human malignant cells (Brittingham and Chaplin, 1960; McCredie *et al.,* 1959; Hueper and Russell, 1932; Lindstrom, 1927; Izawa *et al.,* 1966; Dar, 1901; Vidal, 1911; Vaughan, 1912; Murray, 1958; Buinauskas *et al.,* 1959). Generally the results were not convincing, and the usefulness of the method is dubious. On the other hand, attempts have been made to transfer to a leukemic patient, in the acute phase, immunoglobulin taken from another leukemic patient in remission (Sumner and Foraker, 1960). Until now these trials have not given spectacular results except perhaps in the case of Burkitt's lymphoma, where the transfer of 150 ml. of plasma from a patient who had shown tumor regression, to a patient with a progressing tumor, provoked a sudden regression in the latter (Ngu, 1965).

More recently some authors have used antibodies more or less specific for malignant cells. De Carvalho (1963) reported a series of treatments of leukemia and cancer by specific immunotherapy. He used horse and donkey antisera, immunized by "tumor antigens" coming from pools of leukemic or tumor cells. The cell extracts made by the fluorocarbon method are freed of normal antigens by precipitation with anti-normal cell serum; only the supernatant was used. The results reported involved 15 cases of leukemia, and 16 cases of cancer were presented as encouraging, a complete remission being observed following the treatment in one patient.

Sekla *et al.* (1967) have obtained encouraging results with sheep and pig antibodies, specific for different forms of leukemia. They obtained these antibodies in animals rendered tolerant at birth to normal human blood cells and then immunized when adult with leukemic cells. Vial and Callahan (1957) have tried to treat melanomas with ^{131}I-labeled antimelanin antibodies. They observed neither preferential localization of antibodies in the melanoma nor regression of the tumor.

In man, ^{125}I-labeled rabbit antibodies, specific for a brain tumor, have shown a preferential localization in the tumor (Mahaley, 1965).

IV. Conclusion

It is true that passive immunotherapy applied to malignant disease has given more disappointment than encouragement, but it would be imprudent to state positively that nothing useful will come of the method. Today nobody hopes to kill a large number of malignant cells by immunotherapy. The role reserved now for immunotherapy is rather a "clearing" of the last cells. This role could be played by passive immunotherapy, particularly if the recent attempts at using the antibodies as carriers for any type of cytotoxic agent gives the good results expected. It is hoped that coupling with a specific carrier such as an antibody will enable the use of products whose toxicity prevented their use previously.

Consequently we think that antibodies specific for tumor cells could play an interesting role in the treatment of malignant disease, bringing a quality difficult to obtain from other therapy—the specificity against target cells. One part of the problem is to learn how to produce these specific antibodies in great quantity and the other is to be able to attach these antibodies to a potent cytotoxic factor so that they can exert a useful effect.

REFERENCES

Abdou, N. I., and McKenna, J. M. (1969). *Int. Arch. Allergy Appl. Immunol.* **35**, 20.
Ainis, H., Kurtz, H. M., Kramer, P. I., Weiner, H. E., Ryan, R. M., and Jameson, E. (1958). *Cancer Res.* **18**, 1309.
Alexander, P. (1968). *Progr. Exp. Tumor Res.* **10**, 22.

Alexander, P., Connell, D. T., and Mikulska, Z. B. (1966). *Cancer Res.* **26,** 1508.

Allison, A. C. (1970). *Fed. Proc., Fed. Amer. Soc. Exp. Biol.* **29,** 167.

Allison, A. C., Berman, L. D., and Levey, R. H. (1967). *Nature (London)* **215,** 185.

Amiel, J. L., Méry, A. M., and Mathé, G. (1967). *In* "Cell-bound Immunity with Special Reference to Antilymphocyte Serum and Immunotherapy of Cancer," Vol. 43, p. 197. Univ. Liège, Liège.

Andersson, B., Wigzell, H., and Klein, G. (1967). *Transplantation* **5,** 11.

Anigstein, L., Anigstein, D. M., Rennels, E. G., and O'Steen, W. K. (1966). *Cancer Res.* **26,** 1867.

Argyris, B. F. (1969). *J. Reticuloendothel. Soc.* **6,** 498.

Asakuma, R., and Reif, A. E. (1968). *Cancer Res.* **28,** 707.

Avrameas, T., and Uriel, J. (1966). *C. R. Acad. Sci., Ser. D* **262,** 2543.

Back, N., Shields, R. R., Dewitt, G., Branshaw, R. H., and Ambrus, C. H. (1966). *J. Nat. Cancer Inst.* **36,** 171.

Baldwin, R. W. (1967). *Clin. Radiol.* **18,** 261.

Bale, W. F., Spar, I. L., and Goodland, R. L. (1960). *Cancer Res.* **20,** 1488.

Bases, R. (1963). *Cancer Res.* **23,** 811.

Batchelor, J. R. (1968). *Cancer Res.* **28,** 1410.

Batchelor, J. R., Boyse, E. A., and Gorer, P. A. (1960). *Transplant. Bull.* **26,** 449.

Baxter, J. H., and Small, P. A. (1963). *Science* **140,** 1406.

Bennett, B., Old, L. J., and Boyse, E. A. (1964). *Transplantation* **2,** 183.

Bernardini, A., Imperato, S., and Plescia, O. U. (1970). *Immunology* **18,** 187.

Bonatti, A., Rapp, W., and Burtin, P. (1964). *C. R. Acad. Sci.* **258,** 6023.

Boyse, E. A., Old, L. J., and Stockert, E. (1962). *Nature (London)* **194,** 1142.

Bremberg, S., Klein, E., and Stjernsward, J. (1967). *Cancer Res.* **27,** 2113.

Brittingham, T. E., and Chaplin, M., Jr. (1960). *Cancer* **13,** 412.

Broder, S., and Whitehouse, F., Jr. (1968). *Science* **162,** 1494.

Brody, J. I., and Beizer, L. H. (1963). *Blood* **22,** 139.

Brondz, B. D. (1965). *Transplantation* **3,** 356.

Bubenik, J., and Koldovsky, P. (1964). *Folia Biol. (Prague)* **10,** 427.

Bubenik, J., and Turano, A. (1968). *Nature (London)* **220,** 928.

Bubenik, J., Ivanyi, J., and Koldovsky, P. (1965a). *Folia Biol. (Prague)* **11,** 240.

Bubenik, J., Grystofova, H., and Koldovsky, P. (1965b). *Folia Biol. (Prague)* **11,** 415.

Bubenik, J., Ivanyi, J., and Koldovsky, P. (1965c). *Folia Biol. (Prague)* **11,** 426.

Bubenik, J., Turano, A., and Fadda, G. (1969). *Int. J. Cancer* **4,** 648.

Buinauskas, P., McCredie, J. A., Brown, E. R., and Cole, W. H. (1959). *AMA Arch. Surg.* **79,** 432.

Burke, J. F. (1969). *Cancer Res.* **29,** 2363.

Burke, J. F., Mark, V. H., Soloway, A. H., and Leskowitz, S. (1966). *Cancer Res.* **26,** 1893.

Burkitt, D., Hutt, M. S. R., and Wright, H. (1965). *Cancer* **18,** 399.

Burtin, P., Buffe, D., Von Kleist, F., Wolff, E. N., and Wolff, E. T. (1970). *Int. J. Cancer* **5,** 88.

Caso, L. V. (1965). *Advan. Cancer Res.* **9,** 47.

Cerilli, G. J., and Treat, R. C. (1969). *Transplantation* **8,** 774.

Chard, T. (1968). *Immunology* **14,** 583.

Chard, T., French, M. E., and Bachelor, J. R. (1967). *Transplantation* **5,** 1266.

Cinader, B. (1963). *Proc. Can. Cancer Res. Conf.* **5,** 279.

Cruse, J. M., Germany, W. W., and Dulaney, A. D. (1965). *Lab. Invest.* **14,** 1554.

Daniels, C. A., Borsos, T., Rapp, M. J., Snyderman, R., and Notkins, A. L. (1970). *Proc. Nat. Acad. Sci. U. S.* **65,** 528.

Dar, L. (1901). *Gaz. Hebd. Med. Chir.* [N. S.] **6**, 73.

Day, E. D., Planinsek, J. A., and Pressman, D. (1959a). *J. Nat. Cancer Inst.* **22**, 413.

Day, E. D., Planinsek, J. A., and Pressman, D. (1959b). *J. Nat. Cancer Inst.* **23**, 799.

De Carvalho, S. (1963). *Cancer* **16**, 306.

De La Pava, S., Nigogosyan, G., and Pickeren, J. W. (1962). *Arch. Intern. Med.* **109**, 391.

Deodhar, S. D., and Crile, J. G. (1969). *Cancer Res.* **29**, 776.

Deodhar, S. D., Crile, J. G., and Schofield, P. F. (1968). *Lancet* **1**, 168.

Dixon, F. J., Jacot-Guilarmot, H., and McConahey, P. J. (1967). *J. Exp. Med.* **125**, 1119.

Doré, J. F., Motta, R., Marholev, L., Hrsak, Y., Colas de la Noue, H., Seman, G., de Vassal, F., and Mathé, G. (1967). *Lancet* **2**, 1396.

Editorial. (1969). *Lancet* **1**, 505.

Eilber, F., and Morton, D. (1970). *Nature (London)* **225**, 1137.

Fass, L., and Herberman, R. B. (1969). *J. Immunol.* **102**, 140.

Fass, L., and Herberman, R. B. (1970). *Proc. Soc. Exp. Biol. Med.* **133**, 286.

Fauci, A. S., Frank, M. M., and Johnson, J. S. (1970). *J. Immunol.* **105**, 215.

Fefer, A. (1969). *Cancer Res.* **29**, 2177.

Fefer, A. (1970). *Int. J. Cancer* **5**, 327.

Fefer, A., McCoy, J. L., Perk, K., and Glynn, J. P. (1968). *Cancer Res.* **28**, 1577.

Fenyö, E. M., Klein, E., Klein, G., and Swiech, K. (1968). *J. Nat. Cancer Inst.* **40**, 69.

Ferrer, J. F., and Mihich, E. (1968). *Cancer Res.* **28**, 245.

Fisher, B., Soliman, O., and Fisher, E. R. (1969). *Proc. Soc. Exp. Biol. Med.* **131**, 16.

Freedman, S. O., Gold, P., Krupey, J., Machado, H., and Da, C. (1969). *Proc. Can. Cancer Res. Conf.* **8**, 407.

Furusawa, M., Adachi, H., and Asayama, S. (1965). *Exp. Cell Res.* **40**, 151.

Gerson, R. K., and Carter, R. L. (1970). *Nature (London)* **226**, 368.

Ghose, T., Cerini, M., Carter, M., and Nairn, R. C. (1967). *Brit. Med. J.* **1**, 90.

Gold, P. (1967). *Cancer* **20**, 1663.

Gold, P., and Freedman, O. (1965). *J. Exp. Med.* **122**, 467.

Gorer, P. A., and Kaliss, N. (1959). *Cancer Res.* **19**, 824.

Grace, J. T., Gollan, F., Taylor, W. L., and Carlson, R. I. (1957). *Surg. Forum* **8**, 185.

Graham, J. B., and Graham, R. M. (1955). *Cancer* **8**, 409.

Grant, G. A., and Roe, J. C. (1969). *Nature (London)* **223**, 1060.

Hamard, M., Cannat, A., and Seligmann, M. (1964). *Rev. Fr. Etud. Clin. Biol.* **9**, 716.

Harder, F. H., and McKhann, C. F. (1968). *J. Nat. Cancer Inst.* **40**, 231.

Hellmann, K., Hawkins, R. I., and Whitecross, S. (1968). *Brit. Med. J.* **2**, 533.

Hellström, I., Hellström, K. E., Pierce, G. E., and Bill, A. M. (1968). *Proc. Nat. Acad. Sci. U. S.* **60**, 1231.

Hellström, I., Hellström, K. E., Evans, C. A., Heppner, G. M., Pierce, G. E., and Yang, J. P. (1969). *Proc. Nat. Acad. Sci. U. S.* **62**, 362.

Hellström, K. E., and Möller, G. (1965). *Progr. Allergy* **9**, 158.

Henry, C., and Jerne, N. K. (1968). *J. Exp. Med.* **128**, 133.

Herbut, P. A., and Kraemer, W. H. (1956). *Cancer Res.* **16**, 408.

Hericourt, J., and Richet, C. (1895). *C. R. Acad. Sci.* **21**, 373.

Hirsch, M. S. (1970). *Fed. Proc., Fed. Amer. Soc. Exp. Biol.* **29**, 169.

Hirsch, M. S., and Murphy, E. A. (1968). *Lancet* **2**, 37.

Holeckova, E., Sekla, B., Cumlivski, B., Kout, M., and Janele, J. (1963). *Acta Unio Int. Contra Cancrum* **19**, 107.

Hoyer, L. W., and Trabold, N. C. (1970). *J. Clin. Invest.* **49,** 87.

Hueper, W. C., and Russell, M. (1932). *Arch. Intern. Med.* **49,** 113.

Hutchin, P., Amos, D. B., and Prioleau, W. H. (1967). *Transplantation* **5,** 68.

Izawa, T., Sakurai, M., Atsuta, Y., and Yoshizumi, T. (1966). *Ann. Paediat. Jap.* **12,** 346.

Jacquet, J., and Steeg, L. (1966). *C. R. Soc. Biol.* **160,** 279.

Jameson, E., Ainis, H., and Ryan, R. M. (1958). *Cancer Res.* **18,** 866.

Kaliss, N. (1966). *Ann. N. Y. Acad. Sci.* **129,** 155.

Klein, E., and Sjögren, H. O. (1960). *Transplant. Bull.* **26,** 442.

Klein, G., Klein, E., and Clifford, P. (1968). *Cancer* **21,** 587.

Kodovsky, P. (1966). *Lancet* **1,** 654.

Kolar, V., Kadlecova, D., Mechl, Z., Sakalova, J., and Svabenikova, L. (1967). *Neoplasma* **14,** 67.

Kröger, H., Stutz, E., Rother, M., and Niemoff, S. (1966). *Experientia* **22,** 300.

Kröger, H., Stutz, E., Rother, M., and Niemoff, S. (1967). *Eur. J. Cancer* **3,** 165.

Krupey, J., Gold, P., and Freedman, S. O. (1967). *Nature (London)* **215,** 67.

Landy, M., and Pillemer, L. (1956a). *J. Exp. Med.* **103,** 823.

Landy, M., and Pillemer, L. (1956b). *J. Exp. Med.* **104,** 383.

Laszlo, J., Buckley, C. E., and Amos, D. B. (1968). *Blood* **31,** 104.

Law, L. W. (1970). *Fed. Proc., Fed. Amer. Soc. Exp. Biol.* **29,** 171.

Law, L. W., Ting, R. C., and Stanton, M. F. (1968). *J. Nat. Cancer Inst.* **40,** 1101.

Levi, E. (1963). *Nature (London)* **199,** 501.

Levi, E., and Schechtman, A. M. (1963). *Cancer Res.* **23,** 1566.

Levi, E., and Zerubavel, R. (1966). *Cancer Res.* **26,** 668.

Levi, E., Golden, R., Zerubavel, R., and Fisher, J. (1966). *Cancer Res.* **26,** 659.

Lewis, M. G. (1967). *Lancet* **2,** 921.

Lindstrom, G. A. (1927). *Acta Med. Scand.* **22,** 1.

Linscott, W. D., and Levinson, W. E. (1969). *Proc. Nat. Acad. Sci. U. S.* **64,** 520.

McCredie, J. A., Brown, E. R., and Cole, W. H. (1959). *Proc. Soc. Exp. Biol. Med.* **100,** 31.

McKenzie, D., Colsky, J., and Hetrick, D. L. (1967). *Cancer Res.* **27,** 2386.

McKhann, C. F. (1969). *Transplantation* **8,** 209.

Mahaley, M. S. (1965). *Pa. Med. J.* **68,** 45.

Mardiney, M. R., Block, J. B., and Serpick, A. A. (1969). *Cancer Chemother. Rep.* **53,** 3.

Mathé, G. (1965). *Eur. J. Cancer* **1,** 1.

Mathé, G., and Tran Ba Loc (1959). *In* "L'action antimitotique et caryoclasique de substances chimiques," Vol. 1. C.N.R.S., Paris.

Mathé, G., Tran Ba Loc, and Bernard, J. (1958). *C. R. Acad. Sci.* **246,** 162.

Mathé, G., Schwarzenberg, L., and Amiel, J. L. (1967). *Nouv. Rev. Fr. Hematol.* **7,** 721.

Mazurek, C., and Duplan, J. F. (1963). *Bull. Cancer* **50,** 545.

Mihich, E. (1969). *Cancer Res.* **29,** 848.

Mildenhall, P., and Nelson, D. S. (1968). *Brit. J. Exp. Pathol.* **49,** 170.

Miller, D. G., Moldovanu, G., Kaplan, A., and Tocci, S. (1968). *Cancer* **22,** 1192.

Miller, G. L., and Wilson, J. E. (1968). *J. Immunol.* **101,** 1078.

Möller, E. (1965). *J. Exp. Med.* **122,** 11.

Möller, E., and Möller, G. (1962). *J. Exp. Med.* **115,** 527.

Möller, G. (1963a). *J. Nat. Cancer Inst.* **30,** 1177.

Möller, G. (1963b). *J. Nat. Cancer Inst.* **30,** 1205.

Möller, G. (1964). *Nature (London)* **204**, 846.
Moolten, F. L., and Cooperband, S. R. (1970). *Science* **169**, 68.
Motta, R. (1970a). *Eur. J. Clin. Biol. Res.* **15**, 161.
Motta, R. (1970b). *Eur. J. Clin. Biol. Res.* **15**, 510.
Murray, G. (1958). *Can. Med. Ass. J.* **79**, 249.
Narcissov, N. V., and Abelev, G. I. (1959). *Neoplasma* **6**, 353.
Ngu, V. A. (1965). *Brit. J. Cancer* **19**, 101.
Nigro, N. (1967). *In* "Relazione al XXXII Congresso Italiano di Pediatria menaggio," Vol. 1, p. 263. Como.
Old, L. J., Stockert, E., Boyse, E. A., and Geering, G. (1967). *Proc. Soc. Exp. Biol. Med.* **124**, 63.
Oravec, C., and Cambelova, J. (1969). *Neoplasma* **16**, 677.
Parigot, J., Lacour, F., and Lacour, J. (1958). *Bull. Cancer* **45**, 454.
Pasanen, V. J., and Mäkelä, O. (1969). *Immunology* **16**, 399.
Perper, R. J., Yu, T. Z., and Kooistra, J. B. (1970). *Int. Arch. Allergy Appl. Immunol.* **37**, 418.
Pfordte, K., and Ponsold, W. (1969). *Neoplasma* **16**, 609.
Phillips, M. E., and Stetson, C. A. (1962). *Proc. Soc. Exp. Biol. Med.* **111**, 265.
Pilch, Y. H., and Riggins, R. S. (1966). *Cancer Res.* **26**, 871.
Pillemer, L., and Ross, O. A. (1955). *Science* **121**, 732.
Reif, A. E., and Kim, C. A. (1969). *Nature (London)* **223**, 1377.
Rottino, A., and Levy, A. L. (1957). *Cancer* **10**, 877.
Sedallian, J. P. (1966). *C. R. Soc. Biol.* **160**, 2092.
Sedallian, J. P., and Jacob, G. (1967). *Nature (London)* **215**, 156.
Sekla, B., and Holeckova, E. (1962). *Acta Unio Int. Contra Cancrum* **18**, 76.
Sekla, B., Holeckova, E., Janele, J., Libansky, J., and Hnevkovsky, O. (1967). *Neoplasma* **14**, 641.
Slettenmark, B., and Klein, E. (1962). *Cancer Res.* **22**, 947.
Southam, C. M. (1958). *J. Clin. Invest.* **37**, 933.
Southam, C. M. (1961). *Cancer Res.* **21**, 1302.
Southam, C. M., and Pillemer, L. (1957). *Proc. Soc. Exp. Biol. Med.* **96**, 596.
Sumner, W. C., and Foraker, A. G. (1960). *Cancer* **13**, 79.
Tamura, N. (1970). *Immunology* **18**, 203.
Tokuda, S., and McEntee, F. (1967). *Transplantation* **5**, 606.
Troup, G. M., and Walford, R. L. (1965). *Cancer* **18**, 1079.
Uhr, J. W., and Baumann, J. B. (1961). *J. Exp. Med.* **113**, 935.
Uriel, J., de Nechaud, B., Birencwajg, M. S., Masseyeff, R., Leblanc, L., Quenum, C., Loisillier, F., and Grabar, P. (1967). *C. R. Acad. Sci.* **265**, 75.
Vaughan, J. W. (1912). *J. Amer. Med. Ass.* **59**, 1764.
Vial, A. B., and Callahan, W. (1957). *Cancer* **10**, 999.
Vidal, E. (1911). *In* "2e conference international pour l'étude du Cancer," Vol. 1, p. 293. Paris.
Voisin, G. A. (1963). *Rev. Fr. Etud. Clin. Biol.* **8**, 927.
Voisin, G. A., Kinsky, R., Jansen, F., and Bernard, C. (1969). *Transplantation* **8**, 618.
Von Kleist, F., and Burtin, P. (1969). *Cancer Res.* **29**, 1961.
Wahren, B. (1968). *J. Nat. Cancer Inst.* **41**, 931.
Winn, H. J. (1960). *J. Immunol.* **84**, 530.
Winn, H. J. (1962). *Ann. N. Y. Acad. Sci.* **101**, 23.
Witz, I., Yagi, Y., and Pressman, D. (1968). *J. Immunol.* **101**, 217.
Witz, I., Klein, G., and Pressman, D. (1969). *Proc. Soc. Exp. Biol. Med.* **130**, 1102.

Woodruff, M. F. (1964). *Lancet* **2,** 265.
Woodruff, M. F., and Smith, L. H. (1970). *Nature (London)* **225,** 377.
Woods, D. A., (1969). *Nature (London)* **224, 276.**
Yamada, M., Yamada, A., and Hollander, V. P. (1969). *Cancer Res.* **29,** 1420.
Zilber, L. A., and Ludogovskaya, L. A. (1967). *Folia Biol. (Prague)* **13,** 331.
Zitnan, D., Cebecauer, L., and Ujhazy, V. (1968). *Experientia* **24,** 1057.

HUMORAL REGULATORS IN THE DEVELOPMENT AND PROGRESSION OF LEUKEMIA

Donald Metcalf

Cancer Research Unit, Walter and Eliza Hall Institute, Melbourne, Australia

I. Introduction

The demonstration that tumors of certain organs in mice and rats could be induced by disturbances in specific hormones regulating these organs was the first evidence that prolonged imbalance in regulator levels could be carcinogenic. The subsequent demonstration that in at least one case, cancer of the breast in mice, the hormones probably act by facilitating the action of a tumor virus (the Bittner mammary tumor virus) has done nothing to detract from the importance of hormones in the etiology of endocrine tumors or tumors of endocrine target organs. Furthermore, many such tumors have been shown to be highly responsive to regulation by specific hormones and to have their subsequent progression substantially modified by alterations of levels of these hormones.

Speculation that some leukemias might be deficiency diseases or examples of regulatory imbalance was initially given impetus by the demonstration that the gross disturbances of proliferation and differentiation in hematopoietic cells seen in pernicious anemia were correctable by vitamin B_{12}. However, interest in such speculations dwindled when the known hormones and vitamins failed to modify substantially the progression of leukemia.

Since production of the various blood cells is precisely regulated in the normal body despite the fact that the deposits of hematopoietic tissue are diffusely scattered throughout the body, it is probable that specific humoral regulators operate to control hematopoietic cell proliferation. If this is the case, there seems no good reason why the situation with the development of at least some types of leukemia might not be essentially similar to endocrine tumor development, and Furth (1954) speculated that many leukemias might well be due to prolonged disturbances in levels of humoral white cell regulators. The current enthusiasm for viruses as the etiological agents of leukemia, although soundly based, has tended to stifle efforts to determine the real nature of the underlying cellular disturbances in the various leukemias and the role of regulatory factors in the development and progression of these diseases.

Studies in animals, particularly mice, have made it clear that the common types of leukemia are genuine transplantable neoplasms, but in humans increasing awareness of the erratic proliferative behavior of leukemic cells during the course of the disease has again raised serious doubts whether these leukemias are really autonomous neoplasms. Technical advances in recent years have now begun to allow the identification, characterization and precise assay of various specific humoral regulators controlling hematopoiesis and it is becoming possible to reexamine the role played by humoral regulators in leukemia.

Some of the questions at issue in this subject may be phrased as follows: Do specific humoral regulators exist for the various types of hematopoietic cells? Do abnormalities in the levels of these regulators or in the responsiveness of target cells to these regulators occur either before leukemia development or during the disease? Do abnormalities in regulator-target cell interaction ever cause leukemia development or substantially modify the progression of the disease?

It must be stated at the outset of this review that complete answers cannot yet be given to any of these questions. Indeed, it is probably premature to attempt a review of this field at the present time. However, work in this area is at last beginning to develop momentum and it may serve as a useful catalytic process to review the present situation and indicate some of the intriguing straws in the wind which are becoming apparent.

II. General Principles Established with Endocrine Tumors

Much of the background of this field has been reviewed by Furth (1969). Tumors can be induced to develop in endocrine target organs by establishing a protracted imbalance in the level of normal regulatory hormones. The earliest documented example was the work of Biskind and Biskind (1944) who demonstrated that transplantation of an ovary into the spleen of a gonadectomized recipient led to tumor development in the ovary. Subsequent work demonstrated that this process occurred because the ovarian hormones released by the graft entered the portal circulation and were inactivated by the liver. The pituitary responded to the apparent deficiency of ovarian function with an increased production of gonadotropin, which in time produced ovarian hyperplasia. Persistence of this situation of interrupted feedback inhibition led ultimately to tumor development in the target ovarian tissue.

Similar situations can be created in the pituitary-thyroid axis by treatment with toxic doses of radioiodine or the use of thiouracil. Both procedures disrupt the normal feedback inhibition of thyrotropin (TSH) production by thyroid hormone and lead to the development of neoplasms of TSH-secreting cells in the pituitary and, in the case of thiouracil, also to tumors of the thyroid.

Furth and his colleagues demonstrated another fundamental phenomenon regarding tumor development in such situations by showing that the tumor cells progressed through a graded series of characterizable changes before reaching a fully autonomous state. Initially such tumor cells were completely dependent for their neoplastic behavior on maintenance of the state of hormonal imbalance which initiated the tumor (Gadsden and Furth, 1953; Furth and Clifton, 1957). Thus transplanted thyroid tumor cells initially could produce progressively growing tumors only if transplanted to recipients with excessive levels of TSH and proliferation of these cells ceased if they were grafted to normal recipients.

Such tumors were termed "dependent." Subsequently, tumor cells progressed to a stage in which preferential growth occurred in animals
with excess levels of TSH but some tumor growth was possible in normal
recipients. These tumors were termed "responsive." Finally, abrupt
changes occurred in the tumor population with the emergence of clones
of cells whose proliferative behavior was independent of the level of
TSH and these autonomous tumors proliferated equally well in animals
with normal or elevated levels of TSH. Changes in functional capacity
and differentiation of the tumor cells paralleled changes in proliferative
capacity. Thus dependent tumors were typically highly functional,
whereas the acquisition of autonomy was usually paralleled by a profound or total loss of specific functional capacity.

These concepts of progression of tumor cells from dependency to
autonomy with respect to normal regulators have been widely confirmed
with other endocrine tumors in animals and man and have provided
useful therapeutic measures for the control of breast and prostatic
cancer in man.

The demonstration that viruses play a role in tumor development
in mammals led to a reassessment of the role of hormones. So far, only
one model situation exists for such studies—that of breast tumor development in mice, in which viruses of the MTV complex have been demonstrated as causative agents. The MTV virus appears able only to induce
a low incidence of breast cancer development in hypophysectomized or
gonadectomized mice and studies have shown that hormonal stimulation
of the breast epithelial cells greatly potentiates transformation by the
virus of normal cells to neoplastic cells. The exact cellular processes
operating in this situation are still uncertain but it seems clear that the
hormones, particularly prolactin, play a critical accessory role in tumor
development in this one situation known to involve a tumor virus.

The principles emerging from endocrine tumorogenesis are 2-fold;
(a) that prolonged disturbances in the level of normal regulators, either
by themselves or in collaboration with tumor viruses, can lead to tumor
development in target organs, and (b) that tumors which develop in
such situations initially are not autonomous but progress through a
series of stages to autonomy, during which the behavior of the tumor
cells can often be profoundly modified by normal regulators for that
cell type.

What analogies exist between endocrine tumorigenesis and leukemia
development? Can similar principles be demonstrated to apply to the
development of leukemia? Before discussing these questions, it is necessary to review briefly what is currently known about the humoral regulators of hematopoiesis and their possible modes of action.

III. Regulation of Hematopoiesis

It is clear from experiments of many types that hematopoiesis is regulated by the combined interaction of humoral regulators and specific hematopoietic tissue microenvironments. This subject has been reviewed recently by Metcalf and Moore (1971). The involvement of organ microenvironments in the regulation of hematopoiesis must be emphasized here before passing on to a discussion solely of humoral regulators. Although microenvironments have been shown to exist and some of their functional properties characterized in quantitative terms, virtually nothing is known regarding the cellular mechanisms that create and maintain microenvironments. This present ignorance is unfortunate as it is probable that at least some types of microenvironments are more important in regulating cell differentiation and proliferation than are humoral factors. In the discussion to follow, mention will be made of microenvironments on the few occasions where some information is available.

The mouse is the species in which most is known about the organization and regulation of the hematopoietic system, but it is likely that the basic features are similar in all mammals including man. In the mouse, the hematopoietic system has a pyramidal organization in which three functional compartments are recognizable:

1. *Stem cells,* which are few in total numbers, have an extensive but not unlimited capacity for self-replication and are also capable of generating progenitor cells. Most stem cells in a normal animal are in a noncycling (G_0) state but when required can feed into a smaller population of stem cells in active cell cycle. Most stem cells are multipotential and have the capacity to generate cells of all blood classes.

2. *Progenitor cells,* are more numerous than stem cells and, like the stem cells, have not been identified morphologically. They differ from stem cells in that most are in continuous cell cycle, are not self-generating, and have been modified by a microenvironmental inductive influence to be capable of entering only one pathway of differentiation, e.g., erythroid, granulocytic, lymphoid, etc. The progenitor cells are the target cells of the humoral regulators which "commit" them to begin actively expressing their differentiated state and to generate morphologically recognizable members of a specific cell class, e.g., to transform erythropoietin-sensitive cells (ESC's) to proerythroblasts.

3. The *morphologically recognizable cells* of the various blood cell classes are again arranged in a pyramidal population structure and generate the mature end cells, e.g., red cells or polymorphs, in each cell class. Within each cell class there is a graded sequence of proliferating

cells, each subclass being more numerous and more highly differentiated than the preceding, e.g., myeloblast to myelocyte to metamyelocyte to polymorph. Usually the penultimate stage in this sequence of immature cells, e.g., the metamyelocyte, is incapable of division, and by further maturation, these cells become end cells.

As was mentioned above, the major action of the known humoral regulators is confined to the progenitor cell class. Other humoral regulators may well exist with actions on stem cells or morphologically recognizable hematopoietic cells but, with the exception of CSF action on granulocytic cells (see later) so far these have not yet been recognized. Since progenitor cells appear to be precommitted to one pathway of differentiation, the known humoral regulators have their activity restricted to one cell class and any influence they may have on leukemic cells can also be assumed to be restricted to leukemias of the appropriate cell class. The known humoral regulators will now be briefly described.

A. Erythropoietin

This regulator is a neuraminic acid-containing glycoprotein of molecular weight approximately 60,000 (Lowy et al., 1960; Winkert and Gordon, 1960; Goldwasser and Kung, 1968) whose site of production is uncertain. The kidney plays a highly important role in its production (Jacobson et al., 1957; Mirand and Prentice, 1957; Mirand, 1968a) possibly by producing a renal erythropoietic factor (REF) which converts an erythropoietin precursor in the plasma to erythropoietin (Kuratowska et al., 1964; Contrera and Gordon, 1968). Erythropoietin is a normal regulator of erythropoiesis and its production is increased by anoxia, blood loss, or excessive red cell destruction. Erythropoietin levels in the plasma or urine are assayed in mice or rats whose erythropoietic tissues have been suppressed by hypertransfusion-induced polycythemia, anoxia, starvation, or hypophysectomy (Fried et al., 1957; Hodgson et al., 1958; Jacobson et al., 1961; Cotes and Bangham, 1961). The end point measurement of erythropoietin action is an increase in ^{59}Fe uptake into hematopoietic organs and elevations of reticulocyte or red cell levels.

The major action of erythropoietin appears to be a derepression of the genome of the erythropoietic progenitor cell (ESC) during the G_1 period of the cell cycle, leading successively to messenger-RNA, RNA, and protein synthesis and culminating in the specific initiation of hemoglobin synthesis (Alpen and Cranmore, 1959; Jacobson et al., 1961; Alpen et al., 1962; M. Gross and Goldwasser, 1969; Pavlov, 1969). Erythropoietin can also be shown to have an effect on more differentiated erythropoietic cells in vitro as measured by increased heme synthesis in an action essentially similar to its action on ESC's (Krantz, 1968). There is no evidence that erythropoietin actually increases the rate of division of erythropoietic cells (that is, shortens their cell cycle times) nor does it need to initiate mitosis in ESC's since these cells are already in cell cycle. Indeed, it has been suggested by Stohlman *et al.* (1968) that cytoplasmic hemoglobin content may actually be the regulator of proliferative activity in erythropoietic cells and when the concentration of hemoglobin reaches approximately 20%, this finally terminates mitotic activity in the mature erythroblast, followed by nuclear extrusion and the formation of the reticulocyte.

The features of relevance in what is known of erythropoietin action are its permanent derepressing action on the genome of the ESC's, the progeny of these cells continuing to behave as specific erythropoietic cells, and its apparent lack of direct action on the proliferative activity of the cells.

B. Colony-Stimulating Factor (CSF)

This regulator is a glycoprotein of molecular weight 45,000 (Stanley and Metcalf, 1969, 1971) which is demonstrable in the serum and urine of normal mice and humans (W. Robinson *et al.*, 1967; Foster *et al.*, 1968a; Chan *et al.*, 1971; Metcalf and Stanley, 1969). This factor is extractable from, and released by, many different tissues, e.g., bone marrow, spleen, thymus, submaxillary gland, lung, kidney, and can also be shown to be produced *in vitro* by some continuous cell lines, e.g., L and L 1210 cells (Pluznik and Sachs, 1966; Bradley and Metcalf, 1966; Ichikawa *et al.*, 1966; Bradley and Sumner, 1968). Although the kidney is a good source of CSF, it does not have the major role in CSF production played by the kidney in erythropoietin production and most urinary CSF represents plasma CSF cleared by the kidney (Chan, 1970). Indirect evidence suggests that CSF is a major regulator of granulopoiesis and monocyte formation in the body (Bradley *et al.*, 1969; Metcalf and Moore, 1971) and production of CSF is increased sharply during infections (Foster *et al.*, 1968b; Metcalf and Wahren, 1968) and in response to antigenic stimulation (McNeill, 1970; Metcalf, 1971). CSF is assayed *in vitro* by its capacity to initiate and sustain the formation by bone marrow cells in agar cultures of colonies of granulocytes and/or macrophages (W. Robinson *et al.*, 1967; Metcalf *et al.*, 1967a; Metcalf and Stanley, 1969). The *in vitro* colony-forming cells (CFC's) appear to be progenitors of the granulocytic and monocyte-macrophage series and, like ESC's, the majority of *in vitro* CFC's are in continuous cell cycle in the normal body (Lajtha *et al.*, 1969; Rickard *et al.*, 1970). *In vitro* CFC's exhibit wide heterogeneity in their sensitivity to stimulation by CSF and the number of cells stimulated to initiate colony formation *in vitro* bears a sigmoid dose-response relationship to CSF concentration (Metcalf and Stanley, 1969; Metcalf, 1970). Analysis of *in vitro* colony formation has provided clear evidence that granulocytes and monocytes share a common progenitor cell and that this progenitor cell (the *in vitro* CFC) probably shares a common ancestor with ESC's (Metcalf, 1969a,b, 1970). There is a lag period *in vitro* before many CFC's commence proliferation and this lag period is shortened progressively by increasing the concentration of CSF (Metcalf, 1970). The mechanisms involved are uncertain in view of the fact that most *in vitro* CFC's are already in continuous cell cycle of length 8–12 hours. There is some evidence for a small compartment of G_0 *in vitro* CFC's (Iscove *et al.*, 1970) and it may be possible that one action of CSF is to initiate entry of G_0 cells into the active cell cycle.

The growth rate of individual colonies is determined to a major degree by CSF concentration, although other factors, e.g., colony crowding, also influence colony growth rates· (Metcalf, 1968). Since colonies contain mixtures of dividing cells and nondividing metamyelocytes, polymorphs and macrophages, it has not yet been possible to determine whether the increased growth rates induced by high CSF concentrations are achieved by shortening cell cycle times or by forcing more progeny cells to remain parental in type and capable of further divisions. However, as cell cycle times are short (less than 12 hours) in dividing colony cells, the latter explanation seems more probable. CSF has a dramatic effect on the proliferation of relatively differentiated granulocytes and macrophages, a type of action not seen with erythropoietin.

In vivo, injected CSF produces a granulocytosis and monocytosis in neonatal mice and a monocytosis in adult mice (Bradley *et al.*, 1969). It also appears to alter some colony-forming cells so that they are able to initiate colony formation immediately after culture *in vitro* (Metcalf and Moore, 1971). This action could be essentially similar to the *in vitro* effects of CSF referred to above.

C. THYMIC HUMORAL FACTOR

In mammals, the thymus has a profound regulatory influence on the production of lymphocytes and antibody-forming cells. However, there is still dispute regarding the mechanisms involved as the thymus is undoubtedly a major source of the lymphocytes found in the spleen, lymph nodes, lymph, and blood (Weissman, 1967). Neonatal thymectomy leads to a great reduction in the cellularity of lymphoid organs and the number of recirculating lymphoid cells (Miller, 1962; Miller and Mitchell, 1969). Immune responses to certain antigens are also depressed by neonatal thymectomy (Miller, 1962; Good *et al.*, 1962; Jankovic *et al.*,

1962). A recent analysis of the mechanisms involved has indicated that for some immune responses collaboration between thymus-derived and bone marrow-derived lymphoid cells is necessary before antibody-forming cells can be generated. The thymus-derived cells proliferate following antigenic stimulation, but do not themselves form antibodies (Davies *et al.*, 1966, 1967; Nossal *et al.*, 1968). However, these proliferating thymus-derived cells are required for some reason to allow bone marrow-derived cells to proliferate and form antibodies (Claman *et al.*, 1966; Miller and Mitchell, 1969).

Lymphopoiesis within the thymus is regulated by the thymic epithelial cells (Metcalf, 1966a) which have the morphology of secretory cells (Arnesen, 1958; Clark, 1966). What remains uncertain is whether a humoral factor is secreted by these epithelial cells and whether such a factor influences thymic lymphopoiesis or the proliferation of lymphocytes in other organs following antigenic stimulation.

Extracts of thymus were shown to induce a lymphocytosis in lymphocyte-depleted neonatal and thymectomized adult mice (Metcalf, 1956c, 1959a,b). The lymphocytosis-stimulating activity of the serum in AKR mice was abolished by prior thymectomy (Metcalf, 1959a). Similar observations on the effects of thymus extracts have been made in irradiated neonatal rats (Camblin and Bridges, 1964) and neonatally thymectomized mice (De Somer *et al.*, 1963; Trainin *et al.*, 1966). More recently, extracts from thymus tissue have been observed to increase tritiated thymidine uptake into DNA of mouse lymphoid cells *in vivo* and rabbit lymph node cells *in vitro* (Klein *et al.*, 1965). The active material, termed "thymosin," has not been characterized but may have a molecular weight of less than 10,000 (Goldstein *et al.*, 1966). Thymosin has also been claimed to increase immune responses in neonatally thymectomized animals to sheep red cells and rejection of skin or tumor allografts (Law *et al.*, 1968; Hardy *et al.*, 1968). In a parallel series of experiments, Trainin and co-workers showed that thymus extracts increased immune responses in neonatally thymectomized mice (Small and Trainin, 1967) and also restored immunological responsiveness to spleen cells from neonatally thymectomized mice (Trainin and Linker-Israeli, 1967; Trainin *et al.*, 1969). In the latter experiments a brief exposure of as little as 1 hour increased the ability of these cells to mount *in vitro* immune responses of the GVH type. The active material in these experiments was heat labile and appeared to be of higher molecular weight than that suggested for thymosin.

Indirect evidence for the existence of a thymic humoral factor has been obtained from the successful use of thymus grafts in cell-impermeable chambers to restore immunological responses in neonatally thymectomized mice (Law *et al.*, 1964a; Osoba and Miller, 1964) and the implantation of at least two types of thymic tumors induced by polyoma virus (Law *et al.*, 1964b) or carcinogens (Stutman *et al.*, 1968, 1969) restored immunological responsiveness in neonatally thymectomized animals.

The overall impression from this work is that a thymic humoral factor does exist and that its action complements the role of the thymus in supplying lymphoid cells to peripheral lymphoid organs, but the mode of action of thymic humoral factor is obscure.

D. THROMBOPOIETIN

A humoral factor stimulating platelet formation has been described by a number of workers (Yamamoto, 1957; De Nicola *et al.*, 1958). Thrombopoietin is detectable in the serum and is elevated in such conditions as acute blood loss, X-irradiation, and acute thrombocytopenia. Its chemical nature is uncertain but it appears to be a heat-labile, nondialyzable glycoprotein moving in the β-globulin region electrophoretically (Yamamoto, 1957; Kelemen *et al.*, 1958; Rak *et al.*, 1960; De Nicola and Gibelli, 1963; Linman and Pierre, 1962). Its site of production is unknown.

Thrombopoietin is assayed *in vivo* by its capacity to stimulate increases in blood platelets and an increased uptake of ^{75}Se-selenomethionine, an isotopic label incorporated in the cytoplasm of immature megakaryocytes (Cohen *et al.*, 1965; Evatt and Levin, 1969). The mechanism of action of thrombopoietin is uncertain but experiments have suggested that thrombopioetin may recruit progenitor cells of megakaryocytes into the identifiable population of immature megakaryocytes and may also increase the rate of progression of these cells through the developmental megakaryocyte series (Odell *et al.*, 1962; Krizsa *et al.*, 1968; Ebbe *et al.*, 1968; Harker, 1968).

E. CHALONES AND ANTICHALONES

The chalone concept introduced by Bullough (1962) envisaged that each cell type in the body possesses an intrinsic capacity for proliferation which is inhibited in most differentiated cells by a specific factor, a "chalone," and it was proposed that the chalone is actually a specific product of the mature cell of that class. Corresponding antichalones were proposed which counteract chalone action and permit cell proliferation. These concepts have been supported by an extensive series of observations on the short-term proliferative behavior of skin cells (Bullough, 1965, 1967) but have not been widely investigated with respect to hematopoietic cells. The concept would suggest, for example, that granulocytes produce a chalone inhibiting granulopoiesis and that this inhibitory action is balanced by a corresponding antichalone permitting limited degrees of granulopoiesis.

Formal proof of the existence of chalones depends on the availability of completely pure populations of differentiated blood cells together with the rigid use of control cell populations to establish the specificity of the actions observed. To date these rigid criteria have not been met and the status of chalones remains in some doubt.

Rytomaa (1969) reported that low molecular weight material from semipurified granulocyte populations inhibited uptake of tritiated thymidine by short-term cultures of bone marrow cells, an effect apparently due mainly to inhibition of proliferative activity of granulocytic cells. Rytomaa (1969) also described a higher molecular weight material which blocked the action of the chalone preparation.

These concepts have not been examined extensively for other blood cell classes although red cells have been claimed to contain an anti-erythropoietin factor (Krzymowski and Krzymowska, 1962; Reynafarje et al., 1964; Whitcomb and Moore, 1968). However Erslev and Thorling (1968) failed to confirm these observations and red cell hemolysates stimulated, rather than inhibited, erythropoiesis (Lambardini et al., 1968).

F. Summary

The hematopoietic regulators have only been partially characterized but appear to operate by affecting differentiation processes rather than cell cycle times. Thus the microenvironments induce differentiation of multipotential stem cells to specific progenitor cells while the humoral regulators activate progenitor cells to enter definitive hematopoietic pathways and to express phenotypically the derepression induced by the microenvironment. Both types of regulator action appear to indicate the capacity of extrinsic agents to modify portions of the hematopoietic cell genome in such a way that the progeny of these cells exhibit the same modifications. This capacity of regulator action to induce a heritable change in cell function is potentially of relevance to leukemogenesis, where changes in the genome of the leukemic cell are clearly passed on to daughter cells.

IV. Nonspecific Humoral Regulators of Hematopoiesis and Their Influence on Leukemia Development

Although the classical hormones cannot be considered to exert specific actions of hematopoietic tissues, several of these hormones have marked influences on these tissues and readily measurable effects on leukemogenesis.

A. CORTISONE

In large doses cortisone causes a dramatic dissolution of lymphocytes, particularly thymic lymphocytes (Dougherty et al., 1964). At lower dose levels, cortisone has also been shown to inhibit mitotic activity in primitive lymphoid cells. Cortisone effects on lymphoid cells are demonstrable at physiological concentrations and it appears in the normal animal that the inhibitory influence of cortisone balances the local factors (thymic environmental or antigenic stimulation) tending to stimulate lymphopoiesis. Cortisone also has been shown to cause a depletion of in vitro colony-forming cells in the bone marrow and to be toxic for these cells in vitro (Metcalf, 1969c). Large doses of cortisone profoundly depress serum levels of CSF within hours of administration, primarily by causing an increased clearance of CSF into the urine (Metcalf, 1969c; Chan, 1970).

Kaplan et al. (1954) pointed out from an analysis of radiation-induced lymphoid leukemia development in mice that a good general correlation exists between the stimulatory or inhibitory effects of various hormones on lymphopoiesis and their effects on the development of lymphoid leukemia. Thus cortisone inhibits lymphopoiesis and was also found to decrease the incidence of lymphoid leukemia following irradiation (Kaplan et al., 1951). Conversely, adrenalectomy tends to result in lymphoid hyperplasia and promoted lymphoid leukemia development (Law, 1947). Upton and Furth (1954) confirmed this influence of cortisone on lymphoid leukemia development by showing that chronic administration of cortisone reduced the incidence of this disease in the high leukemia AKR strain. The mechanisms involved in the inhibition of lymphoid leukemia development by cortisone are not known but the situation could be highly complex. Cortisone action in preventing leukemia might be related to its profound inhibitory effect on lymphopoiesis or might be mediated by damage to the thymic epithelial cells which are involved somehow in the leukemogenesis process within the thymus. Complicating the situation is the fact that leukemogenic viruses (Gross virus in AKR mice, RadLV in irradiated C57BL mice) are involved in initiating the leukemogenesis process and it is possible that cortisone could modify the host-virus relationship in a direction favoring a lytic type of relationship rather than the integrated state thought to be important for neoplastic transformation by viruses.

Cortisone can be shown to be cytotoxic for at least some murine lymphoid luekemic cells but the most dramatic effects of cortisone therapy are seen in acute leukemias in man, particularly in childhood. The administration of cortisone or related synthetic compounds (e.g., prednisone) in large doses can induce a high frequency of temporary remissions in which the bone marrow can return to apparent normality (Fessas et al., 1954; Bernard et al., 1954). The mechanisms involved are unknown but on general grounds it seems improbable that this action is due solely to cytotoxic effects on leukemic cells.

B. Sex Hormones

Testosterone has several measurable effects on hematopoiesis. It has been shown to strongly stimulate erythropoiesis in an action which has some similarities with its anabolic effects on many tissues (Fried and Gurney, 1968; Naets and Wittek, 1968). However it is suspected that the action may be more indirect and Gordon et al. (1968) have shown that testosterone increases erythropoietin levels, possibly by elevating levels of the renal erythropoietic factor. Testosterone has the opposite effect on lymphopoiesis, causing profound thymus atrophy although it has only a minor inhibitory effect on lymph node and spleen lymphoid populations (Kaplan et al., 1954).

Paralleling the demonstration of the thymolytic effects of testosterone, it has been observed that lymphoid leukemia development occurs slightly later in male than in female AKR mice (McEndy et al., 1944) and that the final incidence of lymphoid leukemia is lower in males than in females. McEndy et al. (1944) and Law (1947) observed that orchidectomy increased the incidence of lymphoid leukemia in AKR and C58 strain mice and Gardner et al. (1944) showed that testosterone antagonized the leukemia-inducing effects of estrogens. A more dramatic effect of testosterone can be demonstrated in irradiation-induced lymphoid leukemia in mice and Kaplan et al. (1954) showed that testosterone treatment reduced lymphoid leukemia incidence in irradiated C57BL mice from 71% to 20%.

The situation with granulocytic leukemias in mice is the converse of that with lymphoid leukemia. Following irradiation, granulocytic leukemia occurs with a higher incidence in male RF mice than in females and castration reduces the incidence of granulocytic leukemia in male mice (Upton et al., 1966). Testosterone has also been reported to accelerate the development of plasma cell tumors in female BALB/c mice following injection with mineral oil (Takakura et al., 1967).

The possible role of testosterone in leukemia development in humans has not been studied, but the sex incidence of leukemia in man actually suggests an opposite situation from that existing in mice. Chronic lymphoid leukemia is much commoner in males than in females, acute lymphoid leukemia is slightly more common in males than females, and chronic granulocytic leukemia is distinctly commoner in females than males. The basis for these opposite sex-linked predispositions in man and the mouse is unknown.

Estrogens in large doses have inhibitory effects on lymphopoiesis, although Ross and Korenchevsky (1941) reported that estrogens also caused hyperplasia of the epithelial cells of the thymus. Gardner *et al.* (1944) and Lacassagne (1937) demonstrated that estrogens in moderately large doses are leukemogenic for some strains of mice. Ovariectomy sharply reduced the incidence of lymphoid leukemia in AKR mice (McEndy *et al.*, 1944) and Kirschbaum *et al.* (1953) observed that estrogens slightly increased the incidence of lymphoid leukemia following whole-body irradiation. In line with the predisposition of male RF mice to develop granulocytic leukemia, Jenkins *et al.* (1966) found that estrogens decreased the incidence of this disease in RF mice.

The above actions of the sex hormones on hematopoiesis appear not to be mediated by the adrenal cortex as similar effects have been observed in adrenalectomized animals.

C. Growth Hormone

Growth hormone increases the mass of lymphoid tissue in an action paralleling its general growth-stimulating action on other tissues. Moon *et al.* (1950) reported an increased incidence of lymphoid tumors in rats following the chronic administration of growth hormone and Kaplan *et al.* (1954) found that hypophysectomy slightly reduced the incidence of lymphoid leukemia development in irradiated C57BL mice.

D. Comment

While the above hormones have clearly demonstrable modifying effects on leukemia development and progression both in animals and man, these hormones seem unlikely to have primary roles in these processes. The fine control of hematopoietic differentiation and proliferation requires the operation of specific regulatory mechanisms and it is in these specific regulator-target cell interactions that the fundamental abnormalities in leukemia must be sought.

V. Abnormalities in Humoral Regulators in the Preleukemic Period

If analogies exist between leukemogenesis and the development of endocrine tumors, it should be possible to demonstrate abnormal levels of hematopoietic regulators or abnormal reactivity to these regulators in at least some instances during the preleukemic period.

A. NATURE OF THE PRELEUKEMIC PERIOD

Some clarification of the word "preleukemia" is necessary for the following discussion. Karyotypic analysis of leukemias, particularly in chimeric irradiated mice using the T6 marker chromosome system has indicated that most leukemic populations are probably clones derived from single cells since these leukemias are either T6 + or − and rarely of mixed type. This conclusion is supported by studies analyzing patterns of differentiation in lymphoid leukemia in AKR mice in which each leukemia was found to have a unique pattern of differentiation which was maintained on transplantation (Metcalf and Brumby, 1967). Many subpopulations with differing characteristics can develop in a leukemic population if the course of the disease is sufficiently long or if the life of the leukemic population is artificially extended by transplantation to histocompatible recipients, but these secondary populations can usually be shown to be derivatives of the original leukemic population (see, for example, Warner et al., 1969). Thus for reasons not yet clear, the development of the first leukemic cell appears to signal the end of the preleukemic, or developmental, period in leukemogenesis.

The situation appears to have close analogies with the interesting phenomenon demonstrated by Brand et al. (1967) in an analysis of sarcoma development following the implantation of plastic films in mice. In experiments in which multiple films were implanted, distinct clonal preneoplastic populations of fibroblasts were found to develop on the surface of each film, but the acquisition of fully neoplastic properties by one population appeared to inhibit progression of the changes in the other populations.

Whatever the mechanisms involved in this phenomenon, new populations of leukemic cells apparently do not continue to be generated *de novo* in an animal or human with leukemia. The critical point in leukemia development would seem therefore to be the time at which the very first cells develop fully leukemic properties as this appears to signal the end of progressive changes in the remainder of the preleukemic population. This interpretation of leukemogenesis is based on the assumption that leukemia is a neoplastic disease. While this appears to be true for the common murine leukemias, it must be reiterated that it has yet to be established that a disease like acute leukemia in humans is a neoplastic disease and, if it is not, the nature and duration of the preleukemic period remain open questions.

On the basis that leukemia is a neoplastic disease, it seems more correct to consider the preleukemic period as the period extending from the time of application of the effective leukemogenic stimulus, e.g., irradiation or virus infection, to the time when the very first leukemic cells are detectable.

In mice, the period elapsing between virus infection and clinically apparent leukemia ranged from several weeks to several months when passaged, highly virulent, viruses were used (Friend, 1957; Metcalf et al., 1959; L. Gross, 1963). On the other hand, this period extended to 12–18 months when "wild type" viruses were used (L. Gross, 1951; Kaplan, 1967). In the case of irradiation-induced leukemia, the interval usually ranged from 4 to 12 months (see review by Kaplan et al., 1954). Few studies have attempted to determine in mice the time elapsing between the development of the first detectable leukemic cells (as detected by transplantation) and the development of clinically advanced leukemia, but in an analysis of AKR mice developing lymphoid leukemia this period appeared to range from 3 to 4 weeks to 3 to 4 months (Metcalf, 1966b). Thus by subtraction the preleukemic period in mice, as defined above, would be (a) a few days in the case of the Friend virus, (b) a few weeks in the case of passaged Gross or Moloney viruses, (c) 3–9 months for irradiation-induced leukemia or (d) for an animal like the AKR mouse with a natural vertically transmitted viral infection, the period from conception to the age of 6–12 months (middle age).

For the vast majority of humans developing leukemia, little can be said regarding the probable length of the preleukemic period. In the small percentage of cases in which a definite initiating agent can be characterized, e.g., exposure to ionizing radiations or certain chemicals, the period elapsing between exposure and clinical disease has varied from 1 to at least 10 years (Medical Research Council, 1956). On the other hand, the transition between apparently perfect health and terminal illness in some patients with acute leukemia can be catastrophically short, literally a period of a few days. However, it must be appreciated that the preleukemic state is probably compatible with normal health and that even early leukemia may well be symptom-free if there is a sufficient number of surviving normal hematopoietic cells. For these reasons, even in acute leukemia, the true preleukemic period is probably of extended duration.

Since the kinetics of leukemic cells in humans with acute leukemia do not differ grossly from those in murine leukemias (Metcalf and Wiadrowski, 1966; Astaldi and Mauri, 1953; Gavosto et al., 1964; Clarkson, 1969; Mauer et al., 1969), it can be anticipated that in human acute leukemia the interval between the first appearance of leukemic cells and clinical disease may again range from a few weeks to a few months.

The nature and duration of the preleukemic period have been discussed at some length to emphasize the fact that in searching for regulator abnormalities in the *preleukemic* period it is not sufficient, or possibly even relevant, to cover the period of a few weeks before the onset of clinically apparent disease. The true preleukemic period is of longer duration, usually some months in mice and quite possibly months or years in humans.

B. ERYTHROPOIETIN

Erythroleukemia has not been observed to develop spontaneously in mice and nothing can be said regarding erythropoietin levels in such a situation. However, the Friend virus (Friend, 1957) produces a high incidence of erythroleukemia in many mouse strains and subsequently another virus strain was developed by Rauscher (1962) which produces both erythroleukemia and lymphoid leukemia. Studies have been made with both viruses on the modifying influence of erythropoietin on leukemia development. The induction of low levels of endogenous erythropoietin by hypertransfusion-induced polycythemia has been found to inhibit leukemia initiation by the Rauscher virus, at least as assessed by focus formation, splenomegaly, and increased ^{59}Fe uptake (Pluznik *et al.*, 1966; Mirand, 1968b). However, suppression of erythropoiesis by polycythemia did not inhibit erythroleukemia induction by the Friend virus (polycythemia variant) which was able to produce both splenomegaly and increased ^{59}Fe uptake due presumably to proliferating leukemic cells.

This interesting situation has been interpreted as indicating that the target cell for transformation by the Rauscher virus may be the proerythroblast and that the supply of potential target cells for transformation is therefore dependent on the action of erythropoietin which induces erythropoietin-sensitive cells to develop into proerythroblasts. If this interpretation is correct, the Rauscher virus system would constitute a clear example of a normal humoral regulator acting during the preleukemic period as an essential co-factor for leukemia development. The Friend virus, on the other hand, may induce erythroleukemia in the suppressed animal because the erythropoietin-sensitive cell is the actual target cell for this virus and in such a system, erythropoietin would have no specific involvement in the initiation of the disease. Since the Friend virus induces a neoplasm of hemoglobin-synthesizing cells, this would suggest that the virus may be able to exert an erythropoietin-like inducing effect on erythropoietin-sensitive cells and in this context it is of interest that the initial foci of erythropoietic cells seen in the spleen a few days after Friend virus infection (Metcalf *et al.*, 1959) are identical in location and appearance to the foci of erythropoiesis seen in the spleens of hypertransfusion-induced polycythemic mice a few days after the injection of erythropoietin (Jacobson *et al.*, 1961).

At no stage after infection with Friend virus were increased levels of erythropoietin observed in the plasma or urine and antierythropoietin serum had no influence on the development of the disease (Mirand *et al.*, 1968). These results support the conclusion that the action of the polycythemic variant of the Friend virus in provoking erythroid proliferation is independent of erythropoietin.

Studies on the induction of erythroleukemia in the genetically anemic W and S1 mutants have also confirmed these conclusions but have suggested that an intermediate cell may exist between the erythropoietin-sensitive cell and the proerythroblast which may be the preferred target cell of the Friend virus (Steeves *et al.*, 1968).

The extreme rarity of erythroleukemia in humans has precluded any observations on erythropoietin levels in the preleukemic state.

C. COLONY-STIMULATING FACTOR

Neither granulocytic leukemia nor monocytic leukemia occurs spontaneously in mice with sufficient frequency to make studies feasible on preleukemic levels of CSF. There is, however, one strain of mouse, the RF, in which a 30–40% incidence of granulocytic leukemia can be induced by whole-body irradiation. These mice have not yet been surveyed in the preleukemic period following irradiation, but observations on CSF levels in other mouse strains indicate that the behavior of this regulator may be of some importance for the development of leukemia in RF mice.

Surveys on conventional and germ-free Swiss mice indicated that serum CSF levels were unusually low in germ-free mice. However, germ-free mice are quite capable of developing high serum CSF levels, as evidenced by rises in CSF levels following ureteral ligature (Foster and Mirand, 1970) or the development of lymphoid leukemia (Metcalf *et al.*, 1967b). Conversely, serum CSF levels have been observed to rise sharply following viral or bacterial infections in mice and man (Foster *et al.*, 1968a,b; Metcalf and Wahren, 1968; Wahren *et al.*, 1970) and following the injection of antigens or antigen-antibody complexes, particularly antigens of bacterial origin (McNeill, 1970; Metcalf, 1971). These observations suggest that exposure to subclinical infections and saphrophytic organisms may be a major factor determining CSF levels in the serum.

The intriguing finding relating these observations to leukemogenesis in RF mice is the observation by Upton *et al.* (1966) that germ-free RF mice subjected to whole body irradiation do *not* develop granulocytic leukemia but will do so if subsequently conventionalized, and exposed to viral and bacterial infections. The mechanism of action of irradiation in the initiation of granulocytic leukemia is not clear, but some evidence exists that irradiation may activate a latent leukemogenic virus in a manner similar to that demonstrated to occur in lymphoid leukemia development in mice following irradiation (Kaplan, 1967). If this analysis is correct, it seems possible that the stimulation by saphrophytic or subclinical infections of high serum CSF levels may operate as an accessory cofactor for viral transformation, CSF acting in a manner similar to erythropoietin in erythroleukemia induced by the Rauscher virus.

Recently a myelomonocytic leukemia arising in a BALB/c mouse was described in which the leukemic cells were responsive to stimulation by CSF (Warner et al., 1969; Metcalf et al., 1969). This leukemia arose in a mouse subjected to three intraperitoneal injections of mineral oil— the procedure introduced by Potter and Boyce (1962) to induce a high incidence of plasma cell tumors in BALB/c mice and some of their F_1 hybrids. More recent studies in NZB mice and their F_1 hybrids have indicated that these strains are also susceptible to plasma cell tumor development following mineral oil injections (Warner, 1970). However, analysis of the types of neoplasm developing in NZB strains has indicated that other tumors arise in addition to plasma cell tumors. These include reticulum cell sarcomas types A and B together with a few granulocytic and myelomonocytic leukemias. There is no obvious reason why plasma cell tumors should be related to tumors of granulocytic or monocytic cells, and the association may be accidental. However, McIntyre and Princler (1969) have reported that germ-free BALB/c mice do not develop plasma cell tumors following mineral oil treatment but instead develop a high incidence of atypical reticulum cell sarcomas, some of which are probably neoplasms of monocytes or macrophages. Furthermore, Osserman (1967) has described a clinical association of plasma cell tumors and reticulum cell sarcomas in the same patient. These isolated observations suggest that possibly these various diseases may have initiating factors in common or that differing cofactors may divert the impact of the carcinogenic stimulus from one cell type to another in the hematopoietic target population. Whether this be so or not, the observation of a CSF-dependent myelomonocytic leukemia developing in BALB/c mice following mineral oil treatment prompted a study of the long-term effects of mineral oil on CSF levels in BALB/c mice during the preneoplastic period before plasma cell tumor development (2–8 months of age). Analysis showed that three injections of mineral oil induced a permanent elevation of serum CSF levels together with rises in the spleen and bone marrow content of in vitro colony-forming cells (the target cells of CSF) (Hibberd, 1970).

These observations are still inconclusive but they indicate that situations which result in elevated serum levels of CSF are those in which neoplasms of granulocytic cells have been observed to develop. This suggests that CSF might constitute a significant cofactor in leukemia development, either by increasing the number or turnover of target cells (the progenitors of granulocytes and monocytes) or by providing an accessory influence on the differentiation of these cells.

In humans, analysis of serum and urine levels of CSF are technically feasible and large-scale surveys have been made (Metcalf and Stanley, 1969; Chan et al., 1971; Metcalf et al., 1971). However, the rarity of granulocytic leukemia in humans again precludes a survey of populations in the hope of accidentally observing a person in the preleukemic period of this disease. Several conditions are known to be associated with an abnormally high risk of development of granulocytic leukemia, e.g., aplastic anemia, myelosclerosis and polycythemia vera, but it is uncertain whether observations made on these patients would necessarily be relevant to the preleukemic situation in typical acute granulocytic leukemia. To date only limited studies have been made on CSF levels in patients with aplastic anemia and polycythemia vera. In both diseases, elevated CSF levels have been observed in the serum and urine of some, but not all, patients. Sequential studies on patients with aplastic anemia have indicated that CSF levels fluctuate in the course of the disease but can be elevated over long periods (Metcalf et al., 1971). Much more survey work over longer time intervals will be needed before any clear correlation can be expected to emerge between consistently high or low CSF levels and subsequent leukemia development. One serious problem complicating studies on aplastic anemic patients is their susceptibility to infections. These patients respond to infections by developing high serum levels of CSF, as do normal subjects with infections. Recurrent episodes of infection make it difficult to assess basal levels of CSF in these patients, but this does not necessarily detract from the view that CSF may be a significant coleukemogenic factor since, because of these infections, aplastic anemic patients will experience prolonged periods of high CSF levels.

D. THYMIC HUMORAL FACTOR

Lymphoid leukemia development in the mouse is dependent on the presence of the thymus, and thymectomy in (a) AKR and C58 mice, (b) the C57BL irradiation induction system, and (c) mice infected with the Gross leukemia virus greatly decreases the final incidence of lymphoid leukemia (McEndy et al., 1944; Kaplan et al., 1956; Miller, 1959; L. Gross, 1959). The first detectable leukemic cells arise in the thymus (Furth and Boon, 1945) and subsequently progeny of these leukemic cells disseminate to other organs. The reasons underlying the critical role played by the thymus in lymphoid leukemia development are complex and not fully understood. Thymic lymphoid cells differ from other lymphoid cells in size, antigenic content, and cell cycle times (Metcalf, 1966a) and may simply represent a population highly susceptible to viral transformation. Furthermore, it has been suggested that the susceptibility of a given lymphoid target population to transformation may be dependent on local intraorgan leukemia virus titers and that the highest viral titers are to be found in the thymus (see review by Kaplan, 1967). Alternatively, a considerable body of evidence indicates that the epithelial and reticular elements of the thymus are of primary importance in determining susceptibility to leukemia development (Law, 1957; Metcalf, 1966b). Studies on thymus grafts have shown that such grafts become chimeric organs with the epithelial and reticular elements remaining donor in type but the lymphoid population becoming replaced by cells of host origin (Metcalf and Wakonig-Vaartaja, 1964). Parental thymus grafts placed in F_1 hybrid hosts (where one parent was of a high leukemia strain and the other a low leukemia strain) show unequivocally that the development of thymic lymphomata is determined by the nature of the thymic epithelial and reticular cells (Law, 1952; Metcalf, 1964; Metcalf et al., 1966). Similar data have been obtained from an analysis of thymic lymphoma development in irradiated and virus-infected mice (Kaplan et al., 1956; Kaplan, 1967). Studies on thymus graft behavior and on the fine structure of the thymus have indicated that the proliferation and differentiation of thymic lymphoid cells is largely determined by the thymic epithelial and reticular meshwork in the thymus cortex (Metcalf, 1962a, 1963, 1966b) although the nature of this interaction (whether cell contact or short-range humoral factors) is unknown. Of interest here is the fact that lymphopoiesis in the AKR thymus is excessive when compared with low leukemia strain thymuses. Analysis of thymic lymphoma development indicates that leukemia development may well depend at least in part on disturbances in this normal regulatory interaction between the thymic epithelial and reticulum cells and the target lymphoid cell population (Metcalf, 1966b). Whatever the exact mechanisms involved in the initial transformation, microenvironmental influences on the target thymic lymphoid cells play a critical role in determining the incidence and latent period of leukemia development.

Even in mice, not all lymphoid leukemias initiate in the thymus and, from the point of view of the present discussion, one important question is whether the thymus can influence lymphoid leukemia development in extrathymic lymphoid organs. In preleukemic AKR mice, the serum was shown to have exceptional lymphocytosis-stimulating activity when assayed in neonatal mice. Thymectomy of young adult AKR mice led to a fall in the lymphocytosis-stimulating activity of the serum when assayed several months after operation (Metcalf, 1959a). Similarly, the serum of C57BL mice subjected to a leukemogenic schedule of whole-body irradiation was found to exhibit increased lymphocytosis-stimulating activity (Metcalf, 1959b). These observations suggested that a humoral factor regulating some aspects of lymphopoiesis, and of possible thymic origin, may be present in elevated concentrations in the pre-leukemic period in AKR and irradiated C57BL mice. On the other hand, AKR thymus grafts in Millipore diffusion chambers were unable to restore susceptibility to leukemia development in thymectomized (AKR $\times$ C3H) F_1 mice (Metcalf et al., 1966) a finding which has also been obtained by other workers.

The inability to confer susceptibility to leukemia development on thymectomized animals using thymus tissue in diffusion chambers appears to eliminate a thymic humoral factor as being a cofactor in leukemogenesis. It should be pointed out, however, that survival of thymic tissue in diffusion chambers is extremely poor. The short-lived persistence of viable tissue may be adequate for short-term immunological reconstitution experiments (Osoba and Miller, 1964; Law et al., 1964a) but after a few weeks such chambers commonly contain only a monolayer of cells of dubious origin lining the chamber. If leukemogenesis is influenced by a thymic humoral factor, it is probable that such a factor would need to be produced for several months and the present type of diffusion chamber is quite inadequate to support the survival of significant amounts of thymic tissue for such time periods. Until more effective cell-impermeable chambers are developed, the present negative experiments carry little weight.

Since antigenic stimulation is the major proliferation stimulus for thymus- and bone marrow-derived cells in the lymph nodes or spleen, it is pertinent to consider whether antigens or humoral factors released by cells making contact with antigens (e.g., blastogenic factor) might be important coleukemogenic factors in lymphoid leukemia development. Unlike the situation with granulocytic leukemia development in germ-free mice, the axenic state does not appear to be inhibitory for lymphoid leukemia development in AKR mice. Although germ-free mice are certainly not free of antigenic stimulation (due to antigens in food or vertically transmitted viral infections), the ability of germ-free AKR mice to develop lymphoid leukemia suggests that antigenic stimulation may not be a major cofactor in lymphoid leukemia development. A study of C3H mice receiving massive antigenic stimulation for life with either BSA or Salmonella flagellar antigens revealed that a slightly higher incidence of lymphoid leukemia occurred in such mice along with a higher incidence of reticulum cell sarcomata and plasma cell tumors, although the overall incidence of these tumors was only 2-fold higher than in control mice (Metcalf, 1961).

The situation with respect to humoral regulators in lymphoid leukemia remains ambiguous. Lymphoid leukemia development in mice is clearly dependent on abnormalities in the microenvironmental regulation of lymphopoiesis within the thymus which can be demonstrated to exist in the preleukemic period. However, no firm evidence exists for abnormalities of circulating regulators of lymphopoiesis in the preleukemic period or for the involvement of such regulators in lymphoid leukemia development.

E. Humoral Factors in Irradiated Mice

Before leaving the question of the preleukemic period, mention must be made of several unusual observations with respect to the induction of lymphoid leukemia by whole-body irradiation. Fractionated doses of whole-body irradiation induce a very high incidence of lymphoid leukemia in C57BL mice and as mentioned above, disease development has been shown to be due probably to activation of a latent leukemogenic virus in these mice. Kaplan and Brown (1952) and Kaplan et al. (1953) demonstrated that shielding a limb during irradiation or the injection of normal bone marrow cells following irradiation greatly reduced the subsequent incidence of lymphoid leukemia development. The most likely basis for this phenomenon is the prompt restoration of immunological competence following irradiation, thus preventing in some manner the activation of the lymphoid leukemia virus (Haran-Ghera, 1967).

On the other hand, some workers have suggested that the phenomenon may be due to active repopulation of the thymus by normal bone marrow stem cells with the restoration of normal thymic lymphopoiesis. Irradiation induces chromosome abnormalities in lymphoid cells (Ilbery et al., 1963) and cells with abnormal karyotypes accumulate in the thymus during the preleukemic period (Joneja and Stich, 1963). However, it is difficult to envisage how normal stem cells repopulating the thymus would actively suppress or displace populations of cells with abnormal karyotypes. Furthermore, infection of thymic lymphoid cells by leukemia virus has the unusual effect of interrupting the normal repopulation of the thymus by bone marrow cells which should occur continuously throughout life (Kaplan, 1967). On this basis the striking ability of injected bone marrow cells to prevent leukemia development following irradiation is a puzzling phenomenon which cannot really be explained by a cellular repopulation hypothesis.

An alternative suggestion has been that the injected bone marrow cells may produce, or allow the production of, a radiation-protection factor which allows prompt thymic regeneration and somehow prevents or suppresses the leukemogenic effects of irradiation. Berenblum *et al.* (1965) and Hodes *et al.* (1966) reported that the injection of sheep spleen extracts or sheep serum inhibited the development of lymphoid leukemia in C57BL mice following whole-body irradiation. The active component in the spleen extracts was nondialyzable and heat labile and it has been suggested that it may be an α_2-macroglobulin (Berenblum *et al.*, 1968). Whole body irradiation of C57BL mice was found to depress trypsin esterase binding activity in the serum and this fall could be prevented by injections of sheep serum with radiation-protection activity (Yip and Hodes, 1970). At the present time the nature and mechanism of action of this radiation-protection factor are not known, but the factor may promote hematopoietic regeneration like the α_2-macroglobulin described by Hanna *et al.* (1967). Even if this is so, it remains uncertain whether the leukemia-preventing action is due to improved immune responses or to displacement of preleukemic cells from the thymus.

VI. Humoral Regulator Levels in Leukemia

In animals or humans with established leukemia, there are two general reasons why regulator levels might be abnormal: (a) abnormalities present in the preleukemic period may persist after leukemia develops, or (b) preexisting abnormalities may be accentuated or new abnormalities develop secondary to the presence of leukemia. For example, leukemia is usually associated with varying degrees of anemia which might disturb erythropoietin levels and the high susceptibility of some leukemic patients to infections may lead to secondary changes induced by these infections on CSF levels. The situation is potentially highly complex and it may prove difficult to determine whether some regulator abnormalities are an integral part of the leukemic process or common indirect effects of the leukemic state.

A. Erythropoietin

Assays on erythropoietin levels in mice with erythroleukemia induced by the Friend virus have not revealed abnormally high or low levels of erythropoietin in the plasma or urine (Mirand, 1968b). Injected erythropoietin increased the rate of spleen enlargement and the rise in hematocrit levels in this disease. On the other hand, antierythropoietin antisera did not substantially modify the development of the disease (Mirand *et al.*, 1968). Extensive surveys do not appear to have been made on erythropoietin levels in other types of leukemia.

B. Colony-Stimulating Factor

Surveys have been made on serum CSF levels in mice with various types of leukemia. CSF levels were elevated in most AKR mice with lymphoid leukemia (W. Robinson *et al.*, 1967) and were elevated also in germ-free AKR mice with this disease (Metcalf *et al.*, 1967b). The latter observations suggest that although infections are known to elevate serum CSF levels, secondary bacterial or protozoal infections in leukemia AKR mice are not responsible for the elevated levels observed. However, the possibility cannot be eliminated that vertically transmitted viral infections might become activated in the leukemic state even in germ-free AKR mice.

Similar elevations of serum CSF levels were observed in Swiss mice with lymphoid leukemia induced by the Buffett virus (Metcalf and Foster, 1967) and in BALB/c mice with lymphoid leukemia induced by the Moloney virus (Metcalf and Bradley, 1970). In both these latter types of viral-induced leukemia, some parallelism was observed between the extensiveness of the leukemic process and the degree of elevation of CSF levels. Elevated CSF levels were also observed in DBA/1 mice with erythroleukemia induced by the Friend virus. Here serum levels appeared to rise within 24 hours of infection and remained high throughout the leukemic period (Metcalf and Bradley, 1970). In other studies, moderate elevations of serum CSF levels were observed in mice bearing transplanted lymphoid leukemias, reticulum cell sarcomas, and plasma cell tumors (Hibberd and Metcalf, 1971).

It may appear strange that mice with lymphoid or erythroleukemia should exhibit elevated serum levels of a factor stimulating granulopoiesis and monocyte formation. However, studies on conventional and germ-free AKR mice with lymphoid leukemia have shown all such mice to have elevated levels of granulocytes in the peripheral blood and kinetic studies with tritiated thymidine have revealed an increased rate of production of granulocytes in such mice (Hibberd and Metcalf, 1971). Similarly, in Friend virus-induced erythroleukemia, the disease is accompanied by elevated granulocyte and monocyte levels in the blood (Metcalf *et al.*, 1959). Most tumor-bearing mice also exhibit elevations of granulocytes or monocytes in the peripheral blood (Hibberd and Metcalf, 1971). Studies on C57BL mice with transplanted lymphoid leukemia have shown that these mice also excrete abnormally high levels of CSF in the urine and this can be accentuated by treatment with cytosine arabinoside (Chan, 1971).

Studies on humans showed that elevated CSF levels were present in a portion of sera from patients with acute leukemia, chronic granulocytic and lymphoid leukemia, Hodgkin's disease, Burkitt lymphoma, and reticulum cell sarcoma. Some correlation was noted in patients with chronic lymphoid leukemia, Hodgkin's disease, and reticulum cell sarcoma between the extensiveness of the disease, its clinical activity, and the frequency of elevated CSF levels (Foster *et al.*, 1968a). In a serial study of children with acute leukemia, serum CSF levels were found to be elevated in all patients at some stage in the disease but levels fluctuated during the course of the disease and were often within normal limits (Foster *et al.*, 1971). In these children, no correlation was observed between the hematological status of the patient (that is, whether the patient was in remission or relapse) and serum CSF levels, although levels tended to rise terminally, often in association with terminal secondary infections.

A more extensive study has been made of 24 patients with acute granulocytic leukemia in which serum and urine levels of CSF were followed from periods varying from a few days to 18 months (Metcalf *et al.*, 1971). During the course of this study, it was shown that CSF levels in normal serum were higher than formerly believed owing to the fact that inhibitors are present in all normal serum which block CSF action in stimulating colony formation *in vitro* and thus mask the detection of CSF (Chan and Metcalf, 1970). Results using a modified assay procedure for CSF involving preliminary removal of inhibitors indicated that serum CSF levels were elevated in only 25% of serum samples from these leukemic patients but again elevated levels did not correlate with the clinical state of the patient. Paradoxically, patients with acute granulocytic leukemia tended to excrete excessive amounts of CSF in the urine and elevated levels (sometimes up to 50 times normal) were observed in 60% of 984 urines assayed. Patients with high serum CSF levels tended to excrete high levels of CSF in the urine, but on the other hand, 50% of patients with normal or subnormal serum CSF levels also excreted excessive amounts of CSF in the urine (Metcalf *et al.*, 1971). As mentioned earlier, in normal animals and man, bacterial and viral infections cause elevations in serum and urine levels in CSF. In patients with acute granulocytic leukemia, the development of infections caused similar changes in patients who were in partial or complete remission but patients in relapse seemed less able to develop elevated CSF levels.

Thus the state of patients with acute granulocytic leukemia appears to be roughly characterizable as often being a "CSF-loss syndrome," the patients losing excessive amounts of CSF in the urine and being less able than normal persons to develop high CSF levels in response to infections. It is of interest in this context that in at least one infectious disease in man (infectious mononucleosis) the capacity to develop high serum CSF levels correlated well with resistance to the disease as assessed by a brief duration of fever and mild clinical course (Metcalf and Wahren, 1968). The hypersusceptibility of the acute leukemic patients to infections may be related to their apparent inability often to develop high serum CSF levels following infection.

In these patients it was also observed that the administration of certain cytotoxic drugs, particularly cytosine arabinoside, led to periods of increased urinary excretion of CSF. The basis for this phenomenon is not known but appears to be essentially similar to that observed in mice with transplanted leukemia. In normal mice cytosine arabinoside elevated serum and urine levels of CSF, but this response occurred earlier in leukemic mice and CSF levels were considerably higher in the urine than in normal mice (Chan, 1971). Chemical studies on CSF in leukemic and normal human urine have demonstrated that CSF from both sources has the same general properties, electrophoretic mobility, and behavior on column chromatography (Stanley and Metcalf, 1969). Furthermore, anti-human urine CSF antisera prepared in rabbits were capable of blocking the action of CSF from both normal and leukemic urine (Stanley et al., 1970). It appears therefore that the CSF in these leukemic patients is not an abnormal molecule but simply present in abnormal concentrations.

Work with CSF has emphasized a major difficulty in assessing the significance of plasma or urine levels of a regulatory factor in a particular disease state. With a classical hormone, the production site of the hormone is at a distance from the target tissue and the plasma level of the hormone can be assumed to indicate the level of the hormone impinging on the target cells. A more complex situation exists if there are multiple production sites of a regulator, including cells surrounding or adjacent to the target cells. Here the possibility exists that there may be high local tissue concentrations of a regulator which may not be reflected in circulating regulator levels, particularly if regulator breakdown or clearance is excessively rapid.

In the specific case of CSF, the origin of this factor is certainly widespread in the body, and bone marrow cell populations themselves can produce CSF in liquid cultures (Metcalf, 1970, 1971). Furthermore, the half-life of CSF in the serum is less than 3 hours (Metcalf and Stanley, 1971) with CSF rapidly being cleared by the kidney. In this situation it is difficult to assess the CSF "load" on target colony-forming cells in the bone marrow. The target cells may actually utilize CSF during the stimulation process, though CSF concentration, rather than total amount, is the factor determining the level of stimulation (Metcalf, 1970). The commonest situation observed in acute leukemic patients is that of a normal or low serum CSF level associated with excessive excretion of CSF in the urine. This suggests that the target cells in the bone marrow may be subjected to normal or subnormal levels of CSF stimulation. However, as assessed from total CSF output, the body may in fact be producing more CSF than normal, and if diffusion is slow across the tissue fluid compartment and bone marrow cells are a significant source of CSF, the target cells in this location could actually be exposed to higher concentrations of CSF than in the normal bone marrow.

The situation is analogous to a transport terminal in which people are arriving in Room A and being transferred to Room B by a moving footpath. The number of people on the footpath at any one time (serum CSF concentration) gives no indication of the number of people arriving in Room A or the crowding in Room A (tissue CSF concentration). If the system is in balance, the number of people leaving Room B (urine CSF output) will give an index of the number arriving in Room A (CSF production) but will again not give an indication of the crowding in Room A. An increased delivery of people to Room B can be achieved by increasing the number on the moving footpath (serum CSF concentration) or by increasing the speed of the footpath (shortening serum CSF half-life) but measurements of these parameters can only establish a minimum estimate of the crowding in Room A, and not the true level. If on the other hand, Room A is a closed room of fixed size and the people are actually being created in the room, then an increased arrival in Room B means an increased crowding in Room A.

In the case of the target cells for CSF in the leukemic bone marrow, the assessment of the true tissue concentration of CSF depends on the degree to which the bone marrow is self-supporting in terms of CSF production and the degree to which CSF enters from other locations in the body. Until this can be assessed, it is not possible from the present data to determine the level of stimulation impinging on these cells in acute leukemia. If all body tissue spaces are in equilibrium, the increased output of CSF in the urine may well indicate an increased target cell stimulation by CSF, despite the normal or subnormal serum levels of CSF.

The serum of many normal mice and of all normal humans has the capacity to inhibit, to a greater or lesser degree, colony formation *in vitro* stimulated by CSF. Analysis of such sera has shown that the inhibitors are lipoprotein in nature and that at least two electrophoretically separable types are present in normal human serum (Stanley *et al.*, 1968; Chan and Metcalf, 1970; Chan *et al.*, 1971). This material does not appear to be firmly complexed with CSF in the serum, shows some species specificity, and is not toxic for the bone marrow cells in the assay cultures. Brief incubation of mouse bone marrow suspensions with inhibitory material followed by removal and washing of the cells appears to modify the colonies subsequently produced by these treated cells, all colonies being macrophage in composition rather than granulocytic and/or macrophage (Chan, 1971).

The *in vivo* function of these inhibitors is quite unknown but it has been observed that normal human serum contains uniformly high inhibitor levels (Chan *et al.*, 1971). In sharp contrast, inhibitor levels were subnormal and often undetectable in 60% of sera in patients with acute granulocytic leukemia (Chan and Metcalf, 1970). No correlation was observed between serum inhibitor levels and CSF levels in either serum or urine (Metcalf *et al.*, 1971). However, a slight correlation was observed between clinical status of the patient and serum inhibitor levels, patients in relapse tending to have lower inhibitor levels than those in remission. Low serum inhibitor levels have not been observed in other types of leukemia or in advanced neoplastic disease not involving the hematopoietic system, but the significance of the low levels in acute granulocytic leukemia and the effects these inhibitors have on leukemic cells have yet to be determined.

C. Serum Factors in Lymphoid Leukemia

No direct information exists on levels of thymic humoral factor in leukemia. In the initial studies on the response of neonatal mice to injections of thymus extracts, it was observed that injections of serum from patients with chronic lymphoid leukemia and lymphosarcoma elevated blood lymphocyte levels in neonatal mice. This response was not observed following the injection of serum from patients with acute leukemia, chronic granulocytic leukemia, or a variety of other neoplastic diseases (Metcalf, 1956a,b). The nature and origin of the lymphocytosis-stimulating activity in the sera of these patients was not established, but serum activity was observed to fall following the transfusion of fresh whole blood and to rise following the injection of adrenaline (Metcalf, 1956b).

It was initially reported by Astaldi *et al.* (1965) that serum from patients with chronic lymphoid leukemia inhibited the transformation of normal peripheral blood lymphocytes by PHA, but this was subsequently retracted (Astaldi and Airo, 1967).

VII. Production of Humoral Factors by Leukemic Cells

One proposal regarding the nature of leukemic cells has suggested that such cells may be characterizable by one or all of the following properties: (a) production of growth-stimulating substances, (b) failure to produce growth-inhibitory substances and (c) relative insensitivity to growth inhibition by such inhibitory substances (Sachs, 1968). These proposals in essence are an elaboration of the general chalone-antichalone concept of the regulation of tissue growth.

Some of these questions have been investigated recently using the agar culture system for growing colonies of granulocytes and macrophages from hematopoietic progenitor cells. Paran et al. (1968) demonstrated that cells from transplantable lymphoid, granulocytic, and erythroleukemias could release or secrete a nondialyzable factor capable of stimulating macrophage and granulocyte colony formation by normal hematopoietic cells of mouse embryo liver. Similarly, underlayers of lymphoid leukemic cells from AKR mice were found to be capable of stimulating colony formation in vitro by mouse bone marrow cells (Bradley and Metcalf, 1967). Cells from a myelomonocytic leukemia (WEHI-3) of BALB/c mice had the highly unusual ability to stimulate granulocyte and macrophage colony formation by normal cells when mixed in agar cultures with normal bone marrow cells (Metcalf et al., 1969). This property was not shown by other leukemias and lymphomas tested in the same manner, although when cultured in liquid medium many of these leukemias were able to secrete or release active material (probably CSF) which could stimulate colony formation. Again, the myelomonocytic leukemia (WEHI-3) was unusual as medium conditioned by these cells stimulated a unique giant colony composed entirely of loosely dispersed granulocytic cells in addition to the normal types of granulocytic and macrophage colonies. The active factor released by the WEHI-3 cells has not been fully characterized chemically but initial studies have suggested that it may be a variant type of CSF.

This capacity of leukemic cells to condition medium and stimulate hematopoietic colony growth in vitro is by no means unique to leukemic cells. Conditioned medium of similar potency can be prepared from suspension cultures of cells from many tissues, e.g., kidney, embryo, bone marrow, spleen, lymph node and thymic cells and even continuous cell lines (Ichikawa et al., 1966; Bradley and Sumner, 1968; Metcalf, 1970, 1971). On a cell-for-cell basis, normal cells appear to produce concentrations of CSF equivalent to that produced by leukemic cells. Furthermore, W. A. Robinson et al. (1971) have shown that normal peripheral white cells have an outstanding capacity to stimulate colony formation in agar by human hematopoietic cells, a property not possessed by the blast cells in the blood of patients with acute granulocytic leukemias.

A second type of active material was reported to be present in medium conditioned by lymphoid, granulocytic, and erythroleukemic cells. This factor was dialyzable and although it was unable to stimulate colony formation by normal hematopoietic cells, it did stimulate the growth of colonies of the three types of leukemic cells (Ichikawa *et al.*, 1969; Pluznik, 1969). As was the case for the CSF-like factor, the dialyzable factor was also shown to be produced by cultures of normal mouse embryo fibroblasts (Pluznik, 1969). Of considerable interest was the observation that this dialyzable factor also appeared capable of inducing differentiation of myeloblasts growing in colonies in agar to nondividing metamyelocytes, polymorphs, and macrophages (Ichikawa, 1969, 1971).

So far therefore there has been little evidence to support the suggestion that leukemic cells are distinguishable from normal hematopoietic cells with regard to their ability to secrete or release growth-promoting factors.

Ichikawa *et al.* (1967) demonstrated that partially purified preparations of peritoneal or spleen macrophages were able to inhibit macrophage and granulocyte colony formation in agar when incorporated in an underlayer below the target cells. This inhibitory activity was also detectable in culture fluid from such cells and appeared to be of low molecular weight since it was freely dialyzable. Rytomaa (1969) extracted similar low molecular weight inhibitory material from semipurified preparations of granulocytes and claimed this was a specific granulocytic chalone. In his assay system, this material caused a temporary reduction in the incorporation of isotopically labeled thymidine by cultures of bone marrow cells, an effect due mainly to an influence on proliferating granulocytic cells. Unfortunately, inadequate control tissues were used to justify the claim that this was a specific product of granulocytic cells. Extracts of chloroleukemic tissue from transplanted Shay chloroleukemia in rats were stated to be deficient in this inhibitory material (Rytomaa and Kiviniemi, 1968).

In this laboratory we have demonstrated the elaboration or release of low molecular weight inhibitory material in liquid cultures of normal bone marrow, spleen, lymph node, and thymic cells. This material is dialyzable, relatively heat-stable (inactivated above 90°C.) and ether resistant. It appears to inhibit CSF-stimulated formation of both granulocytic and macrophage colonies. The only indication of specificity of origin of this inhibitory material has been the observation that thymic and lymph node cells are much poorer sources of this inhibitor than are bone marrow or spleen cells, suggesting that possibly lymphoid cells may not be the origin of this inhibitor. Contrary to the suggestion that leukemic cells might not produce such inhibitors, we have in fact found that myelomonocytic leukemic (MML) cells produce higher concentrations of this inhibitor than do normal cells (inhibitory titers of fluid from cultures of 10×10^6 cells/ml. were 1:32 for MML fluid versus 1:2 for normal fluid). Similarly, cultures of reticulum cell sarcomas and lymphoid leukemias have also been found to release high concentrations of this inhibitor.

Our experience with these inhibitors has left us with the strong impression that they are not specific antagonistic molecules for CSF and are not necessarily products of specific mature cells. Furthermore, it is evident that generalizations can be very misleading if based on a single leukemia. Where some authors have found a particular leukemia to be a poor source of inhibitors, the survey of a wider range of leukemias and allied tumors has revealed that in general, most are very good sources of such inhibitors. It must be added that little evidence exists for the existence *in vivo* of such inhibitors. Repeated tests on serum from normal and leukemic humans and mice have failed to detect the presence of dialyzable inhibitors of *in vitro* colony growth but the same procedures have little difficulty in demonstrating the existence of high molecular weight inhibitory material which is present in most normal sera. There is considerable doubt therefore whether the low molecular weight inhibitory factors released from cultured cells and found in tissue extracts are really produced *in vivo* and have any important role in the regulation of hematopoiesis.

Paran *et al.* (1969) reported that partially purified preparations of rat granulocytes produced a nondialyzable inhibitor blocking macrophage and granulocyte colony formation *in vitro*. A myeloid leukemic cell line was reported not to produce this inhibitor. This inhibitory material may well be similar to the inhibitory lipoproteins which can be demonstrated in normal mouse and human serum. These were discussed in detail earlier, but in the context of the present discussion, it is worth repeating that inhibitor levels have been observed to be abnormally low in many sera from patients with acute granulocytic leukemia (Chan and Metcalf, 1970).

It is common in patients with leukemia to show anemia, thrombocytopenia, and depressed immune responses. With the exception of the hemolytic anemias sometimes seen as a complication of chronic lymphoid leukemia, the nature of the abnormal processes leading to these defects is quite obscure. It is tempting to speculate that these abnormalities represent some type of inhibition due to the presence of leukemic cells, but the original explanation of crowding out of the bone marrow by leukemic cells is no longer seriously accepted in its literal sense. Since all hematopoietic cell populations arise from common stem cells, it might be speculated that channeling of stem cells into a leukemic pathway might deplete the stem cell pool to the detriment of other blood cells. However, leukemic populations (at least in mice) are almost certainly clones derived from a single abnormal ancestor and continued

recruitment of stem cells into the leukemic population is extremely unlikely. This process cannot therefore be suggested as the basis for the
depressed erythropoiesis or megakaryocyte formation.

Several possibilities remain to explain the generalized depressions
of hematopoiesis: (a) leukemic cell infiltration may damage the structural cells of the hematopoietic microenvironments which are vital for
the induction and maintenance of erythropoiesis and megakaryocyte
formation, (b) toxic factors similar to toxohormone (Nakahara and
Fukuoka, 1958) may interfere with the metabolism of the rapidly cycling
hematopoietic cells, (c) leukemic cells may preferentially trap important
metabolites, causing a critical deficiency for normal cells, or (d) leukemic
cells may elaborate more specific factors impairing normal hematopoietic
cells. No experimental data exist which can support or eliminate any of
the above suggested mechanisms. The only observation from studies
on animal leukemia which may be relevant to the question is the demonstration with a number of lymphoid leukemia-inducing viruses that
such viruses may be found in large numbers in megakaryocytes and
seem to provoke their disintegration (Dunn *et al.*, 1961). These viruses
can also induce granulocytic leukemia and possibly other types of
reticular neoplasms (L. Gross, 1963). It is possible therefore that other
hematopoietic populations in a leukemic animal may be damaged as
a result of infection by the virus initiating the leukemia.

VIII. Responsiveness of Leukemic Cells to Humoral Regulators

If analogies with the endocrine system are at all valid for leukemia,
then one might anticipate that leukemic cells would exhibit a variety of
patterns of responsiveness to normal humoral regulators, ranging from
full dependency to complete autonomy.

Little can be said regarding erythroleukemia and the responsiveness
of the neoplastic cells to erythropoietin in this condition. However, with
the Friend virus-induced leukemia, Mirand (1968b) has reported that
injection of erythropoietin slightly increased the rate of spleen enlargement and the uptake of ^{59}Fe.

The disease polycythemia vera provides some interesting insights
into abnormal responsiveness of target cells to humoral regulators. This
condition is characterized by excessive production of red cells and often
terminates in leukemia development. Since the terminal leukemia is
usually granulocytic in nature, it is presumed that abnormal cellular
proliferation in polycythemia vera may involve other hematopoietic
cells besides the erythroid class. The response in a normal animal to
polycythemia is an immediate reduction in plasma and urine erythropoietin levels and patients with polycythemia vera do show exceptionally

low plasma and urine levels of erythropoietin (Noyes *et al.*, 1962; De Gowin and Gurney, 1964; Mirand, 1968a; Adamson and Finch, 1968). Since erythropoietin levels rise in a normal fashion in these patients following bleeding, the system regulating erythropoietin production appears to be normal in this disease (Adamson and Finch, 1968). It could be postulated that in polycythemia vera, the erythropoietic cells are exquisitely sensitive to stimulation by the very low levels of erythropoietin which are present. However, Krantz (1968), using cultures of marrow cells, showed that erythropoietic cells from polycythemic patients were in fact abnormally hyporesponsive, or unresponsive, to added erythropoietin. No inhibitor of erythropoietin appeared to be present in the plasma of polycythemia vera patients since normal bone marrow cells responded normally to added erythropoietin in the presence of such plasma. Thus the situation in polycythemia vera appears to be that the erythropoietic cells are abnormally hyporesponsive to erythropoietin yet at the same time total erythropoiesis is in excess of normal. The most likely interpretation is that the erythropoietic cells are in a neoplastic-like state in which commitment of erythropoietin-sensitive cells to erythropoiesis and the subsequent proliferation and differentiation of these cells is independent of erythropoietin action. The basis for this state is not known but the end result is somewhat similar to that following infection of mice by the polycythemic variant of the Friend virus (Mirand, 1968b).

The agar culture system is beginning to provide some intriguing information regarding the responsiveness of leukemic granulocytic and monocytic cells to CSF and associated regulators. In studies made on the myelomonocytic leukemia (WEHI-3) in BALB/c mice, it was demonstrated that certain of the leukemic cells could proliferate in agar and form colonies containing both granulocytic and monocytic cells (Metcalf *et al.*, 1969). The neoplastic nature of these colony cells was confirmed by karyotypic identification of the characteristic 39-chromosome karyotype of this myelomonocytic leukemia in dividing colony cells and by producing transplanted myelomonocytic leukemia in normal BALB/c mice by grafting individual agar colonies under the spleen or kidney capsule.

The leukemic colonies had a gross morphology similar to that of normal hematopoietic colonies and their growth rate was modified by colony crowding as is characteristic of normal hematopoietic colonies (Metcalf, 1968). Of more interest was the fact that, unlike the situation with normal hematopoietic colonies, colony formation could occur in the absence of added CSF. However, when CSF was added, more colonies developed and colonies grew at a more rapid rate than in cultures without added CSF (Metcalf *et al.*, 1969). Assays on column-fractionated CSF indicated that the leukemic cells were responding to the same factor (CSF) that was stimulating normal hematopoietic colonies. The experiments provided clear evidence that at least some stem cells in this freely transplantable myelomonocytic leukemia were still responsive to stimulation by the normal regulator, CSF. It was subsequently demonstrated that myelomonocytic leukemic cells are a good source of CSF. This makes it quite likely that most if not all of the colony-forming cells in the myelomonocytic leukemic population were still responsive to regulation by CSF. The intriguing possibility exists that a vicious circle occurs in animals bearing this particular leukemia. Such mice develop high serum CSF levels either in response to the tumor or because the tumor cells produce CSF (Metcalf *et al.*, 1969). This may result in more rapid multiplication of the myelomonocytic leukemic cells, further elevating CSF levels and thus accentuating leukemic cell growth etc. The cells in WEHI-3 leukemic colonies in agar exhibited some degree of differentiation to metamyelocytes and functional macrophages, but most cells showed abnormalities of nuclear or cytoplasmic differentiation. No effect of CSF was observable on this pattern of differentiation.

Tests on cultures of myelomonocytic leukemic cells using dialyzable inhibitors produced either by myelomonocytic leukemic cells or normal bone marrow cells showed that colony formation *in vitro* by the leukemic cells was as susceptible to inhibition as was normal colony formation and no evidence was obtained to support the suggestion that leukemic cells might be characterizable by resistance to such inhibitors.

It was demonstrated that the myelomonocytic leukemic colonies themselves contained colony-forming cells, i.e., that the colony-forming cells were capable of self-generation. Since single colony-forming cells were able to self-replicate as well as to generate both cell types of this leukemia in individual colonies, these colony-forming cells can be regarded as leukemic stem cells. A series of observations was made on the stem cell content of myelomonocytic leukemic tissue in various organs which clearly indicated the importance of the microenvironment in regulating stem cell proliferation (Metcalf and Moore, 1970). It was found that the incidence of stem cells was always higher in splenic deposits of leukemic tissue than in apparently similar leukemic deposits in the peritoneal cavity or the subcutaneous tissues. The basis for this phenomenon was investigated by grafting randomly selected agar colonies of myelomonocytic leukemic cells either to the spleen or under the kidney capsule. Tumor masses having similar cytological composition and growing at similar rates resulted in both locations, but tumor deposits in the spleen contained far higher numbers of stem cells than kidney or subcutaneous tumors. When spleen tumor cells were grown in agar and randomly chosen colonies transplanted to subcutaneous spleen or thymus grafts, again the tumor population in the spleen grafts contained higher numbers of stem cells than comparable populations in thymus grafts which had the low stem cell content characteristic of extrasplenic deposits of this tumor. These experiments made it evident that stem cell self-replication in this leukemic population was not a fixed genetic trait of the stem cells nor were certain leukemic stem cells with high self-replicative capacity selected by the spleen. Rather, the spleen microenvironment was able to modify profoundly the self-replicative capacity of the stem cells in this leukemic population. The experiments therefore provided further evidence of the responsiveness of a leukemic population to growth regulation by normal regulatory factors, in this case microenvironmental factors.

Somewhat similar observations have been made on a transplantable murine granulocytic leukemia by Ichikawa (1969). This leukemia grows in conventional liquid cultures as a uniform population of undifferentiated blast cells and, when grown in agar, forms discrete colonies which can be cloned repeatedly from single colony cells. In the presence of conditioned medium, the colonies in agar developed differentiating populations of granulocytic and macrophage cells. The system used was more complex than the above studies with CSF, since the conditioned medium probably contained other regulators besides CSF. In this context, subsequent work by Ichikawa (1970) demonstrated that a *dialyzable* factor from the conditioned medium was capable of inducing dramatic changes in developing colonies of leukemic cells, transforming many of the myeloblasts to phagocytic macrophages.

In their investigations, Pike and Robinson (1970) adapted the basic agar culture technique to allow the growth of granulocytic or mixed colonies from human bone marrow or peripheral blood cells. Human colonies grew poorly when stimulated by human urine CSF but grew to a large size when incubated over feeder layers of normal peripheral white cells. Normal human blood contained approximately one colony-forming cell per 2×10^6 nucleated blood cells. Suggestive evidence was obtained that the colony-stimulating activity of the peripheral white cells was due to the granulocytic cells. White cells from patients with acute granulocytic leukemia having high numbers of circulating myeloblasts, when cultured over feeder layers of normal white cells, formed up to 700 colonies per 2×10^5 peripheral white cells. Although these colonies have not been shown beyond doubt to be derived from the leukemic blast cells, such an origin seems highly probable. The important aspect of such colonies is that by day 20 of incubation a high proportion of colony cells are well-differentiated metamyelocytes and polymorphs.

It is likely that the action of the normal white cell feeder layers in stimulating colony formation by leukemic cells is highly complex and more than one factor may be released from such feeder layers (probably including CSF and the dialyzable factor of Ichikawa).

These series of observations are exciting in that they suggest it may be possible with the agar culture technique eventually to characterize with some precision the factors regulating the growth and differentiation of leukemic cells of the granulocytic and monocytic series. The preliminary evidence that maturation to nondividing cells can be induced in leukemic blast cells is in urgent need of extension and analysis. One practical problem with this technique is the discrimination of normal from leukemic colonies. In the case of the myelomonocytic leukemic studies, this was achieved by karyotypic analysis and transplantation tests. With human leukemic cells, it should be possible in many cases to use similar karyotypic analysis and this must certainly be done to document any situations in which differentiation is achieved. For more general studies on colony growth characteristics, it may be feasible to use discriminatory stimuli to induce colony formation. For example, in the studies of Ichikawa et al. (1969) a dialyzable stimulus was detected which could stimulate the growth of leukemic cells but not that of normal colony-forming cells and if this type of situation applies more generally to human leukemic cells, parallel cultures can be envisaged, one set designed to culture only leukemic cells, another to culture both normal and leukemic colony-forming cells. One study which obviously needs to be attempted is to characterize the nature of the colonies grown from patients with chronic granulocytic leukemia, for here, the Philadelphia chromosome should provide a workable marker system. At the present time no information exists regarding the comparative growth characteristics in agar of leukemic blast cells from patients in relapse and remission but such studies now seem close to being technically feasible and should provide important information on the puzzling behavior of residual leukemic cells during prolonged periods of remission.

While the agar culture system has proved to be a great technological advance for studying granulocytic and monocytic leukemias, unfortunately no comparable system has yet been devised for analyzing the lymphoid leukemias. Some lymphoid leukemic cell lines have been adapted to grow in liquid cultures, e.g., L1210 cells and some Burkitt lymphoma cell lines, and these will also form colonies in agar, but the problem is that such cultures are not primary cultures taken recently from the animal or patient. It is improbable that analyses of the growth characteristics of such cells will offer much relevant information regarding the status of leukemic lymphoid populations in the patient, since long-term cultured cells have almost certainly undergone significant changes and selection from their original state. The situation is particularly regrettable with chronic lymphoid leukemia, for in this disease the low proliferative capacity of the cells and their abnormally long life span make it highly probable that abnormal responsiveness to regulators or disturbances in regulator levels could well be important facets of the disease process. Short-term cultures of normal peripheral blood lymphocytes can be achieved using phytohemagglutinin and similar agents, but the response of chronic lymphoid leukemic cells to these agents is poor (Astaldi and Airo, 1967) and this approach does not seem to offer an adequate system for comparing growth characteristics.

As was mentioned earlier, lymphoid leukemia development in several mouse systems (e.g., AKR mice or irradiated C57BL mice) is dependent on the presence of the thymus and there is some evidence for the existence of a thymic humoral factor regulating lymphoid cells. Studies have shown that leukemic lymphoid cells in AKR mice grow equally rapidly in thymectomized and sham-operated recipients (Metcalf, 1962b), although the situation is potentially complicated by the fact that leukemic cells contain antigens not represented in the host and the growth of such cells might be partially held in check by immune responses. If such were the case, thymectomy might have two mutually antagonistic effects on leukemic cells: (a) it might allow a greater proliferation of leukemic cells by causing some immunodepression, but (b) it might remove a thymic humoral influence tending to stimulate proliferation of leukemic cells. In contrast, in studies on AKR lymphoid cells during the late preleukemic period, evidence was obtained that transplantation of these cells to young adult thymectomized animals slowed the rate of progression of these cells to the leukemic state and delayed death from lymphoid leukemia in the recipients compared with sham thymectomized recipients (Metcalf, 1962b). However, these latter observations do not necessarily indicate that lymphoid leukemic cells are initially responsive to growth regulation by the thymus, for thymectomy may only have delayed the conversion of preleukemic to leukemic cells. Leukemic populations in the AKR thymus do not exhibit higher mitotic indices or shorter cell cycle times than corresponding populations in the lymph node and spleen. This is in sharp contrast to the situation in normal mice where the mitotic indices and cell cycle times of lymphoid cells within the thymus indicate a much higher average level of proliferative activity than in lymphoid cells in the lymph node or spleen (Nakamura and Metcalf, 1961). These data suggest that lymphoid leukemic cells may no longer be responsive to the stimulating influence of the thymic microenvironment but it may equally well be that the massive leukemic infiltration of the thymus which characterizes the disease in such mice disturbs or destroys the delicate meshwork of epithelial cells responsible for maintaining the thymic microenvironment.

IX. Nature of Remissions in Acute Leukemia

The remissions seen in acute leukemia, particularly in children, are one of the most intriguing, yet puzzling, aspects of leukemia. Unfortunately, comparable remissions do not appear to occur in leukemic animals and no satisfactory model systems exist for a detailed analysis of this phenomenon. Essentially, a complete remission is characterized by the disappearance of leukemic cells from the blood, a return of the bone marrow to the normal pattern, restoration of red cell and platelet levels, and increased resistance to infections. Even complete remissions do not represent a return to complete normality, since in the vast majority of cases, recurrence of the disease occurs. The leukemic cells involved in the relapse often resemble the original leukemic population, making it probable that the original leukemic population was suppressed, rather than eliminated, during remission. One puzzling aspect of remissions is that the duration of a remission can be exceedingly long in relation to the known population doubling times for leukemic cells. This makes untenable the original explanation that remissions simply represent the subtotal destruction of the leukemic population with a lag period before relapse, due to the time required for exponential reexpansion of the leukemic population. Remissions therefore have two facets (a) elimination of virtually all of the existing leukemic population, and (b) suppression for varying periods of regeneration of surviving leukemic cells.

It has been demonstrated both in man and the mouse that some leukemic cells normally can enter a G_0 (nondividing) state (Clarkson, 1969; Mauer et al., 1969; Rosen and Perry, 1970) and it is natural to speculate that remissions may represent an exaggeration of this process. Even if this is so, the problem remains as to what mechanisms are responsible for forcing cycling leukemic cells to enter the null, G_0, state. Obviously if this process is manipulable, such an approach might constitute a highly effective therapeutic measure in leukemia.

At the present time three mechanisms can be considered as being possibly involved in the induction of remissions: (a) an unpredictable effect of some cytotoxic drugs falling short of actual cell destruction, (b) the activation of an immune response, possibly by antigens released from leukemic cells destroyed by chemotherapy, with antibody- or cell-mediated destruction or inhibition of leukemic cells, (c) suppression of leukemic cells by normal regulatory mechanisms. While it is easy to document a return to normality in measurable hematopoietic parameters during remissions, these observations *per se* do not provide any clues as to the mechanisms involved in restoring normal cell proliferative functions. On the analogy with chorionepitheliomas and Burkitt lymphomas, the most reasonable hypothesis is to suggest that somehow normality is restored by the combined action of cell killing with cytotoxic drugs and an immune response which may previously have been present but have been unable to cope with the large numbers of leukemic cells. However, little positive evidence yet exists in human leukemia that specific immune responses occur or are effective in limiting leukemic cell proliferation.

The alternative is to suggest that massive cell destruction either triggers a readjustment of regulators within the body or, as was postulated for immune responses, reduces the size of the abnormal population to one more effectively regulatable by these control mechanisms. Even more likely is the possibility that both immune responses and regulators collaborate to achieve a temporary return to near-normal hematopoiesis.

The antigenic nature of leukemic cells allows responses in regulators to be initiated which may act synergistically with immune responses in controlling leukemic populations. Antigenic stimulation has been observed to elevate serum CSF levels (McNeill, 1970; Metcalf, 1971) and similar responses have been observed in animals grafted with antigenic syngenic tumor cells or allogenic tumor cells (Hibberd and Metcalf, 1971). Elevation of serum CSF levels can be expected to result in an increased production of monocytes and macrophages and increases in the levels of progenitor cells of these two cells have also been observed in leukemic mice. In the presence of specific antibody, the macrophages would be available for cell-mediated attack on leukemic cells. This example of a synergistic regulator-immune response is theoretically operative in any situation in which the leukemic cells are antigenic.

X. General Discussion

The experiments reviewed in the preceding discussion have made it likely that hormones and humoral regulators are involved both in the development and progression of some types of leukemia. However, a complete picture has not yet emerged for any one of these agents and at present this subject very much resembles a partially filled-in jigsaw in which outlines are beginning to emerge but many details are still missing. Some of the missing information which is essential for a proper understanding of the effects of the various regulators on target cell proliferative behavior can be phrased in the following questions. Is the conversion of G_0 to a cycling cell under regulator action? Are cell cycle times shortened by regulators? Does the action of one regulator modify the responsiveness of a target cell to another? In what way does regulator action modify the response of the host cell to infection by a leukemia-inducing virus? What is the exact action of a regulator when it induces differentiation or the expression of differentiation in a cell? Is this action a type of induced "somatic mutation" passed on to the offspring of that cell in the absence of further exposure to the regulator?

Until information on the above questions becomes available, it is possible only to speculate in broadest terms on the reasons why regulators can act as cofactors in leukemogenesis or modify the progression of the disease. Some of the suggestions raised to explain hormone action in tumor development in target tissues seem improbable or not fully adequate when considered in the context of leukemogenesis.

It has been suggested that regulators or hormones act as cocarcinogens by increasing the number of target cells available to the primary inducing agent—which in the case of many leukemias must be presumed to be one of the group of leukemia viruses. Certainly a regulator like erythropoietin increases the number of ESC's being committed to pro-erythroblasts and with the Rauscher virus this increase in susceptible target cells leads to an increase in the number of neoplastic foci initiated by the virus. Conversely, testosterone in inhibiting lymphoid leukemia development in the thymus certainly reduces the total number of target thymic lymphoid cells. However, this simplistic reasoning is unlikely to provide a full explanation for the action of regulators. For example, multiple grafts of up to 50 thymuses have been placed in individual C57BL mice, thereby grossly increasing the number of potential lymphoid target cells for the latent Rad LV virus, without leading to an increase in the incidence of lymphoid leukemia (Metcalf, 1965). Conversely, irradiation induces thymus atrophy which is at least superficially similar to that induced by testosterone or cortisone, yet irradiation increases the incidence of lymphoid leukemia whereas testosterone and cortisone tend to prevent the development of this disease.

An alternative suggestion, related to the concept of total numbers of available target cells, has been that regulators may increase the "mitotic activity" of target cells, thereby rendering them more susceptible to somatic mutations in a situation where some genetic instability has been induced by virus infection or irradiation. In its extreme form, this hypothesis must contain some elements of truth, for if target cell proliferation is completely suppressed by regulator action, the primary characteristic of neoplastic cells (unrestrained proliferation) is unlikely to be expressed and no leukemia would develop. Again however, this is unlikely to be a complete explanation of cocarcinogenesis because, if neoplastic somatic mutations or transformation in a virus-infected target cell population occurred solely at random, a moderate increase in the number of mitotic cells should lead to a proportional increase in the incidence of neoplastic transformations. From the type of observation referred to above, this explanation does not really fit the observed facts. Similarly, hematopoietic regulators are unlikely to force errors in replication by shortening cell cycle times and forcing the cells to "rush" gene replication. This type of explanation may be relevant for carcinogenesis in other tissues with slowly turning over cell populations, but cell cycle times in hematopoietic cells are already minimal (6–12 hours) in the normal animal and do not appear to be shortened significantly by humoral regulators, e.g., erythropoietin or CSF.

What may be a more likely basis for regulator action in leukemogenesis is the apparent capacity of regulators to modify the phenotypic expression of genetic material in the cell—the type of process associated with derepression of specific portions of the genome occurring during the induction and activation of differentiation in hematopoietic cells. It is conceivable that if this type of action occurs in a target cell where the genetic apparatus has been altered or rendered unstable by virus action, derepression may result in the activation of a cell with abnormal properties—specifically with abnormalities in responsiveness to the same regulator. On this basis, infection of a stem cell or progenitor cell by a leukemia virus might modify or damage the cell but these changes would only be recognized as a neoplastic transformation if regulator action subsequently activated these cells by derepressing the faulty part of the genome. This type of action might be particularly relevant where the target cell is usually in a G_0 state, as is the case for most hematopoietic stem cells.

In this view of regulator action in leukemogenesis it is conceived that the primary leukemogenic agent may produce many gene abnormalities, but only those affecting differentiation of progeny to a nondividing state are relevant for leukemogenesis. These genes might initially be under repressor control in a leukemogen-altered cell, the repressor acting as a lid for what is now a Pandora's box. The normal derepressing role of the humoral regulator can then be likened to opening the lid of this Pandora's box, allowing expression of the modified abnormal genes. An hypothesis such as this would explain why initially tumors of endocrine target tissues or hematopoietic cells might exhibit responsiveness to growth control by the appropriate regulator.

A quite different view of regulator action in leukemogenesis is to propose that regulators have nothing whatsoever to do with the initiation of leukemic cells but that they can suppress or promote the emergence of fully transformed leukemic populations simply because the leukemic cells initially still exhibit some vestiges of responsiveness to control by these regulators. Emergence and progressive growth of a leukemic population would then depend either on deficiencies or abnormalities in the level of regulators or on the progressive loss of responsiveness of the leukemic cells to these regulators. This hypothesis would place regulator control mechanisms in the same category as immune responses, namely as components of a safeguard system for eliminating or suppressing abnormal hematopoietic cells. Certainly this type of regulator action must be operating during the course of leukemia development and this hypothesis is probably the most commonly accepted view of the involvement of regulators in carcinogenesis.

However, it may be unwise to regard the role of hematopoietic regulators in leukemia simply as control mechanisms which may sometimes be able to restrict the proliferation of leukemic cells. To do so is to ignore the lessons of endocrine tumorogenesis where it has been shown clearly that prolonged disturbances in regulator levels precede the onset of neoplasia and are intimately involved in the initiation of some target cell neoplasms. Comparable information for hematopoietic regulators is as yet fragmentary, but what evidence exists suggests that a similar situation may well apply in some leukemias, e.g., with CSF in granulocytic leukemia or myelomonocytic leukemia.

Even if human leukemia is viral-induced, experience with animal leukemia viruses suggests that such viruses are probably vertically transmitted and that active immunization procedures in postnatal life cannot materially affect the outcome of such prior virus infections. What is apparent from the example of thymectomy in AKR mice is that modification of target cells and/or regulators subsequent to virus infection can effectively modify the duration of the latent period and the final incidence of leukemia.

Finally, the major reason for resisting at present the concept of leukemia as a neoplastic disease which is initiated independently of regulator action is the possibility that leukemia in animals may not be a valid model for leukemia in humans. For human diseases like acute leukemia or chronic lymphoid leukemia, there is no compelling evidence that leukemic cells are autonomous neoplastic cells and to regard them as such is to approach the analysis of leukemia development wearing mental blinkers. Human leukemic cells may well be abnormal but recent results suggest that some are dependent on and responsive to normal regulators and possibly what appear to be abnormalities intrinsic to the leukemic cells may be externally directed by abnormal regulator action.

The past few years have seen some exciting advances in the knowledge of specific humoral regulators of hematopoietic cells. Techniques are now available which allow a study of some human hematopoietic cells and regulators *in vitro* and, with the exception of certain specific types of murine leukemia, there now seems more virtue in making a direct analysis of these human leukemias rather than continuing to use the highly artificial model systems in mice. The agar culture system provides an effective method for analyzing granulocytes and monocytes and recent developments in agar and fibrin gel culture of erythropoietic cells seem likely to allow similar studies on cells of the erythroid series. Because of the small numbers of leukemic patients available for extensive study by any one group and the variability of leukemia, what is now needed is the exploitation of the present techniques by a much larger number of groups to establish the basic abnormalities in regulator levels and responsiveness of leukemic cells in preleukemic and leukemic patients.

References

Adamson, J. W., and Finch, C. A. (1968). *Ann. N. Y. Acad. Sci.* **149**, 560–563.

Alpen, E. L., and Cranmore, D. (1959). *In* "Kinetics of Cellular Proliferation" (F. Stohlman, ed.), pp. 290–300. Grune & Stratton, New York.

Alpen, E. L., Cranmore, D., and Johnston, M. E. (1962). *In* "Erythropoiesis" (L. O. Jacobson and M. Doyle, eds.), pp. 184–188. Grune & Stratton, New York.

Arnesen, K. (1958). *Acta Pathol. Microbiol. Scand.* **43**, 339–349.

Astaldi, G., and Airo, R. (1967). *In* "The Lymphocyte in Immunology and Haemopoiesis" (J. .M. Yoffey, ed.), pp. 73–80. Arnold, London.

Astaldi, G., and Mauri, C. (1953). *Rev. Belge Pathol. Med. Exp.* **23**, 69–82.

Astaldi, G., Costa, G., and Airo, R. (1965). *Lancet* **1**, 1394–1396.

Berenblum, I., Cividalli, G., Trainin, N., and Hodes, M. E. (1965). *Blood* **26**, 8–19.

Berenblum, I., Burger, M., and Knyszynski, A. (1968). *Nature (London)* **217**, 857–859.

Bernard, J., Bilski-Pasquier, G., and Deltour, G. (1954). *Bull. Soc. Med. Hop. (Paris)* **70**, 579–589.

Biskind, M. S., and Biskind, G. R. (1944). *Proc. Soc. Exp. Biol. Med.* **55**, 176–179.

Bradley, T. R., and Metcalf, D. (1966). *Aust. J. Exp. Biol. Med. Sci.* **44**, 287–300.

Bradley, T. R., and Metcalf, D. (1967). Unpublished data.

Bradley, T. R., and Sumner, M. A. (1968). *Aust. J. Exp. Biol. Med. Sci.* **46**, 607–618.

Bradley, T. R., Metcalf, D., Sumner, M., and Stanley, R. (1969). *In Vitro* **4**, 22–35.

Brand, K. G., Buoen, L. C., and Brand. I. (1967). *J. Nat. Cancer Inst.* **39**, 663–679.

Bullough, W. S. (1962). *Biol. Rev.* **37**, 307–342.

Bullough, W. S. (1965). *Cancer Res.* **25**, 1683–1727.

Bullough, W. S. (1967). "The Evolution of Differentiation." Academic Press, New York.

Camblin, J. G., and Bridges, J. B. (1964). *Transplantation* 2, 785–787.

Chan, S. H. (1970). *Proc. Soc. Exp. Biol. Med.* 134, 733–737.

Chan, S. H. (1971). Unpublished data.

Chan, S. H., and Metcalf, D. (1970). *Nature (London)* 227, 845–846.

Chan, S. H., Metcalf, D., and Stanley, E. R. (1971). *Brit. J. Haematol.* 20, 329–341.

Claman, H. N., Chaperon, E. A., and Triplett, R. F. (1966). *Proc. Soc. Exp. Biol. Med.* 122, 1167–1171.

Clark, S. L. (1966). *Thymus: Exp. Clin. Stud., Ciba Found. Symp., 1965* pp. 3–30.

Clarkson, B. D. (1969). *Nat. Cancer Inst. Monogr.* 30, 81–119.

Cohen, P., Cooley, M. H., and Gardner, F. H. (1965). *J. Clin. Invest.* 44, 1036–1037.

Contrera, J. F., and Gordon, A. S. (1968). *Ann. N. Y. Acad. Sci.* 149, 114–119.

Cotes, P. M., and Bangham, D. R. (1961). *Nature (London)* 191, 1065.

Davies, A. J. S., Leuchars, E., Wallis, V., and Koller, P. C. (1966). *Transplantation* 4, 438–451.

Davies, A. J. S., Leuchars, E., Wallis, V., Marchant, R., and Elliott, E. V. (1967). *Transplantation* 5, 222–231.

De Gowin, R. L., and Gurney, C. W. (1964). *Arch. Intern. Med.* 114, 424–433.

De Nicola, P., and Gibelli, O. (1963). *Hemostase* 3, 47–57.

De Nicola, P., Soardi, F., and Cappelletti, G. A. (1958). *Haematologica* 43, 779–796.

De Somer, P., Denys, P. J., and Leyten, R. (1963). *Life Sci.* 2, 810–819.

Dougherty, T. F., Berliner, M. L., Schneebeli, G. L., and Berliner, D. L. (1964). *Ann. N. Y. Acad. Sci.* 113, 825–843.

Dunn, T. B., Moloney, J. B., Green, A. W., and Arnold, B. (1961). *J. Nat. Cancer Inst.* 26, 189–221.

Ebbe, S., Stohlman, F., Overcash, J., Donovan, J., and Howard, D. (1968). *Blood* 32, 383–392.

Erslev, A. J., and Thorling, E. B. (1968). *Ann. N. Y. Acad. Sci.* 149, 173–178.

Evatt, B. L., and Levin, J. (1969). *J. Clin. Invest.* 48, 1615–1626.

Fessas, P., Wintrobe, M. M., Thompson, R. B., and Cartwright, G. E. (1954). *Arch. Intern. Med.* 94, 384–401.

Foster, R. S., and Mirand, E. A. (1970). *Proc. Soc. Exp. Biol. Med.* 133, 1223–1227.

Foster, R. S., Metcalf, D., Robinson, W. A., and Bradley, T. R. (1968a). *Brit. J. Haematol.* 15, 147–159.

Foster, R. S., Metcalf, D., and Kirchmyer, R. (1968b). *J. Exp. Med.* 127, 853–866.

Foster, R. S., Cortner, J., and Metcalf, D. (1971). *Cancer* (in press).

Fried, W., and Gurney, C. W. (1968). *Ann. N. Y. Acad. Sci.* 149, 356–365.

Fried, W., Plzak, L. F., Jacobson, L. O., and Goldwasser, E. (1957). *Proc. Soc. Exp. Biol. Med.* 94, 237–241.

Friend, C. (1957). *J. Exp. Med.* 105, 307–318.

Furth, J. (1954). *Leuk. Res. Ciba Found. Symp., 1953* pp. 38–41.

Furth, J. (1969). *Harvey Lect.* 63, 47–71.

Furth, J., and Boon, M. C. (1945). *A.A.A.S. Res. Conf. Cancer, 1944* pp. 129–138.

Furth, J., and Clifton, K. (1957). *Cancer* 10, 842–853.

Gadsden, E. L., and Furth, J. (1953). *Proc. Soc. Exp. Biol. Med.* 83, 511–514.

Gardner, W. U., Dougherty, T. F., Williams, W. L. (1944). *Cancer Res.* 4, 73–87.

Gavosto, F., Pileri, A., Bachi, C., and Pegoraro, L. (1964). *Nature (London)* 203, 92–94.

Goldstein A. L., Slater, F. D., and White, A. (1966). *Proc. Nat. Acad. Sci. U. S.* **56**, 1010–1017.

Goldwasser, E., and Kung, C. K. H. (1968). *Ann. N. Y. Acad. Sci.* **149**, 49–53.

Good, R. A., Dalmasso, A. P., Martinez, C., Archer, O. K., Pierce, J. C., and Papermaster, B. W. (1962). *J. Exp. Med.* **116**, 773–795.

Gordon, A. S., Mirand, E. A., Wenig, J., Katz, R., and Zanjani, E. D. (1968). *Ann. N. Y. Acad. Sci.* **149**, 318–335.

Gross, L. (1951). *Proc. Soc. Exp. Biol. Med.* **76**, 27–32.

Gross, L. (1959). *Proc. Soc. Exp. Biol. Med.* **100**, 325–328.

Gross, L. (1963). *Acta Haematol.* **29**, 1–15.

Gross, M., and Goldwasser, E. (1969). *Biochemistry* **8**, 1795–1805.

Hanna, M. G., Nettesheim, P., Fisher, W. D., Peters, L. C., and Francis, M. W. (1967). *Science* **157**, 1458–1461.

Haran-Ghera, N. (1967). *Brit. J. Cancer* **21**, 739–749.

Hardy, M. A., Quint, J., Goldstein, A. L., State, D., and White, A. (1968). *Proc. Nat. Acad. Sci. U. S.* **4**, 875–882.

Harker, L. A. (1968). *J. Clin. Invest.* **47**, 458–465.

Hibberd, A. D. (1970). Unpublished data.

Hibberd, A. D., and Metcalf, D. (1971). *Isr. J. Med. Sci.* **7**, 202–210.

Hodes, M. E., Clewell, D. B., Hubbard, J. D., and Yu, P-L. (1966). *Cancer Res.* **26**, 1780–1786.

Hodgson, G., Perreta, A., Yudilevich, D., and Eskuche, I. (1958). *Proc. Soc. Exp. Biol. Med.* **99**, 137–142.

Ichikawa, Y. (1969). *J. Cell. Physiol.* **73**, 43–48.

Ichikawa, Y. (1970). *J. Cell. Physiol.* **76**, 175–184.

Ichikawa, Y., Pluznik, D. H., and Sachs, L. (1966). *Proc. Nat. Acad. Sci. U. S.* **56**, 488–495.

Ichikawa, Y., Pluznik, D. H., and Sachs, L. (1967). *Proc. Nat. Acad. Sci. U. S.* **58**, 1480–1486.

Ichikawa, Y., Paran, M., and Sachs, L. (1969). *J. Cell. Physiol.* **73**, 43–48.

Ilbery, P. L. T., Moore, P. A., Winn, S. M., and Ford, C. E. (1963). *In* "Cellular Basis and Aetiology of Late Somatic Effects of Ionizing Radiation" (R. J. C. Harris, ed.), pp. 83–92. Academic Press, New York.

Iscove, N. N., Till, J. E., and McCulloch, E. A. (1970). *Proc. Soc. Exp. Biol. Med.* **134**, 33–36.

Jacobson, L. O., Goldwasser, E., Fried, W., and Plzak, L. F. (1957). *Nature (London)* **179**, 633–634.

Jacobson, L. O., Goldwasser, E., and Gurney, C. W. (1961). *Haemopoiesis: Cell Prod. Regul., Ciba Found. Symp., 1960* pp. 423–445.

Jankovic, B. D., Waksman, B. H., and Arnason, B. G. (1962). *J. Exp. Med.* **116**, 159–175.

Jenkins, V. K., Odell, T. T., and Upton, A. C. (1966). *Cancer Res.* **26**, 454–458.

Joneja, M. G., and Stich, H. F. (1963). *Exp. Cell Res.* **31**, 220–223.

Kaplan, H. S. (1967). *Cancer Res.* **27**, 1325–1340.

Kaplan, H. S., and Brown, M. B. (1952). *Science* **116**, 195–196.

Kaplan, H. S., Marder, S. N., and Brown, M. B. (1951). *Cancer Res.* **11**, 629–633.

Kaplan, H. S., Brown, M. B., and Paull, J. (1953). *J. Nat. Cancer Inst.* **14**, 303–316.

Kaplan, H. S., Nagareda, C. S., and Brown, M. B. (1954). *Recent Progr. Horm. Res.* **10**, 293–333.

Kaplan, H. S., Carnes, W. H., Brown, M. B., and Hirsch, B. B. (1956). *Cancer Res.* **16**, 422–425.

Kelemen, E., Cserhati, I., and Tanos, B. (1958). *Acta Haematol.* **20**, 350–355.

Kirschbaum, A., Shapiro, J. R., and Mixer, H. W. (1953). *Cancer Res.* **13**, 262–268.

Klein, J. J., Goldstein, A. L., and White, A. (1965). *Proc. Nat. Acad. Sci. U. S.* **53**, 812–817.

Krantz, S. B. (1968). *Ann. N. Y. Acad. Sci.* **149**, 430–436.

Krizsa, G., Gergely, G., and Rak, K. (1968). *Acta Haematol.* **39**, 112–117.

Krzymowski, T., and Krzymowska, H. (1962). *Blood* **19**, 38–44.

Kuratowska, Z., Lewartowski, B., and Lipinski, B. (1964). *J. Lab. Clin. Med.* **64**, 226–237.

Lacassagne, A. (1937). *C. R. Soc. Biol.* **126**, 193–195.

Lajtha, L. G., Pozzi, L. V., Schofield, R., and Fox, M. (1969). *Cell Tissue Kinet.* **2**, 39–49.

Lambardini, J., Sanchez-Medal, L., Arriaga, L., Lopez, D., and Smyth, J. F. (1968). *J. Lab. Clin. Med.* **72**, 419–428.

Law, L. W. (1947). *J. Nat. Cancer Inst.* **8**, 157–159.

Law, L. W. (1952). *J. Nat. Cancer Inst.* **12**, 789–805.

Law, L. W. (1957). *Ann. N. Y. Acad. Sci.* **68**, 616–635.

Law, L. W., Trainin, N., Levey, R. H., and Barth, W. F. (1964a). *Science* **143**, 1049–1051.

Law, L. W., Dunn, T. B., Trainin, N., and Levey, R. H. (1964b). *In* "The Thymus" (V. Defendi and D. Metcalf, eds.), pp. 105–119. Wistar Inst. Press, Philadelphia, Pennsylvania.

Law, L. W., Goldstein, A. L., and White, A. (1968). *Nature (London)* **219**, 1391–1392.

Linman, J. W., and Pierre, R. V. (1962). *Proc. Soc. Exp. Biol. Med.* **110**, 463–466.

Lowy, P. H., Keighley, G., and Borsook, H. (1960). *Nature (London)* **185**, 102–103.

McEndy, D. P., Boon, M. C., and Furth, J. (1944). *Cancer Res.* **4**, 377–383.

McIntyre, K. R., and Princler, G. L. (1969). *Immunology* **17**, 481–487.

McNeill, T. A. (1970). *Immunology* **18**, 61–72.

Mauer, M. M., Saunders, E. F., and Lampkin, B. C. (1969). *Nat. Cancer Inst., Monogr.* **30**, 63–79.

Medical Research Council (1956). "The Hazards to Man of Nuclear and Allied Radiations." H. M. Stationery Office, London.

Metcalf, D. (1956a). *Brit. J. Cancer* **10**, 169–178.

Metcalf, D. (1956b). *Brit. J. Cancer* **10**, 431–441.

Metcalf, D. (1956c). *Brit. J. Cancer* **10**, 442–457.

Metcalf, D. (1959a). *Proc. Can. Cancer Res. Conf.* **3**, 351–366.

Metcalf, D. (1959b). *Radiat. Res.* **10**, 313–322.

Metcalf, D. (1961). *Brit. J. Cancer* **15**, 769–779.

Metcalf, D. (1962a). Leukaemogenesis in AKR mice. *Tumour Viruses Murine Origin, Ciba Found. Symp., 1961* pp. 233–253.

Metcalf, D. (1962b). *Nature (London)* **195**, 88–89.

Metcalf, D. (1963). *Aust. J. Exp. Biol. Med. Sci.* **41**, 437–448.

Metcalf, D. (1964). *Cancer Res.* **24**, 1952–1957.

Metcalf, D. (1965). Unpublished data.

Metcalf, D. (1966a). "The Thymus." Springer, Berlin.

Metcalf, D. (1966b). *J. Nat. Cancer Inst.* **37**, 425–442.

Metcalf, D. (1968). *J. Cell. Physiol.* **72**, 9–20.

Metcalf, D. (1969a). *Brit. J. Haematol.* **16**, 397–407.

Metcalf, D. (1969b). *J. Cell. Physiol.* **74**, 323–332.

Metcalf, D. (1969c). *Proc. Soc. Exp. Biol. Med.* **132**, 391–394.

Metcalf, D. (1970). *J. Cell. Physiol.* **76**, 89–100.

Metcalf, D. (1971). *Immunology* (in press).

Metcalf, D., and Bradley, T. R. (1970). *In* "Regulation of Hematopoiesis" (A. S. Gordon, ed.), pp. 187–215. Appleton, New York.

Metcalf, D., and Brumby, M. (1967). *Int. J. Cancer* **2**, 37–42.

Metcalf, D., and Foster, R. (1967). *J. Nat. Cancer Inst.* **39**, 1235–1245.

Metcalf, D., and Moore, M. A. S. (1970). *J. Nat. Cancer Inst.* **44**, 801–808.

Metcalf, D., and Moore, M. A. S. (1971). "Haemopoietic Cells." North-Holland Publ., Amsterdam (in press).

Metcalf, D., and Stanley, E. R. (1969). *Aust. J. Exp. Biol. Med. Sci.* **47**, 453–466.

Metcalf, D., and Stanley, E. R. (1971). *Brit. J. Haematol.* **20**, 547–554.

Metcalf, D., and Wahren, B. (1968). *Brit. Med. J.* **3**, 99–101.

Metcalf, D., and Wakonig-Vaartaja, R. (1964). *Proc. Soc. Exp. Biol. Med.* **115**, 731–735.

Metcalf, D., and Wiadrowski, M. (1966). *Cancer Res.* **26**, 483–491.

Metcalf, D., Furth, J., and Buffett, R. F. (1959). *Cancer Res.* **19**, 52–58.

Metcalf, D., Wiadrowski, M., and Bradley, R. (1966). *Nat. Cancer Inst. Mongr.* **22**, 571–583.

Metcalf, D., Bradley, T. R., and Robinson, W. (1967a). *J. Cell. Physiol.* **69**, 93–108.

Metcalf, D., Foster, R., and Pollard, M. (1967b). *J. Cell. Physiol.* **70**, 131–132.

Metcalf, D., Moore, M. A. S., and Warner, N. L. (1969). *J. Nat. Cancer Inst.* **43**, 983–1001.

Metcalf, D., Chan, S. H., Gunz, F. W., Vincent, P., and Ravich, R. B. A. (1971). *Blood* (in press).

Miller, J. F. A. P. (1959). *Nature (London)* **183**, 1069.

Miller, J. F. A. P. (1962). *Proc. Roy. Soc. Ser. B* **156**, 415–428.

Miller, J. F. A. P., and Mitchell, G. F. (1969). *Transplant. Rev.* **1**, 3–42.

Mirand, E. A. (1968a). *Ann. N. Y. Acad. Sci.* **149**, 94–106.

Mirand, E. A. (1968b). *Ann. N. Y. Acad. Sci.* **149**, 486–496.

Mirand, E. A., and Prentice, T. C. (1957). *Proc. Soc. Exp. Biol. Med.* **96**, 49–51.

Mirand, E. A., Steeves, R. A., Lange, R. D., and Grace, J. T. (1968). *Proc. Soc. Exp. Biol. Med.* **128**, 844–849.

Moon, H. D., Simpson, M. E., Li, C. H., and Evans, H. M. (1950). *Cancer Res.* **10**, 297–308.

Naets, J. P., and Wittek, M. (1968). *Ann. N. Y. Acad. Sci.* **149**, 366–376.

Nakahara, W., and Fukuoka, F. (1958). *Advan. Cancer Res.* **5**, 157–177.

Nakamura, K., and Metcalf, D. (1961). *Brit. J. Cancer* **15**, 306–315.

Nossal, G. J. V., Cunningham, A., Mitchell, G. F., and Miller, J. F. A. P. (1968). *J. Exp. Med.* **128**, 839–853.

Noyes, W. D., Domm, B. M., and Willis, L. C. (1962). *Blood* **20**, 9–18.

Odell, T. T., McDonald, T. P., and Asano, M. (1962). *Acta Haematol.* **27**, 171–179.

Osoba, D., and Miller, J. F. A. P. (1964). *J. Exp. Med.* **119**, 177–194.

Osserman, E. F. (1967). *In* "Gamma Globulins" (J. Killander, ed.), pp. 573–581. Almqvist & Wiksell, Uppsala.

Paran, M., Ichikawa, Y., and Sachs, L. (1968). *J. Cell. Physiol.* **72**, 251–254.

Paran, M., Ichikawa, Y., and Sachs, L. (1969). *Proc. Nat. Acad. Sci. U. S.* **62**, 81–87.

Pavlov, A. D. (1969). *Biochim. Biophys. Acta* **195**, 156–164.

Pike, B. L., and Robinson, W. A. (1970). *J. Cell. Physiol.* **76**, 77–84.

Pluznik, D. H. (1969). *Isr. J. Med. Sci.* **5**, 306–312.

Pluznik, D. H., and Sachs, L. (1966). *Exp. Cell Res.* **43**, 553–563.

Pluznik, D. H., Sachs, L., and Resnitzky, P. (1966). *Nat. Cancer Inst. Monogr.* **22**, 3–12.

Potter, M., and Boyce, C. R. (1962). *Nature (London)* **193**, 1086–1087.

Rak, K., Cserhati, I., and Kelemen, E. (1960). *Magy. Belorv. Arch.* **13**, 22–27.

Rauscher, F. J. (1962). *J. Nat. Cancer Inst.* **29**, 515–543.

Reynafarje, C., Ranos, J., Faura, J., and Villavicencio, D. (1964). *Proc. Soc. Exp. Biol. Med.* **116**, 649–650.

Rickard, K. A., Shadduck, R. K., Howard, D. E., and Stohlman, F. (1970). *Proc. Soc. Exp. Biol. Med.* **134**, 152–156.

Robinson, W., Metcalf, D., and Bradley, T. R. (1967). *J. Cell. Physiol.* **69**, 83–92.

Robinson, W. A., Kurnick, J. E., and Pike, B. L. (1971). *Blood* (in press).

Rosen, P. J., and Perry, S. (1970). *Proc. Amer. Ass. Cancer Res.* **11**, 68 (abstr).

Ross, M. A., and Korenchevsky, V. (1941). *J. Pathol. Bacteriol.* **52**, 349–360.

Rytomaa, T. (1969). Hemic. cells. *In Vitro* **4**, 47–58.

Rytomaa, T., and Kiviniemi, K. (1968). *Eur. J. Cancer* **4**, 595–606.

Sachs, L. (1968). *Proc. Can. Cancer Res. Conf.* **8**, 146–161.

Small, M., and Trainin, N. (1967). *Nature (London)* **216**, 377–379.

Stanley, E. R., and Metcalf, D. (1969). *Aust. J. Exp. Biol. Med. Sci.* **47**, 467–483.

Stanley, E. R., and Metcalf, D. (1971). *Proc. Soc. Exp. Biol. Med.* (in press).

Stanley, E. R., Robinson, W. A., and Ada, G. L. (1968). *Aust. J. Exp. Biol. Med. Sci.* **46**, 715–726.

Stanley, E. R., McNeill, T. A., and Chan, S. H. (1970). *Brit. J. Haematol.* **18**, 585–590.

Steeves, R. A., Bennett, M., Mirand, E. A., and Cudkowicz, G. (1968). *Nature (London)* **218**, 372–374.

Stohlman, F., Ebbe, S., Morse, B., Howard, D., and Donovan, J. (1968). *Ann. N. Y. Acad. Sci.* **149**, 156–172.

Stutman, O., Yunis, E. J., and Good, R. A. (1968). *J. Nat. Cancer Inst.* **41**, 1431–1452.

Stutman, O., Yunis, E. J., and Good, R. A. (1969). *J. Exp. Med.* **130**, 809–820.

Takakura, K., Yamada, H. Weber, A. H., and Hollander, V. P. (1967). *Cancer Res.* **27**, 932–937.

Trainin, N., and Linker-Israeli, M. (1967). *Cancer Res.* **27**, 309–313.

Trainin, N., Bejerano, A., Strahilevitch, M., Goldring, D., and Small, M. (1966). *Isr. J. Med. Sci.* **2**, 549–559.

Trainin, N., Small, M., and Globerson, A. (1969). *J. Exp. Med.* **130**, 765–775.

Upton, A. C., and Furth, J. (1954). *Blood* **9**, 686–695.

Upton, A. C., Jenkins, V. K., Walburg, H. I., Tyndall, R. L., Conklin, J. W., and Wald, N. (1966). *Nat. Cancer Inst. Monogr.* **22**, 329–347.

Wahren, B., Lantorp, K., Sterner, G., and Espmark, A. (1970). *Proc. Soc. Exp. Biol. Med.* **133**, 934–939.

Warner, N. L. (1970). *Abst. Int. Cancer Congr. 10th, 1970* p. 237.

Warner, N. L., Moore, M. A. S., and Metcalf, D. (1969). *J. Nat. Cancer Inst.* **43**, 963–982.

Weissman, I. L. (1967). *J. Exp. Med.* **126**, 291–304.

Whitcomb, W. H., and Moore, M. (1968). *Ann. N. Y. Acad. Sci.* 149, 462–471.
Winkert, J. W., and Gordon, A. S. (1960). *Biochim. Biophys. Acta* 42, 170–171.
Yamamoto, S. (1957). *Acta Haematol. Jap.* 20, 163–182.
Yip, L. C., and Hodes, M. E. (1970). *Proc. Soc. Exp. Biol. Med.* 133, 1285–1288.

COMPLEMENT AND TUMOR IMMUNOLOGY

Kusuya Nishioka

Virology Division, National Cancer Center Research Institute, Tokyo, Japan

I. Introduction

Classical immunological concepts and methods which have been established and conducted by immunologists can now merge with new analytical methods based on molecular reactions. This has resulted in a renascence of immunology; and the precision and sensitivity of antigen-antibody reactions as analytical tools are recognized generally by researchers in the field of biological, physical, and behavioral sciences. Tumor immunology could not stay out of the influence of this renascence.

Information and fundamental knowledge on the nature of neoplasia have been accumulated in various aspects based on these newly developed immunological tools. It is necessary to arrange and classify the problems before getting into detailed discussion.

What is the definition of tumor immunology? From the standpoint of basic principles of immunology, it would be defined as the recognition of the tumor as an antigen by an autochthonous or syngenic host, resulting in production of specific antibody. Although the final purpose of immunotherapy is to suppress the growth of neoplastic cells, the above process in the host does not always induce heightened resistance against tumor cells. On the contrary, a variety of phenomena induced by the antigen-antibody reaction in the host may often result in manifestation of pathological allergic symptoms as observed in hypersensitivity phenomena in infectious diseases. In some other cases which occur more frequently, if the pathological manifestations by themselves are strong compared with the rather weak immunological reaction of the tumor cells by the host, neither heightened resistance nor an allergic phenomenon is observed. Therefore, when the immunological reaction of the host is focused upon, three main projects should be considered: (a) Recognition of tumor cells as antigen. (b) Mechanism of host defense induced by immunological recognition, such as destruction of tumor cells or antigen uptake by macrophages. (c) Mechanism of the immunopathological reaction induced by the antigen-antibody reaction *in vivo*.

For the purpose of investigating host-tumor cell relationships from these standpoints, the characterization of the tumor cell *per se* is required as an essential prerequisite. This will also serve to help understand the mechanism of carcinogenesis, to discover chemotherapeutic agents or to give a specific diagnosis. For these purposes, immunological methods would provide potential tools as they did for infectious diseases because of their methodological uniqueness and superiority in specificity and sensitivity. To analyze tumor immunology employing the complement system, as assigned to the author of this article, it will be proper to describe (a) immunological cell markers which characterize the cells by various complement methods, (b) the principle and mechanism of each immunological reaction employed, and (c) their biological implications.

Complement research began after the first demonstration by Nuttall (1888) that the bactericidal power of immune serum was dependent on a heat-labile component in the serum. Complement had emerged as a complex system comprising four factors which act sequentially; C1, C4, C2, and C3 (Ferrata, 1907; Ritz, 1912; Coca, 1914; Gordon *et al.*, 1926; Ueno, 1938). A comprehensive outline of the experimental method and of theoretical analysis at the molecular level was given by Mayer (1961b) based on studies on the immune hemolysis of sheep erythrocytes by rabbit antibody and guinea pig complement. Starting from this background, six new components were discovered and by now nine distinct proteins and four inhibitors are recognized in the complement system (Nishioka and

Linscott, 1963; Linscott and Nishioka, 1963; K. Inoue and Nelson, 1965, 1966; Tamura and Nelson, 1967; R. A. Nelson and Biro, 1968; Okada *et al.*, 1970a). They are designated as C1, C4, C2, C3, C5, C6, C7, C8, and C9 in their sequence of reaction (World Health Organization Immunology Unit, 1968) and some of the properties of guinea pig complement proteins are listed in Table I.

In 1961, it was first demonstrated that only the first four complement components were necessary for immune adherence (Nishioka and Linscott, 1963) and for immune phagocytosis (R. A. Nelson, 1962). During the past decade, extensive studies were carried out by many investigators in different laboratories on the isolation, purification, reaction mechanism, and submolecular fragmentation of each complement component and of intermediate antigen-antibody complement complexes. Consequently, it becomes clear that complement is not merely a reaction system which kills bacterial and animal cells but an immunopathological mediator or effector system in immunity and allergy (Mayer, 1970). Reviews of general interest in complement have been published by Osler (1961), Mayer (1961b, 1970), R. A. Nelson (1965), Müller-Eberhard (1968a, 1969), and Rapp and Borsos (1966a). Methods for the preparation of

TABLE I

PROPERTIES OF GUINEA PIG COMPLEMENT COMPONENTS

	Sedimentation constant[a]	Molecular weight[b]	Electrophoretic mobility[c]	Isoelectric point[d]	Eluted at ionic strength (μ) from	
					DEAE-cellulose at pH 7.5	CM-cellulose at pH 5.0
C1	19	1,000,000	0.95	5.3	—	—
			0.34	6.0	—	—
			0.08			
C4	7.7	220,000	0.34	5.9	0.14	0.13
C2	5.7	210,000	0.49	5.33	0.025	0.085
C3	8.2	180,000	0.19	6.25	0.07	0.14
C5	7.6	210,000	0.40	5.10	0.12	0.15
C6	5.7	140,000	0.17	6.63	0.02	0.14
C7	5.0	120,000	0.27	5.78	0.06	0.12
C8	7.8	190,000	0.31	6.34	0.03	0.20
C9	4.5	60,000	0.57	5.18	0.09	0.25

[a] Determined by R. Fugman (personal communication).

[b] Calculated by M. Mayumi (personal communication).

[c] Nishioka (1966), Tachibana (1967), Okada *et al.* (1970c). Relative value taking amido black 10B as reference dye. 1.0.

[d] Mukojima (1970).

reagents and separation of component from guinea pig serum were given by R. A. Nelson *et al.* (1966) and from human serum by Vroom *et al.* (1970). Those interested in purified human complement components and their mode of action also should refer to the review of Müller-Eberhard (1968a, 1969).

In this way, as Mayer described in 1961 (1961b), the essential concepts and experimental approaches which have been developed on model systems of immune hemolysis have been amenable to general application and have served as a guide to the study of the various immunological phenomena involving complement. Tumor immunology is not an exceptional part of immunology and possible application of complement research to tumor immunology has been discussed in reviews by R. A. Nelson (1968), and Müller-Eberhard (1968b). In this article, the author will attempt a brief review of theoretical considerations and practical applications of complement research to tumor immunology in each of five projects: (a) the immunological cell receptors, (b) immune adherence, (c) C1 fixation and transfer test, (d) complement fixation test, (f) immune cytotoxicity test.

II. Cell Receptors—New Immunological Cell Markers

The presence of several different receptors on a variety of cells to which antigen (Ag)-antibody (Ab) or antigen-antibody complement (C) complex adhere has been described. A possible role of these receptors participating in immunological reactions, such as immune phagocytosis (Taniguchi *et al.*, 1930; R. A. Nelson, 1953, 1962, 1965; Nishioka, 1965; Lay and Nussenzweig, 1968, 1969; Henson, 1969) or hypersensitivity reaction (Siqueira and Nelson, 1961; D. S. Nelson and Boyden, 1967; Henson and Cochrane, 1969) has been postulated. Because of their characteristic distribution, these receptors have been used as immunological cell markers for cytological classification of cell types for which classification was difficult by other cytological methods (Huber *et al.*, 1969; Nishioka *et al.*, 1971b). Adherence of sensitized sheep erythrocytes to the cells infected with herpes simplex virus was also reported (Watkins, 1964a). The last phenomenon has been considered a result of sensitized sheep erythrocytes and the altered state of the cell membrane which occurs in the early stages of herpes virus infection. Except for the first one, the IA receptor, complement does not participate actually in the reaction but to give a comparative classification of these receptors, the characters of the other receptors will be summarized in this chapter.

A. Receptor for Antigen-Antibody Complement Complex

Since the first description of immune adherence (R. A. Nelson, 1953), the specific receptor site present on primate erythrocytes or nonprimate platelets was described and has been known as immune adherence (IA) receptor which combined with Ag-Ab-C complex. On the other hand, evidence for the lack of immune adherence reactivity of nonprimate erythrocytes and primate platelets have accumulated (see review by D. S. Nelson, 1963). Megakaryocytes of mice or guinea pigs or spindle-shaped cells (thrombocytes) of fowls and other animals not possessing true blood platelets were shown to be reactive (Kritschewsky and Tscherikower, 1925; Grünbaum, 1928).

The nature of immune adherence of polymorphonuclear or mono-nuclear leukocytes has long been unclear (D. S. Nelson, 1963). Since then the necessity of the first four components of complement for immune adherence (Nishioka and Linscott, 1963) as well as for immune phagocytosis (Gigli and Nelson, 1968) was shown and the presence of IA receptor was also demonstrated on both primate and nonprimate leukocytes (van Loghem and van der Hart, 1962). Recently, for the reaction of phagocytic cells with antigen-antibody complement complex, the term of opsonic adherence was proposed by Coombs and Franks (1969) claiming that it is distinct from immune adherence of human erythrocytes and antigen-antibody C1423 complex. Although as pointed out by them, the physicochemical characterization of the receptor on human erythrocytes and on phagocytic cells needs to be carefully studied as do the respective receptors on fixed C3, it is not proper at this moment to conclude that the reaction of human erythrocytes differs from that of phagocytic cells simply because the reaction of antigen-antibody complement complex to human erythrocyte is temperature-dependent and that to phagocytic cells is not. Actually, when rat complement was employed, the immune adherence of human erythrocytes gave highest reactivity at 20°C. and could hardly be recognized at 37°C. (Sakamoto et al., 1967). Temperature requirements for the immune adherence reaction are also quite different according to whether the antibody is IgG or IgM. Some typical experiments are shown in Figs. 1 and 2 (Okuda et al., 1971). Employing the optimal concentrations of both rabbit IgG and IgM antibody against sheep erythrocytes, the reactivity of rat and guinea pig complement was measured at 4°C., 20°C., 30°C., and 37°C. The reactivity of complement was expressed as the final dilution of fresh serum to give a 2+ immune adherence pattern with human erythrocytes. It is clear that when only IgM antibody was used, the guinea pig complement showed the maximum reactivity at 37°C.; thus the reaction is typically temperature-dependent. Except for this case, 37°C. is most unfavorable for obtaining high reactivity of immune adherence pattern in all other cases. A C3 inactivator and other inhibitors might participate in this reaction but these results are quite contradictory to Coombs definition, and I will use the term immune adherence for both reactions to avoid confusion in terminology

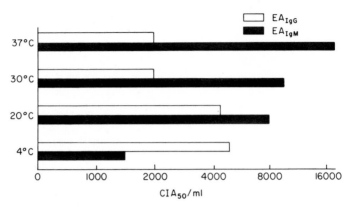

FIG. 1. Comparison of guinea pig complement reactivity in immune adherence hemagglutination with sheep erythrocytes sensitized with IgG or IgM rabbit antibody at different temperatures.

until the essential difference is known. A distinction of the IA receptor from the IgG receptor which reacts with IgG in the absence of complement was made (Huber *et al.*, 1968). Since then, IgM antibody was employed to make Ag Ab C complex as an indicator cell to detect IA receptor.

Interspecies comparative studies (Henson, 1969) have been made, and the presence of IA receptor on macrophages, blood monocytes, and polymorphonuclear neutrophils has been shown, but the reactions differed. Human erythrocytes and polymorphonuclear cells, rabbit macrophage and guinea pig macrophage did not show any interspecies incompatibility with human, rabbit, guinea pig, or equine complements which were

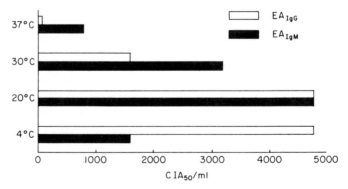

FIG. 2. Comparison of rat complement reactivity in immune adherence hemagglutination with sheep erythrocytes sensitized with IgG or IgM rabbit antibody at different temperatures.

employed to make EA (IgM) C (sheep erythrocytes sensitized by IgM fraction of rabbit antibody and complement) complex. On the other hand, guinea pig polymorphonuclear neutrophils are only compatible with EA (IgM) guinea pig complement, and rabbit polymorphonuclear neutrophils are compatible with rabbit and equine complement. Both rabbit and guinea pig platelets showed some interspecies incompatibility with complement of xenogenic origin. Eosinophils behaved like neutrophils but the adherence of basophils or peritoneal mast cells was not yet observed. A small portion of lymphocytes in blood preparations from man, guinea pig, rabbit (Henson, 1969), and mouse lymphocytes taken from lymph nodes (10–25%) showed receptor sites for EA (IgM) homologous complement complex while none of the thymus lymphocytes of the mice showed the reactivity (Lay and Nussenzweig, 1968).

Mucoids or mucopeptides derived from human erythrocytes have been presumed to be the IA receptor (D. S. Nelson and Uhlenbruck, 1967) but yield and activity is not high enough to convincingly identify these substances as IA receptor. Although the reactivity of normal human erythrocytes was found to be abolished by treatment with trypsin, tannic acid, papain, chymotrypsin, formaldehyde (Koulirsky *et al.*, 1955; D. S. Nelson and Nelson, 1959), and with acetone and other organic solvents (Sekine, 1970), the physicochemical characterization of IA receptor requires further experiment. Immunoglobulin G (IgG) from nonimmunized animals did not inhibit the interaction of IA receptor and antigen-antibody complement complex while distinct inhibition was observed in the adherence of antigen-antibody (IgG) complex with IgG receptor (Huber *et al.*, 1968).

Employing complement of the same species origin, neutrophils, macrophages, and monocytes of mouse, rabbit neutrophils and guinea pig neutrophils were differentiated from a portion of lymphocytes from the mouse lymph node, rabbit macrophages and platelets, guinea pig macrophage and platelets and human neutrophils and erythrocytes. They were classified into the (A) group and the (B) group. Inhibitory effects by EDTA vary according to the type of cells. Adherence of EA(IgM)C complex to the first group (A) was inhibited by addition of EDTA and to the second group (B) was not inhibited by EDTA. Requirement of Mg^{2+} was shown in the reaction of mouse leukocytes (Lay and Nussenzweig, 1968; Henson, 1969). By these semiquantitative measurements, a clear-cut difference between the two types of receptors was demonstrated but some discrepancy was observed when guinea pig platelets were reacted with egg albumin anti-egg albumin-guinea pig C complex which was inhibited by addition of EDTA (Siqueira and Nelson, 1961).

Whether there is an essential difference between (A) type receptor and (B) type receptor, and if so, whether the cells of (B) type contain (A) type receptor sites on the cells should be investigated further by more quantitative methods.

For the indicator cells to detect IA receptor, use of EA(IgM)C43 cells is recommended. In our laboratory, these cells are prepared first by sensitization of the optimal amount of IgM rabbit antibody against sheep E; 1000 SFU of guinea pig C1, 300 SFU of human C4, 200 SFU of guinea pig C2 and 300 CIA_{50} of guinea pig C3 per sheep erythrocyte. Second, C1 and C2 are removed by EDTA and by prolonged incubation at 37°C. Although the chemical nature of the receptor is not yet clarified at this moment, uniform reactivity of ontogenically and phylogenically defined cells with Ag-Ab C complex suggested the usefulness of adopting the IA receptor as one of the immunocytological cell markers.

Therefore, employing these EA(IgM)C43 cells, the distribution of IA receptor on a variety of human cells was examined more quantitatively (Yoshida et al., 1970; Sekine et al., 1970). On the average, 60% of peripheral erythrocytes from healthy adults and 90% of granulocytes and monocytes showed positive adherence. The similar distribution pattern was observed in erythrocytes and erythroblasts of 3-month fetuses. Leukemia cells obtained from chronic myelogenous leukemia showed a positive adherence pattern with EA(IgM)C43. On the other hand, those obtained from chronic lymphatic leukemia, acute lymphatic leukemia, and acute myelogenous leukemia did not react with EA(IgM)C43, indicating lack of IA receptor.

B. Receptors for Antigen-Antibody Complex, IgG Receptor, and IgM Receptor

Without participation of the complement system, antigen-antibody complexes adhere to a variety of cells. Depending upon the immunoglobulin class, the receptors of these cells were classified as IgG receptor (Lo Buglio et al., 1967) and IgM receptor (Lay and Nussenzweig, 1969). Some characteristics of these two receptors will be described, comparing them with the IA receptor.

For detection of IgG receptor, sheep erythrocytes sensitized with IgG fraction of antibody were most widely employed. EA(IgG) was prepared by mixing sheep erythrocytes and optimal amounts of IgG antibody obtained from prolonged hyperimmunization which give the highest rate of rosette formation with target cells. Adherence of EA(IgG) to neutrophils and macrophages or monocytes was known. Adherence to neutrophils of rabbit and guinea pig occurred only with IgG of the same species origin while adherence to human neutrophils and to human, rabbit, and guinea pig macrophages occurred with IgG of all of three species (Henson, 1969). As for the nature of IgG receptor of neutrophils, much remains obscure. The receptor of macrophage or monocytes resembles receptor for cytophilic antibodies (Howard and Benacerraf, 1966; Berken and Benacerraf, 1966). Human monocytes interact at least preferentially with IgG1 and IgG3, showing subclass specificity and the binding of IgG for macrophages resides in the Fc fragment (Huber and Fudenberg, 1968). Ten μg./ml. of free normal IgG could inhibit the reaction (Huber et al., 1969) but essentially no inhibition was observed by addition of EDTA in the interaction of neutrophils and monocytes with EA(IgG) (Henson, 1969). The IgG receptor site on guinea pig macrophages was removed or destroyed by treatment with iodoacetamide, p-chloromercuribenzoate, formaldehyde, isothiocyanate, periodate, nitrite, and lecithinase C. From these results, Howard and Benacerraf (1966) stated that free SH groups play an important part in the reactivity of the IgG receptor site peculiar to the macrophage surface membrane. In contrast to IA receptor, the IgG receptor could not be abolished by treatment with trypsin, organic solvent, or phenol (Nishioka et al., 1971b). The IgG receptor was uniformly lacking on lymphocytes, lymphoid cells, and lymphocytes stimulated with phytomitogens in vitro. Based on these observations and employing the method to measure the IgG receptor per cell more quantitatively with ^{125}I-labeled IgG antibody, Huber et al. (1969) proposed that IgG receptor could be an immunological marker for identification of mononuclear cells. This has been utilized to distinguish monocyte or macrophage from lymphatic cells, and showed a possibility of pursuing the development cycle or differentiation pathway of cells of the monocyte-macrophage system.

Receptor for EA(IgM) complex was very recently described. When the large amount of IgM antibody of the same species origin was used for sensitization of E, EA(IgM) complex adheres to the rabbit macrophages or neutrophils and to mouse macrophage. This reaction required Ca^{2+} and was not inhibited by addition of IgG. The receptor could not be destroyed by trypsin (Lay and Nussenzweig, 1969; Henson, 1969).

C. Hemadsorption after Herpes Simplex Virus Infection

A different type of adherence phenomenon of antigen-antibody (IgG) to the cell membrane infected with herpes simplex virus (HSV) was described (Watkins, 1964a). This phenomenon should be differentiated from IA receptor, IgM receptor, and especially from IgG receptor. HeLa cells do not have IA or IgG receptors but in an early stage after infection with herpes simplex virus, the adherence of EA(IgG) was observed and the adsorption was inhibited by anti-HSV antibody.

Development of profound alteration in the cell surface of HeLa cells was observed after HSV infection. First, within 1 hour, the infected cells lost the ability to spread on the glass; this phenomenon was termed membrane paralysis (Watkins, 1964b). Within 5 to 6 hours, virus antigen appeared at the cell surface and the cell acquired the ability to adsorb EA(IgG) complex. Eight hours after infection, cell fusion and giant cell formation were observed (Bungay and Watkins, 1966). Finally, infective virus appeared in 12 hours. In this timetable, hemadsorption coincided with appearance of viral antigen on the cell surface. From an inhibition study with actinomycin D and 5′-iodo-2-deoxyuridine, Watkins (1965) explained the appearance of hemadsorption of EA(IgG) on the infected cell membrane as follows. Infecting viral DNA codes for RNA, which in turn codes for the antigen that appears at the surface about an hour after the completion of DNA-directed RNA synthesis. The synthesis of complete viral DNA is not necessary for this hemadsorption phenomenon but is required for cell fusion.

Hemadsorption of EA(IgG) to infected cells was not due to the appearance of cross-reacting antigen on the cell surface nor due to the IgG receptor since no inhibition was observed by anti-sheep E(IgM) antibody and normal IgG. Furthermore, some preliminary physicochemical characterization studies showed distinct differences. According to Yasuda and Milgrom (1968), treatment with iodoacetamide or p-chloromercuribenzoate and lecithinase C had no effect, while mercaptoethanol or phenol and methanol abolished the reactivity. These results are quite the reverse of effects of these chemical treatments on IgG receptor of monocytes and on the receptor of HSV-infected cells for antigen-antibody (IgG) complex. Although much more quantitative analysis is required, antiglobulin affinity to the HSV-infected cells was differentiated from the IgG receptor by these experiments. The possibility that it would be analogous to the rheumatoid factor was suggested by Milgrom (1962; Yasuda and Milgrom, 1968).

D. APPLICATION OF IMMUNOLOGICAL CELL MARKERS
   FOR CHARACTERIZATION OF CELLS DERIVED
   FROM TUMOR

Detection of cell markers on the membrane by these new methods made it possible to characterize a different kind of cell recognition of which has been difficult by other methods. Also, detection of different reactive sites on a single type of cell membrane became possible. For example, circulating and tissue mononuclear cells have been classified according to their morphological appearances, but difficulties are encountered even when electron microscopic observation is employed.

Differentiation between lymphoid cells and monocyte-macrophage seems to be essential at this time, employing more precise methods, since evidence has been accumulated indicating that both have synergistic but different functions participating in some immunological reactions. It became possible, by employing IgG receptor as an immunocytological marker, to identify mononuclear cells (Huber *et al.*, 1969). The IgG receptor was quantitated on the cells of the monocyte-macrophage system and not on lymphatic cells, even after blast formation. Huber *et al.* (1968) also demonstrated distinct receptor sites, IA receptor and IgG receptor on a single cell type, human monocytes, indicating that these two receptors on the cell may function either independently or cooperatively in the induction of phagocytosis.

A method using such immunological cell markers was applied to tumor immunology, and our results in differentiating between the cultured cell lines derived from Burkitt's lymphoma (BL) and nasopharyngeal carcinoma (NPC) will be described here briefly (Nishioka *et al.*, 1971b).

Following the discovery of herpes type virus (HTV) by Epstein *et al.* (1964) in tissue culture cells derived from BL, the presence of HTV was demonstrated in tissue culture cells derived from NPC (de Thé *et al.*, 1969; Takada *et al.*, 1971; Sugano *et al.*, 1970). Both cultured cell lines derived from NPC and BL were obtained in the floating state; they resembled each other in morphological appearance and were known to carry HTV as revealed by immunofluorescence and electron microscopic observation. Recently, lack of IA receptor was described by Yoshida *et al.* (1970) on a cultured BL cell line. Therefore, employing the above-mentioned immunological cell markers, adherence of EA(IgM)C43 cells and EA(IgG) cells to a number of cultured BL cell lines and NPC cell lines was examined in collaboration with Drs. de Thé and Klein. All NPC cell lines obtained from Taiwan, Hongkong, and Nairobi showed adherence of EA(IgM)C43, showing the rosette formation as shown in Fig. 3 and all BL cell lines did not show such reaction except for one cell line obtained from an ovarian tumor. On the contrary, EA(IgG) did not show rosette formation with NPC cell lines while IA(IgG) adhered to all BL cell lines tested, including a nonvirus-producing line, Raji (Pulvertaft, 1964). Some of the experiments are shown in Table II and the statistical analysis is shown in Fig. 4.

None of the cell lines have yet been cloned except P3HR1, which was done by Hinuma and Grace (1967). Therefore, cultured cell lines were composed of mixed cell populations. Nonetheless, the cultured cell lines derived from NPC and BL could be classified into two different groups according to their origin. Statistical analysis by ridit (Bross, 1958) confirmed this observation. As for positive interaction with EA(IgM)C43

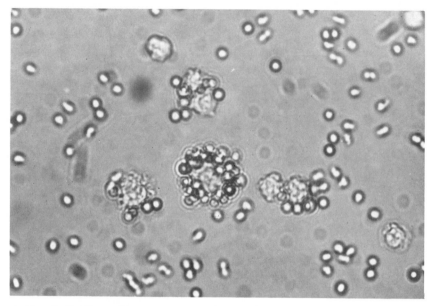

Fɪɢ. 3. Positive adherence pattern of EA(IgM)C43 cells to cultured cell line (No. 204R) derived from nasopharyngeal carcinoma.

and NPC cell line, this was not inhibited by EDTA nor by normal IgG. When these cells were treated with trypsin or acetone, almost all of the reactivity of these cells with EAC43 was lost. As IA receptor was removed by trypsin (D. S. Nelson and Nelson, 1959) and acetone (Sekine, 1970), and no inhibition was observed with normal IgG (Huber *et al.*, 1968), the presence of IA receptor and lack of IgG receptor on the surface of the cultured cell lines derived from NPC were established.

As for the positive reaction of the cells from BL with EA(IgG), two possibilities were considered. First, this may be caused by the presence of IgG receptor on BL cells and second, by the hemadsorption of EA(IgG) owing to altered state of the membrane induced by HTV infection. In both cases, receptor was not digested off by trypsin and no inhibition was observed with addition of EDTA as described above. However, acetone treatment or phenol treatment abolished the reactivity of BL cells with EA(IgG) and no inhibition was observed with the addition of normal IgG. These results did not coincide with the nature of IgG receptor so far described. On the other hand, the hemadsorption activity in the early stage of HSV infection was removed by acetone (Hayashi *et al.*, 1970) or phenol (Yasuda and Milgrom, 1968) and normal IgG preparations did not inhibit the reaction. It is most plausible that the interaction of BL cell lines with EA (IgG) fit into the category of hemad-

TABLE II

PERCENTAGE OF FREQUENCY DISTRIBUTION OF NUMBER OF EA(IgM)C43 CELLS
OR EA(IgG) CELLS ADHERING TO CULTURED CELL SURFACE

Number of EA(IgM)C43/cells	0	1	2	3	4	≥ 5
NPC: Lyll	28	12	5	17	10	28
NPC: 204 R	15	14	6	19	15	30
NPC: 204 M	29	15	5	10	16	26
BL: P3HRl	94	5	1	0	0	0
BL: Raji	93	7	0	0	0	0
BL: Maku	97	2	1	0	0	0
Number of EA(IgG)/cells	0	1	2	3	4	≥ 5
BL: P3HRl	55	6	6	4	2	27
BL: Raji	43	11	5	4	3	34
BL: Maku	71	1	1	1	6	26
NPC: Lyll	93	6	1	0	0	0
NPC: 204 M	100	0	0	0	0	0
NPC: 204 R	98	1	0	1	0	0

sorption after HSV infection and not of IgG receptor. Therefore, EA(IgG) may adhere to the membrane of BL cell lines in a way similar to the altered cell membrane which occurs in the early stage of herpes simplex virus infection. In case of herpes simplex virus infection, the virus particles were liberated and the host cells underwent lysis, resulting in lytic infection. On the other hand, through the entire course of HTV-BL cell line interaction, no lytic infection occurred, but showed the form of persistent infection. It is an interesting finding that these BL cell lines showed a reaction with EA(IgG) similar to cells in the early stage of herpes simplex virus infection and it is most plausible that this reaction might be a manifestation of biological activity of HTV harbored in the host cells. A possibility was suggested that the receptor for EA(IgG) which was induced after HSV infection on the infected cell membrane would be analogous to the rheumatoid factor (Yasuda and Milgrom, 1968; Milgrom, 1962). A relationship could be considered with the phenomenon described by Capra et al. (1969) that cold reactive rheumatoid factor appeared in 72% of sera of patients with infectious mononucleosis, in which HTV is considered to be the etiologic agent (Niederman et al., 1968).

Not only the cultured BL cells, which are known as typically HTV-producing cells, but a non-virus-producing cell line, Raji, isolated from a Burkitt lymphoma showed the same type of reaction, the phenomenon being similar to the early stage of HSV infection in this persistent infection. These findings are in line with the results which demonstrated the

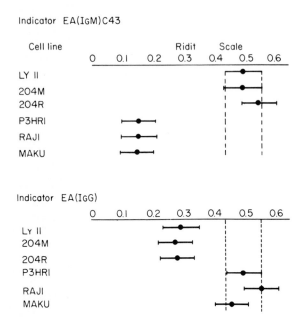

Fig. 4. Relative identified distribution of cultured cell lines in reference to adherence of EA(IgM)C43 cells and EA(IgG) with range of 95% confidence interval.

presence of HTV nucleic acid homology in a "virus-free" line of BL, indicating that HTV has features of known DNA tumor viruses (zur Hausen and Schulte-Holthausen, 1970).

For further analysis, comparative studies of NPC cells with those of BL cells are considered to be of importance. In comparing cultured BL and NPC cell lines, it was clearly demonstrated that these two types of host cells harboring the HTV were discriminated from each other by employing these immunological cell markers. In parallel with biochemical markers or immunoglobulin production, the application of such immunocytological markers can now be considered to give a useful tool for classification of these lymphoid cells or reticulum cells carrying HTV.

Besides the question of the nature of individual cell lines in respect to the malignant character, tumor-host relationships should be considered in regard to the manifestation of oncogenesis. From this point, it is noteworthy that viruses harbored in lymphocytes or reticulum cells have been known to play essential roles in immunological reaction *in vivo*. The fact that the virus is lymphotropic in nature might result in the impairment of the immune reaction of the host, resulting in misrecognition of antigen information or weakness of the immunological surveillance system against malignant transformed cells. If we could consider the appearance of antinuclear antibody as an expression of a misrecognition of antigen due to immunological impairment, it is to be noted that antinuclear antibody appeared in patients' sera of infectious mononucleosis to some extent (Kaplan and Tan, 1968) and more apparently in the sera of nasopharyngeal carcinoma (Yoshida, 1971) both of which were characterized by high anti-HTV titer in the patients' sera (Old *et al.*, 1968; Henle *et al.*, 1968; Niederman *et al.*, 1968; Ito *et al.*, 1969; Kawamura *et al.*, 1971).

III. Cellular Antigen as an Immunological Marker—General Considerations

After the spectacular success achieved against infectious diseases, immunological approaches to cancer were vigorously attempted. However, because of critical opinions on the lack of proper control of immunogenetic aspects in early experiments (Spencer, 1942; Hauschka, 1952), immunologists despaired of their previous optimism, and most characterizations of tumor cells have been performed at the morphologic or biochemical level. Despite these initial disappointments, tumor immunology was restored to its position after remarkable progress occurred in transplantation immunology, based on genetically controlled animals and improvements in quantitative and sensitive immunochemical techniques. Along this line, attempts to distinguish between genuine tumor-specific phenomena and transplantation artefacts, employing syngenic or autochthonous tumor-host relationships, were successful and much evidence has accumulated to indicate that neoplastic cells carry antigenic determinants not possessed by the normal cells of the individual. (See the reviews by G. Klein, 1966; Old and Boyse, 1964; Sjögren, 1965.) Progress in the immunochemical approach to the problem of cancer could provide the most fundamental understanding of how tumor cells differ from normal tissue as a result of the neoplastic transformation induced by various carcinogens, including viruses. Antigens of cells or cellular components could be used as immunological markers for characterization of tumor cells.

Of a number of parameters of tumor cell antigens, the transplantation antigen plays an essential role in host-tumor relationship. The transplantation antigen is considered as the new antigen present on the cell surface, induced by either a chemical carcinogen or coded for by the viral genome in the transformed cell. By definition, the antigen should be responsible for rejection of tumor transplanted in a syngenic host. Transplantation antigens of chemically induced tumors, especially those induced by polycyclic hydrocarbons, are specific for each tumor and the antigens of virus-induced tumor are common to tumors induced by the same virus, indicating that they are coded for by the viral genome. Besides the transplantation antigens, T-antigens or neoantigens common to tumors induced by the same DNA viruses and type-specific or group-specific structural virus antigens are important parameters in pursuing the fate of the virus, or analyzing virus-host-cell relationships in the oncogenic process. Further, to analyze the genetic origin of a tumor or more dynamically, to pursue the gain or loss of antigens in relation to the abilities of tumor cells to grow progressively and kill their host, histocompatibility antigens and other alloantigens (Boyse *et al.*, 1968; Rubin *et al.*, 1970; Aoki *et al.*, 1970; T. Takahashi *et al.*, 1970; Harris *et al.*, 1969; Tachibana *et al.*, 1970) have been employed as markers. Although their direct relationships to oncogenic processes have not yet been proved, a high incidence of association of some carcinoembryonic (Gold and Freedman, 1965; Thomson *et al.*, 1969; von Kleist and Burtin, 1969) and embryonal serum α-globulin (Abelev, 1963, 1968; Uriel *et al.*, 1967) or Australian antigens (Blumberg *et al.*, 1965; Sutnik *et al.*, 1970) in some types of human neoplasia have been described. These associated antigens can be considered as possible useful tools for diagnostic purposes or for expression of immunological impairment of the tumor-bearing host. Detailed critical reviews covering very recent developments on the significance and charácterization of these antigens were given by Pasternak (1969), Deichman (1969), Hellström and Hellström (1969), and Habel (1969). For that reason, no attempt will be made to cover these entire problems again. In this chapter, more emphasis will be given to review of methods for detection of antigens, employing complement as an immunochemical amplifier of the antigen-antibody reaction.

For detection of transplantation antigens induced by chemical carcinogens or oncogenic viruses, the antibody should be prepared in syngenic hosts to avoid repetition of the damaging despair which tumor immunologists experienced in the first five decades of this century. For the detection of other cellular or related subcellular antigens, it is preferable to employ the syngenic animals as a source of antibody donor to avoid nonspecificity; but preparation of potent antibody in syngenic or autochthonous host is often difficult. In general, larger amounts of antibody are produced against the more heterogeneous substance as revealed by accumulated observations in transplantation immunology. Heterogeneity of tumor cells with respect to the host cells of syngenic or autochthonous systems has been indicated to be minor as compared with that of an xenogenic system. Therefore the amount of antibody produced against syngenic or autochthonous tumor is assumed to be very small. Preexisting immunological disability in the tumor-bearing host as manifested by antibody synthetic activity also makes it difficult to detect antibody in such a system. The urgent problem in immunochemical approaches to cancer which is revealed by these facts is the need to increase the sensitivity of the immunological method to detect antibody or antigen in small amounts. Practically, except for detection of tumor transplantation antigens, antibodies were often produced in the experimental animals of different strains or species. In such cases, however, the genetic heterogeneity should be sufficiently controlled to permit the proper interpretation of the experimental results, necessarily excluding the nonspecific reaction due to immunogenetic heterogeneity.

For detection of transplantation antigens *in vivo*, the basic format was given in simplest terms by Prehn (1968). That is, exposure to antigen followed by challenge with live tumor cells. The survival after the tumor challenge determined by properly controlled experiments was taken as "rejection." To analyze the responsible factors for the rejection mechanism, passive transfer of cells or serum from immunized animals to the nonimmunized histocompatible animal (Old *et al.*, 1962; Zbar *et al.*, 1970a,b) or delayed type of hypersensitivity reactions (Oettgen *et al.*, 1968; Hoy and Nelson, 1969) were employed. Further immunotherapy experiments have been attempted employing syngenic animals (Kronman *et al.*, 1970).

To make progress in the analysis of host-tumor relationships, to isolate and purify the antigens, and to find a possible application to human tumor, various *in vitro* techniques have been employed to detect the antigens. As for all the results obtained by these *in vitro* methods, we could not find definitive evidence that the detected antigens are of the transplantation type, and the results should be reevaluated by the transplantation and rejection experiment, namely the basic format.

As *in vitro* techniques, immunocytotoxicity (Gorer and O'Gorman, 1956), membrane immunofluorescence (Möller, 1961; E. Klein and Klein, 1964), mixed cell agglutination (Barth *et al.*, 1967; Tachibana and E. Klein, 1970), clone reduction by antibody and complement or by lymphocytes (Hellström and Sjögren, 1967), and inhibition of migration of normal macrophages (George and Vaughan, 1962; Kronman *et al.*, 1969) have been employed. A concise and critical review of these methods was given by Habel (1969).

As demonstrated, complement plays a role as an immunochemical amplifier or effector system of the antigen-antibody reaction. If the antibody belongs to a class of complement-fixing nature (IgG1, IgG2, IgG3, or IgM), the reaction of antigen and antibody will be visualized as magnified by the activity of complement concerned. Therefore, the immunological reaction using complement is in general more sensitive than methods based on the mere binding of corresponding antigen or antibody without the amplifier or effector.

In the reaction concerned with serological methods involving complement with a constant amount of antigen, there is a reciprocal relationship between the concentration of antibody and complement. When the concentration of antibody decreased, much more complement was required and when the concentration of complement decreased, much more antibody was required for manifestation of the immunological reaction as observed in immune hemolysis (Mayer, 1961a) and in immune adherence (Nishioka, 1963). Therefore, as required in the present situation, when higher sensitivity of antibody measurement is necessary, it is preferable to use as high a concentration of complement as possible. Serological methods in which complement participates can be classified into two types: (a) To measure complement activity left after consumption by a preceding antigen-antibody reaction; (b) to measure activity of complement directly combined in the antigen-antibody reaction. The first group of reactions is represented by conventional complement fixation. The second group is represented by immune adherence, $C\overline{1}$ fixation and transfer, or immunocytotoxicity tests which will be described later. In the first type, the complement activity left after the preceding antigen-antibody reaction is measured by immune hemolysis of sensitized sheep erythrocytes added afterward. Therefore, the higher the concentration of complement added to the antigen-antibody reaction mixture, the greater will be the amount of uncombined complement left. Since the antigen-antibody reaction is measured by consumption of complement as indicated by negative immune hemolysis, to increase the sensitivity of the antibody measurement, the amount of complement to be added should be kept down to the limit which could avoid nonspecific anticomplementary effect. Although this ingenious technique, conventional complement fixation, has contributed much toward detection of antigen or antibody in many cases, one encounters the limitation that the antigen-antibody reaction should be carried out in the presence of limited complement. This is contradictory to the principle that to detect small amounts of antibody one needs the presence of excess complement, based on the reciprocal relation between the concentrations of antibody and complement as described above.

On the other hand, if we could directly measure the activity of complement combined with the antigen-antibody complex, we could increase the amount of complement to the limit that permits us to avoid the activity of natural antibodies present in the serum of the complement source. In this way, we could increase the sensitivity in measurement of antibody greatly, since the larger amounts of complement permit us to detect smaller amount of antibody.

In this way, recent advances in complement research and progress in basic immunochemical methods have contributed further precise and sensitive methods that have been required for detection of very small amounts of antigen or antibody, an urgent problem in the current status of tumor immunology. These methods of immune adherence and C1 transfer fixation will be reviewed together with the conventional complement fixation test and the immune cytotoxicity test.

IV. Immune Adherence

A. PRINCIPLE AND METHODS

Immune adherence was defined by R. A. Nelson (1953) as adherence of specific antigen-antibody and complement complex to primate erythrocytes or to nonprimate platelets. When this reaction has been carried out in the presence of excess complement, it has been proven to be one of the most sensitive methods currently available for the titration of antigen and antibody. When the antigen-antibody complex reacts with the complement system, the uptake of C1, C4, C2, and C3 occurs sequentially. Antigen particles or cells carrying C3 on their surface exhibit the reaction with immune adherence receptor of various indicator cells (practically, in most cases, human erythrocytes have been employed) resulting in immune adherence (Nishioka and Linscott, 1963). This reaction has been utilized as a sensitive indicator for the presence of antigen-antibody complexes on the cell surface or on cellular components. As shown in Table III, this method is capable of detecting 0.0005 μg. of IgM antibody nitrogen (AbN) and 0.017 μg. of IgG AbN against salmonella typhi 0.901. With IgM antibody, it was 130 times more sensitive than C' fixation and 1000 times more sensitive than agglutination and with IgG antibody it was 15 times more sensitive than agglutination (Nishioka et al., 1967a).

It has been suggested by Müller-Eberhard et al. (1966) that several hundred molecules of C3 could bind to the antigenic cell membrane by

TABLE III

MINIMAL AMOUNT OF ANTIBODY NITROGEN REQUIRED FOR POSITIVE REACTION OF ANTI-S. TYPHI ANTIBODY

Antibody	Agglutination[a]	C fixation	Immune adherence
Unfractionated	0.37 (176)	0.11 (52)	0.0021
IgG fraction	0.26 (15)	0.13 (8)	0.0170
IgM fraction	0.50 (1000)	0.065 (130)	0.0005

[a] Figures in parentheses indicate the ratio of AbN required for positive reaction of test to that of IA.

a single site of AgAbC142, and multiplication of a single site of antibody molecules will occur in a sequential reaction at a step of C3. Recently, it was clearly demonstrated that only C3 molecules or subfragments of C3 (C3IA) present on the antigen cell membrane are essential, and other complement component molecules or antibody molecules are not required for the reaction with IA receptor of the indicator human erythrocytes to cause the immune adherence reaction (Sekine *et al.*, 1970; Okada *et al.*, 1970b; Nishioka, 1971). Therefore, the high sensitivity of the immune adherence test in measuring the small amounts of antibody can be explained on a molecular basis by the following facts: (a) a high concentration of complement permits the smallest amount of antibody to react with antigen in the presence of excess complement, (b) there is adherence of a large number of C3 molecules per single antibody C142 site, and (c) these C3 molecules are the only complement components to react with the immune adherence receptor on human erythrocytes.

1. *Immune Adherence with Free Cells*

Because of high sensitivity, carefully controlled experiments are required to avoid nonspecific reactions. Despite our success and that of others in detection of antibodies against cellular or subcellular antigens (Melief *et al.*, 1967; de Planque *et al.*, 1969), Weir (1967) reported in his review that the immune adherence test does not appear to have been used successfully for particulate tissue antigens although in principle the technique should be applicable. He quoted failures to detect antibodies against rat liver cells (Pinckard and Weir, 1966) or antibodies against thyroid microsomes (Roitt *et al.*, 1964). Therefore, it is necessary to mention some technically important points.

All glassware should be cleaned by immersion for at least 4 hours in concentrated H_2SO_4 with dichromate, followed by rinsing at least 10 times with tap water and 6 times with deionized water. Microplates of Plexiglas are cleaned by immersion in 0.4% Hemosol solution for at least 4 hours or the disposable type in H_2SO_4 for a half hour, followed by rinsing by jet into each hole, immersion in deionized water overnight, rinsing with deionized water 10 times, and drying.

As diluents, GVB^{2+} as described by Mayer (1961a) was employed. Care should be taken to avoid contamination with bacteria or fungi which sometimes act as antigen against natural antibody present in the reaction mixture. The pH should be controlled to 7.5 carefully to avoid acid adhesion, and veronal buffer is recommended as most preferable. When it is required to keep the integrity of nucleated cells, 0.2 gm. of KCl and 1.0 gm. of glucose were added to 1 liter of GVB^{2+}. As indicator erythrocytes for immune adherence, human 0 Rh$^+$ red cells are used. There is not much individual difference in immune adherence reactivity of human erythrocytes, but it is preferable to test the reactivities of several donors preliminarily and to select the most reactive one. As a routine method for screening erythrocytes, 2×10^8/ml. cell suspension in GVB^{2+} were prepared and 0.1 ml. of erythrocyte suspension was added to the reaction mixture containing 1×10^7 of optimally sensitized sheep erythrocytes antibody complex and a series of diluted guinea pig complement in a total reaction volume of 1.0 ml. in a special test tube 13 by 75 mm. with a perfectly round bottom (IA tube). After 15 minutes shaking at 37°C. and settling at 37°C. for 60 minutes, the hemagglutination pattern is read. A lot of human erythrocytes giving a positive pattern at the highest dilution of guinea pig serum is selected.

As a source of complement, both guinea pig complement, preferably from young animals, or human complement, preferably from AB Rh$^+$ type, can be employed. Because of its high sensitivity, it is necessary to preclude the participation of natural antibody against target cells or indicator human erythrocytes present in the complement sera. This is done either by diluting out or by absorption. Dilution is not preferable when the reaction requires high sensitivity for detection of antibodies. In such a case, absorption of complement serum should be performed. The principle of absorption of natural antibodies from complement serum is quite different from the absorption of conventional antibodies. When natural antibody is present in high concentration, more complement will be consumed as a result of antigen-antibody-complement interaction during the procedure of absorption. Therefore, in such a case the time should be short and the temperature should be low (at 0°C.) to minimize the consumption of complement. If the natural antibody is present in low concentration or its avidity is low, the absorption should be prolonged and repeated. Considering these factors, the serum of the complement source is to be absorbed with 1/20 volume of packed target cells (in the case of guinea pig, together with indicator human erythrocytes) at 0°C. once for 1 minute, twice for 5 minutes, three times for 10 minutes and then three times for 15 minutes (Fujii and Nelson, 1963). If the amount of natural antibody is considered to be less, the absorption procedure can be done first for 1 minute, second for 3 minutes and third for 10 minutes (Takeuchi et al., 1969). If we cannot obtain sufficient target cells for the absorption test, it can be absorbed with the bulk of cells which are considered to be most closely related antigenically. In this way, natural antibodies can be absorbed, leaving complement unabsorbed in the supernatant. The absorbed sera are centrifuged at high speed after the last absorption procedure to remove the debris of antigen cells, and stored in small portions at $-70°C$. or below. In this way, excess complement can be added to the reaction mixture at a properly high concentration, thus avoiding the participation of nonspecific reactions due to natural antibodies. Assays are carried out in IA tubes or in U type Plexiglas microplates to develop the hemagglutination pattern. The tubes should be kept in a horizontal position in a proper test tube rack. During the time of addition of each reagent and reaction, the test tube or U plate should be shaken gently by hand or mechanically by a micromixer. To develop the hemagglutination pattern, the total reaction volume should not exceed 1.1 ml. in a IA tube and 125 μl. in a U type microplate. Sometimes when antiserum contains strong anticomplement activity, the mixture of antigen-antibody in the test tube or microplate was first allowed to react then washed by centrifugation to remove nonreacted serum components, and then complement and human erythocytes were added. An obvious control for each antigen consisted of measurements of the interference with a negative pattern upon mixture of antigens with human erythrocytes only. With heavy particles or with the antigens which form large clumps in the presence of excess antibody, the particles sometimes settle more rapidly than the erythrocytes and produce irregular patterns. In our experiences, the optimal amount of antigen to give the most proper hemagglutination patterns decreased according to the size of antigen particles. Employing 2×10^7 human erythrocytes as indicator in the total reaction mixture, the optimal number of antigen particles was found to be $4–5 \times 10^7$ for erythrocytes, and $5–10 \times 10^5$ for small lymphocytes or Burkitt lymphoma cells. When the reaction is carried out in a microplate, the optimal ratio of the number of antigen particles to indicator human erythrocyte does not change. With cells larger than this, it is difficult to obtain good hemagglutination patterns and we have to examine them under the microscope. The results are usually read after 15 minutes of shaking at $37°C$. followed by standing at $37°C$. for an additional 60 minutes. In some cases the indicator erythrocytes did not settle completely by this time and the pattern was read again after another 10 minutes of standing at room temperature. The results were expressed as in the usual hemagglutination pattern. Unagglutinated indicator cells collected in a neat central ring or button and this was recorded as negative. Agglutinated erythrocytes formed an even and diffuse deposit and were recorded as from $1+$ to $4+$. When the new antigen-antibody system is employed, the developed hemagglutination pattern should be examined under the microscope to confirm the adherence pattern of antigen particles to human erythrocytes. In most cases good agreement is obtained between the hemagglutination pattern and the results observed under the microscope. In many cases, when the size of the cells is too large, development of the hemagglutination pattern was disturbed and we could read the results only under the microscope. When mouse mammary tumor, MM2 was treated with its syngenic antibody, a positive immune adherence pattern was graded from 4+ to ± as described by Nishioka et al. (1969b).

The positivity was also graded by these patterns from 0–4 or by counting the number of rosette-forming tumor cells with more than two human erythrocytes. The percentage of target cells showing rosette formation was graded as 0% = 0, 1–5% = 1, 6–15% = 2, 16–25% = 3, more than 25% = 4. The specificity of this reaction can be examined by the absorption test. Identification of the results as immune adherence can be confirmed by (a) a nonadherence pattern with nonprimate erythrocytes; (b) inhibition by EDTA which is added before addition of complement to the antigen-antibody complex; (c) conversion of the positive immune adherence pattern to negative after treatment with C3 inactivator (Tamura and Nelson, 1967).

If the reaction mixture was left for extended periods, the agglutinated human erythrocytes often rolled inward and could not be distinguished easily from the button of the unagglutinated erythrocytes. Also, when examined under a microscope after completing the reaction time, the positive reaction sometimes turned into a negative pattern. This occurred more frequently when the amount of specific antigen or antibody was very small and the amount of serum material was present in excess in the reaction mixture. This has been a limitation of the IA technique and we have to read the pattern at a limited time. These limitations need to be overcome to improve the quantitativeness and sensitivity of the test and this has been the problem in trying to detect small amounts of antibody employing cultured cells derived from nasopharyngeal carcinoma or Burkitt's lymphoma as target cells reacting in this system.

Negative conversion of the IA pattern has been considered to be due to the action of C3 inactivator present in the serum sample which inactivates the active C3 site reacting in immune adherence. Therefore, we screened for inhibitors of C3 inactivator first. We found dithiothreitol (DTT) was a most effective inhibitor of the action of C3 inactivator, keeping the positive IA pattern unchanged. It was shown that DTT acted on the C3 site of the antigen-antibody complement complex and rendered the C3 site unsusceptible to the action of C3 inactivator (Nishioka et al., 1971a). Based on these observations, a method for carrying out immune adherence was established as follows. An appropriate dilution of serum in 0.025 ml. in GVB^{2+} was added with 0.025 ml. of 5×10^6/ml. of cultured cells and 0.025 ml. of 1/15 dilution of human C or 1/40 dilution of absorbed guinea pig C. After reaction at 37°C. for 30 minutes, 0.025 ml. of 0.015 M DTT solution in GVB^{2+} was added followed by immediate addition of 0.025 ml. of 1×10^8/ml. of a human erythrocyte suspension. After shaking at 37°C. for 20 minutes and standing at 20°C. for 60 minutes, the immune adherence pattern was read under the microscope. This procedure avoids completely the conversion of a positive immune adherence reaction into a negative pattern. Employing nasopharyngeal patient sera (No. 204) at 1/20 or 1/40 dilutions, 14,6 or 11.0% of rosette formation of an immune adherence positive pattern was observed when reacted with cultured NPC cells 204 of autochthonous origin. When the experiments are carried out with these facts in mind, IA is one of the most useful methods for detecting surface antigens present on free tumor cells. The limitation is that observations are made microscopically or by reading hemagglutination patterns. More quantitative analytical methods are required.

Another advantage of the immune adherence test is that it can be observed with nonliving cells. As shown in Table IV, if antigen is removed from the cell surface or is denatured by various physical or chemical procedures, the pretreated cells will not react with specific antibody and will not give positive immune adherence. Information on the nature of antigenic substances present on mouse mammary tumor cells was obtained through these procedures together with partial degradation of the cell surface as shown in Tables V and VI.

For further physicochemical characterization of the surface antigens, specific inhibition of the immune adherence test has been employed.

TABLE IV

CHARACTERIZATION OF CELL SURFACE ANTIGEN BY IMMUNE ADHERENCE[a]

Immune Adherence	Result
Tumor cells + antibody//complement//human erythrocytes	+
Detection of antigen on cell surface	
Pretreated tumor cells + antibody//complement//human erythrocytes	
if antigen removed	−
if antigen remained	+
Detection of antigen in fractions	
Fraction + antibody//tumor cells + complement//human erythrocytes	
if antigen present	−
if antigen absent	+

[a] // signifies sequential steps of experimental procedure, i.e., mix tumor cells and antibody first, add complement next, and add human erythrocytes last.

TABLE V
IMMUNE ADHERENCE REACTIVITY OF MM2 TUMOR WITH TUMOR-SPECIFIC
ANTIBODY FOLLOWING TREATMENT WITH VARIOUS AGENTS

Untreated		+++
UV-irradiated	20 W, 20 cm, 20 minutes	+++
Frozen and thawed	−78°C. and −20°C.	+++
Lyophilization		++
Heated	100°C., 15 minutes	−
	62°C., 15 minutes	+++
	37°C., 60 minutes	++++
Ethanol	37°C., 15 minutes	−
Methanol	37°C., 15 minutes	−
Ethanol–ether (1:1)	20°C., 60 minutes	−
Acetone	0°C., 60 minutes	++
	20°C., 30 minutes	−
	37°C., 10 minutes	−
Chloroform–		
methanol (2:1)	0°C., 60 minutes	++
	20°C., 30 minutes	+
	37°C., 60 minutes	−

Inhibition tests have been widely employed for detecting specific antigens in various immunological reactions. First, a sample of the fraction is mixed with a limited, predetermined amount of antibody. If antigen is present in the fraction, it combines with antibody and thus inhibits the reaction of antibody with subsequently added tumor cells. This results in a negative immune adherence pattern and human erythrocytes do not adhere to the tumor cells. If antigen is absent in the fraction, antibody left in the free state will produce a positive immune adherence pattern after addition of fresh tumor cells, complement, and human erythrocytes. Thus, by observing the immune adherence pattern, the presence of antigen in the fraction can be detected and the character of antigen can be pursued further. Employing this method, extraction and solubilization of transplantation antigen of mouse mammary tumors were performed (Irie *et al.*, 1969, 1971). The presence of antigen of mouse mammary tumor (MM2 or MM102) was detected in 0.2% deoxycholate extract which reacted specifically with syngenic antibody. After the removal of deoxycholate by dialysis, most antigens were precipitated by centrifugation at 105,000 g for 60 minutes. Hyperimmunization of C3H/He mice with these antigen fractions induced heightened resistance against living tumor challenge. Employing this method and the cytotoxic inhibition test as an indicator, antigens were solubilized from deoxycholate extracts with distilled water. The soluble antigen inhibited the neutralization activity of the tumor-specific anti-

TABLE VI

IMMUNE ADHERENCE REACTIVITY OF HEATED OR UV-IRRADIATED MM2 TUMOR
FOLLOWING TREATMENT WITH ENZYMES OR CHEMICALS AT 37°C. FOR
60 MINUTES

Enzyme or chemical treatment	Concentration	Immune adherence reactivity	
		Cells heated at 62°C. 15 minutes before enzyme or chemical treatment	Cells irradiated with UV before enzyme or chemical treatment
Deoxyribonuclease	50 μg./ml.	+++	+++
Ribonuclease	100 μg./ml.	+++	
Chymotrypsin	100 μg./ml.	+++	
Trypsin	250 μg./ml.	+++	+++
Pepsin	250 μg./ml.	+++	
Papain	250 μg./ml.	+++	
Elastase	250 μg./ml.	+++	
Neuraminidase	30 units/ml.	+++	+++
Periodate	0.01 M	+++	+++
Sodium deoxycholate	1 mg./ml.	−	−
Triton × 100	10 mg./ml.	−	
Triton × 100	1 mg./ml.	±	
Lysolecithin	1 mg./ml.	−	
	0.5 mg./ml.	++	
Snake venom *Naja jaje*	30 μg./ml.	−	
Snake venom *Naja jaje*	10 μg./ml.	+	
Snake venom *Crotalus adamanteus*	30 μg./ml.	−	
	10 μg./ml.	+	
Phospholipase A	10 μg./ml.	−	
Phospholipase C	30 μg./ml.	+	

body to living tumor and we concluded that transplantation antigens of isografted mammary tumors were present in deoxycholate extracts of the tumor cells. Antigen was further purified by 75% ethanol. Chemical analysis of an antigenically active fraction purified 22-fold showed that it was composed of 11.7% protein, 83.3% lipid, 0.35% sugar, and 3.9% RNA. The lipid analyses presented the possibility that the antigens might be extracted from the plasma membrane.

Another type of immune adherence inhibition test was described by Fujii and Nelson (1963), demonstrating the transfer of antibody from surfaces of cells which have chemically related cross-reacting antigen to a subcellular fraction of antigen used for the immunization. The latter concepts are essential for detection of cell-bound antibody based on the cross reaction.

2. *Immune Adherence with Cell Surface Antigens on Monolayer Cells*

To detect cell surface antigen, a variety of methods have been employed. Immunocytotoxic tests or immunofluorescence tests which have been employed for detection of surface antigens of free cells in suspension could hardly be applied to cells adhering on a glass or plastic surface. Requirements for detection of virus-induced tumor antigen or histocompatibility antigen of these types of cells have been increasing in tissue culture systems. Immune adherence (O'Neill, 1968) and mixed hemagglutination (Fagraeus *et al.*, 1966) are methods of choice in such systems and simple micromethods have been recently developed (Tachibana and E. Klein, 1970; Tachibana *et al.*, 1970). Employing Falcon plastic Micro test plates, 100 to 1000 cells were plated in each well and after attaching and growing on the plain bottom, 10 μl. of antiserum was added. After washings, the indicator system composed of 10 μl. of human erythrocytes suspension (2×10^7/ml.) containing 1–2% absorbed guinea pig complement was added. After 30 minutes at 37°C., unattached human erythrocytes were removed by inverting the plate and the results were read under microscope. A typical immune adherence pattern was observed in histocompatibility (H-2) antigen and the surface antigen induced by the Moloney virus reacting with specific antibody respectively. Based on the reliability of this technique, the difference in antigenic expression between hybrid cells obtained by fusion and the parental cells was demonstrated (Harris *et al.*, 1969). Also, this tissue culture method provided a new useful method to assess Moloney leukemia virus infectivity (Nördenskjold *et al.*, 1970). The JLS-V9 bone marrow cell line cultivated in Microtest plates was infected with Mononey leukemia virus and a new surface antigen was detected on the infected monolayer cells by immune adherence employing the serum of mice immunized by Moloney leukemia virus. Detaching of the cells is not necessary and one could perform the reaction with extremely small amounts to economize reagents.

The reaction conducted in the same tissue culture system was compared with the result employing the micro mixed hemadsorption test. The mixed hemadsorption seems to be more sensitive than the immune adherence when H-2 antigens were tested, but sensitivity of both methods was within the same range when the detection of the surface antigens reactive with anti-Moloney serum was attempted. Immune adherence has the high sensitivity as well as specificity for detection of IgM antibody as opposed to that of IgG antibody (Nishioka *et al.*, 1967a). On the other hand, the sensitivity of the mixed antiglobulin reaction is much higher for IgG antibody than the immune adherence, but much less sensitive for IgM antibody (Sell and Spooner, 1966). Therefore, both methods can be applied to monolayer tissue culture cells with extremely small quantity of reagents. In respect to the sensitivity, it seems likely that immune adherence is suitable for detecting IgM antibody and mixed hemagglutination is preferable for detecting IgG antibody.

3. *Immune Adherence with Particulate Antigens Other than Intact Cells*

Other than intact cell surface antigens, the immune adherence reaction has recently been employed for various antigen-antibody systems, especially for particulate antigens.

Because viral antigen, virus-associated antigen, or other antigens in subcellular fractions have to be measured by employing sensitive methods to analyze tumor-host relationships or to pursue the fate of the viruses in viral oncogenesis, the immune adherence test has been applied for such a purpose. Reducing the ionic strength of the reaction medium to 0.084 supplemented by addition of isotonic sucrose, Ito and Tagaya (1966) observed a positive immune adherence pattern of SV40, adenovirus type 3, 5, herpes simplex viruses, B virus, polioviruses type 1, 2, 3, Coxsackie virus A7, B5 and Echo virus type 3, 9, 14, 19, and 25 reacting with their specific antibodies. The box titration pattern, as shown in Fig. 5, indicates 16 times greater sensitivity for antibody titration as compared with that of complement fixation. Employing this method, the time course of SV40 multiplication in green monkey kidney cells both in culture fluid and in the cells was pursued as shown in

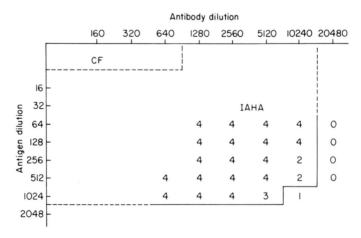

Fig. 5. Box titration of SV40 virus by immune adherence hemagglutination and complement fixation test. Antigen: SV40-GM-8. Antibody: Anti-SV40/green monkey antibody. (From Ito and Tagaya, 1966.)

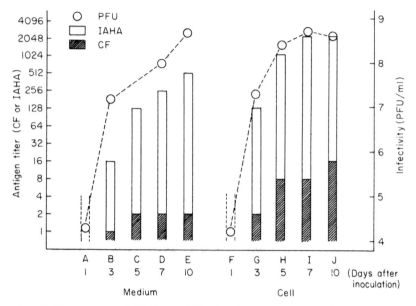

FIG. 6. Time course of SV40 multiplication in green monkey kidney cells. Comparative titration of antigen by immune adherence, complement fixation, and infectivity measurement. (From Ito and Tagaya, 1966.)

Fig. 6 with high sensitivity (Ito and Tagaya, 1966). To obtain more efficient reactivity of C1, C4, C2, C3, and a good sedimentation pattern of nonreacted human erythrocytes, Tamura and Nelson (1968) described a method to carry out the reaction up to C1, C4, C2, and C3 in 3 volumes of glucose-GVB^{2+} (equal volume mixture of GVB^{2+} and 5% glucose, containing optimal amount of Ca^{2+} and Mg^{2+}) at 30°C. for 30 minutes followed by addition of 1 volume of 0.375 M NaCl and then a human erythrocyte suspension in 0.01 M EDTA-GVB was added as indicator cells. After shaking for 5 minutes and incubation at 37°C., the hemagglutination pattern was read about 2 hours after addition of human erythrocytes. To obtain the maximum reactivity with antibody, the ratio of the number of antigen particles to the number of human erythrocytes is important. It should be predetermined by box titration for each antigen-antigen-antibody system concerned. Approximate figures with particulate antigens were given as described before. Employing 2×10^7 human erythrocytes in the reaction mixture, 4.5 to 8×10^{11} of soluble protein such as bovine serum albumin or egg albumin gave the highest reactivity for antibody titration (Nishioka, 1963). As for soluble proteins, the sensitivity is not so strikingly high as compared with particulate antigen, probably owing to spatial restriction, i.e., the lack of enough space in which multiple C3 molecules could adhere to the surface of the soluble antigen molecule.

Australia antigen was found in relatively high frequency in sera of patients with acute leukemia (Blumberg et al., 1965). The association of this serum antigen with serum hepatitis after blood transfusion has been found (Blumberg et al., 1968; Okochi and Murakami, 1968; Prince, 1968) and a direct etiological relationship of leukemia with the antigen is not likely at this moment. When compared with transfused non-leukemic patients, however, the frequency of appearance of Australia antigen in transfused acute lymphocytic leukemia and chronic lympho-cytic leukemia is very high while there are no significant differences in acute and chronic myelogenous leukemia (Sutnik et al., 1970) sug-gesting a persistent infection of serum hepatitis in lymphocytic leukemia due to immune defects induced by virus infection, either on or not on a genetic basis. The phenomena of immunological impairments have been associated with several types of neoplasia due either to chemical carcinogens or oncogenic viruses (Odaka et al., 1966; Salaman and Wedderburn, 1966; Ball, 1970) and it became an important problem both for tumor-host relationships and for the carcinogenic process. De-tection of Australia antigen with more quantitative and sensitive methods would provide information, not only to exclude the blood donor with Australia antigen-positive blood for the prophylaxis of posttrans-fusion hepatitis but as an indicator of some immunological impairment effects in several selected diseases including neoplastic diseases. From a technical point of view, employment of dithiothreitol enabled us to detect small amounts of antigens in excess serum materials which have hitherto interfered with reading of positive patterns of immune ad-herence, owing to the presence of C3 inactivator. Therefore, it would be worthwhile to describe the procedure used in the Blood Transfusion Service of the University of Tokyo Hospital as a typical protocol for detection of virus-related antigen (Mayumi et al., 1971).

As the source of antibody to Australia antigen, sera from patients with liver cirrhosis having received multiple transfusions and a heated plasma protein preparation were employed. The sera were heated at 56°C. for 30 minutes before use. Five units of antibody determined by box titration were employed for detection of antigen. As a test sample for the presence of Australia antigen, serum was separated from donor's blood and was heated at 56°C. for 30 minutes. As a source of complement, serum taken from young guinea pigs and stored at −70°C. was employed. One drop (0.025 ml.) of 1/75 or 1/100 dilution of guinea pig serum did not give any nonspecific hemagglutination pattern with the reagents used. Using a U-type microplate, 0.025 ml. of 2-fold dilutions of test sample in GVB^{2+}

and 0.025 ml. of antibody were mixed with gentle mechanical shaking in a micromixer and incubated at 37°C. for 1 hour. Then 0.025 ml. of fresh guinea pig serum at 1/75 or 1/100 dilution was added and mixed well. After 40 minutes at 37°C., 0.025 ml. of 3 mg./ml. solution of dithio-threitol in 0.04 M EDTA-GVB was added followed by mixing with 0.025 ml. of human erythrocyte suspension (type 0, 1.2×10^8/ml. in 0.04 M EDTA GVB) in a micromixer, keeping up the vibration for 10 minutes. After the plate was left undisturbed at 24°C. for 120 minutes or more, the bottom pattern of the sedimented indicator erythrocytes was observed as described above. By this procedure, the limitation of immune adherence hemagglutination that had hitherto bothered us was overcome, resulting in improvement of sensitivity and reproducibility. The positive pattern persisted unchanged for several days. A comparative experiment of immune adherence with that of conventional microcomplement fixation employing 3CH50 at 37°C. for 60 minutes is shown in Fig. 7. The immune adherence test is 60 times more sensitive than the microcomplement fixation test for detection of Australia antigen and about 10,000 times more sensitive than the agar diffusion precipitin test currently used in many laboratories.

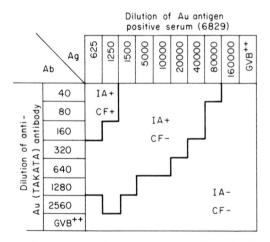

FIG. 7. Box titration of Australia antigen and antibody by immune adherence hemagglutination test and by complement fixation test. (From Mayumi *et al.*, 1971.)

B. MECHANISM AND BIOLOGICAL IMPLICATIONS

Immune adherence (R. A. Nelson, 1953) has been known as a phenomenon in which antigen-antibody complex specifically attaches to IA receptor of indicator cells when the complex has been reacted with the

first four components of complement, i.e., C1, C4, C2, and C3 to form
EAC1423 on the antigen surface (Nishioka and Linscott, 1963). Although
the C2 molecule is released from the complex by a decay reaction with a
half-life of about 23 minutes at 37°C. to give EA143, the immune adherence reactivity of the complex is not decreased (Nishioka and Linscott, 1963). Tamura and Nelson (1967) have shown that EAC43, which
is prepared from EAC143 by treatment with EDTA, also has the immune adherence reactivity unchanged. When EAC43 cells were treated
with 40 µg./ml. of pronase, almost all C4 sites were removed as determined by C4 hemolytic activity or release of isotope-labeled C4. However, these enzyme-treated cells retained immune adherence reactivity
unchanged, showing positive hemagglutination with anti-C3 antibody
(Sekine et al., 1970). A similar phenomenon was shown to occur between
human erythrocytes and tanned sheep erythrocytes coated with highly
purified guinea pig C3 only, i.e., without antibody C1, C4, and C2 (Okada
et al., 1970b). These results indicate that C3 bound on antigen surface is
the sole complement component reacting with IA receptor of indicator
cells. Since highly purified C3 was obtained (Shin and Mayer, 1968;
S. Takahashi et al., 1970), more detailed information has been accumulated on the structure and function of C3 especially concerned with immune adherence reactivity. Purified C3 was radioimmunoelectrophoreti-
cally homogeneous and when examined by electron microscopy with
negative staining using phosphotungstic acid, it gave a uniform homogeneous pattern suggesting high purity of C3 (Suzuki et al., 1971). It had
a circular subunit with a diameter of about 30 Å. When the partial specific
volume of the subunits were assumed to be 0.75 ml./gm., the molecular
weight of the subunit was calculated to be 11,000. When the number of
subunits is assumed to be 17, the whole molecular weight becomes 187,000,
which is very close to that of C3 molecules. On the other hand, concerning
its function, C3 was first found as an essential serum factor reacting in
immune adherence and in immune hemolysis (Nishioka and Linscott,
1963; Linscott and Nishioka, 1963). At present, C3 has been demonstrated to be associated with various biological functions such as immune
phagocytosis (Gigli and Nelson, 1968), peptidase activity (Cooper and
Becker, 1967), generation of anaphylatoxin (da Silva et al., 1967;
Cochrane and Müller-Eberhard, 1968) or chemotactic factor (Ward,
1967), substrate of C3 inactivator (Tamura and Nelson, 1967), con-
glutinogen-activating factor (Lachmann and Müller-Eberhard, 1968),
potentiation of viral neutralization (Yoshino and Taniguchi, 1969; Linscott and Levinson, 1969) or opsonin present in normal mammalian sera
against Diplococcus pneumoniae, and Escherichia coli (Smith and Wood,
1969). A new function of C3 was recently found in the changes in mem-

brane surface reactivity. Although electrophoretic mobility of sensitized sheep erythrocytes increases when reacted with C2, the mobility increases further when reacted with C3 in the sequential reaction of complement component (Kojima et al., 1971). Change in the C2 step is reversible when either C1 or C2 is removed while increase in the C3 step is not reversible when C1 and/or C2 are removed and no other significant change was observed after reaction with other components up to C8; C9 decreases the mobility due to E* formation or rupture of erythrocytes. Molecular anatomy of C3 has been investigated in such a situation and much attention has been paid to elucidating the relationship of molecular structure to these biological activities. We have been engaged in a study on the molecular structure of C3 concerned with its immune adherence activity to clarify the mechanism of this reaction as well as to elucidate the biological activity of C3 on a molecular level.

It has recently been found that dithiothreitol has a remarkable effect on the C3 molecule on EAC43 (Nishioka et al., 1971a,b). The dithiothreitol (DTT)-treated cells became resistant to C3 inactivator as mentioned before. By this treatment, IA reactivity of EAC43 was not changed, although hemolytic reactivity of DTT-treated EAC43 was suppressed further by treatment with monoiodacetate while further treatment with ferricyanide or p-chloromercuribenzoate restored partially the hemolytic reactivity and susceptibility to C3 inactivator. Through these treatments, IA reactivity of EAC43 was not changed. A new inhibitor recently found by Okada et al. (1970a), C5 site generation inhibitor, fixes on C3 of EAC43 and inhibits the hemolytic reactivity of EAC43 with C1, C4, C2 C5, C6, C7, C8, and C9. It does not inhibit the IA reactivity at all.

These results point to differences between the IA reactive site and the hemolytic site on C3 molecules bound to EAC43 cells. The portion of the molecule acting as the hemolytic site and the site susceptible to C3 inactivator have some dependence on disulfide bonds but the IA reactive site has little relationship to disulfide bonds. Moreover, C5 site generation inhibitor may fix on the adjacent part of the hemolytic site which may be a receptor for the C5 molecule and which may be distant from the IA reactive site on the same molecule. Partial enzymic degradation of C3 bound on EAC43 cells and its cross absorption agglutination study showed similar results, indicating a difference between the hemolytic site and the immune adherence reactive site.

Further elucidation of the molecular structure of C3 in relation to its immunological activity was obtained. Cleavage of the C3 molecule on EAC43 was carried out by trypsin digestion and C3 inactivator treatment. Three antigenically different submolecular fragments were obtained from

C3 bound on EAC43 as determined by cross-absorption-agglutination employing rabbit antibody against the whole C3 molecule. The possible relationship of these molecular fragments to immune hemolysis, immune adherence, and binding activity on the cell membrane was suggested (Nishioka, 1971).

As mentioned above, the immune adherence test has proved to be a highly sensitive serological technique in detection of antigen or antibody. Since the first description of immune adherence, the phenomenon also has been considered in relation to the body defense reaction and a hypothesis that primate erythrocytes participate in the body defense mechanism was presented by R. A. Nelson (1956). Such an assumption has been supported by the finding that both immune adherence and immune phagocytosis phenomena are induced by the same complement component, i.e., C1, C4, C2, and C3 and immune adherence receptors on the cell surface.

Moreover, participation of complement, especially of C3 as an essential factor in opsonization of normal serum has been demonstrated (Smith and Wood, 1969). In such a way, the immune adherence reaction or the reaction of IA receptor and antigen-antibody-C1423 complex is considered to be one of the prototypes of the body defense reaction. The direct enhancement of immune phagocytosis as well as the enhancement of antibody production induced *in vivo* could be based on a similar principle.

It has been generally considered that two kinds of cell systems, macrophages and lymphatic cells, are involved in Ab formation. Recognition of antigens occurs in "macrophages" which are thought to pass on information to Ab-producing "lymphatic cells." It is generally known that after administration of a specific antigen (Ag) to a host in which a small amount of Ab coexists, a much greater amount of Ab is produced. This phenomenon may be explained as follows. Ag forms a complex with coexisting Ab, C1, C4, C2, and C3. The adherence rate of this complex to macrophages increases considerably because of the presence of an immune adherence receptor on the cell surface of macrophages. This is the case in enhanced phagocytosis of Ag by Ab and C1, C4, C2, and C3, analogous to immune adherence (Nishioka and Linscott, 1963; Gigli and Nelson, 1968). The macrophages consequently receive a much larger quantity of Ag and pass on more extensive information to lymphatic cells. This would then result in a much higher rate of production of Ab. The process postulated above can explain enhanced antibody production in secondary response or anamnestic reaction because of the coexistence of Ab *in vivo*, even if only a very small amount is left after the initial administration of Ag. This assumption is compatible with the following findings. (a) Enhanced protective immunity was induced by the simultaneous injection of living anthrax vaccine with the antiserum (Sobernheim, 1902, 1904). (b) After the combined injection of antigens with immunoglobulins, antibody formation against heterologous immune globulins was enhanced (Adler, 1956). (c) By the simultaneous injection of Ag and specific antiserum, the immunological sensitization of mice was enhanced (Terres and Wilson, 1961; Morrison and Terres, 1966). (d) There was localization of antigen, antibody (IgM or IgG), and C3 complex in germinal center of lymph nodes presumably on the surface of dendritic macrophage (Gajl-Peczalska et al., 1969) in germinal center of lymph nodes.

Our attempts to induce heightened resistance against isografts of C3H/He mouse mammary tumor (MM2) in syngenic mice were started on this working hypothesis (Nishioka et al., 1969a). When a rabbit antibody is prepared by immunization with MM2, two kinds of antigenic sites must be considered in MM2. They are common antigens to normal tissue components of C3H/He mice, and tumor antigens characteristic to MM2 distinct from nonmalignant components. Both antigens are sensitized by rabbit Ab. In the course of immune cytolysis and immune phagocytosis of MM2 tumors in recipient C3H/He mice, the breakdown products, consisting of material common to normal tissue components, would be metabolized through the host system without being recognized as "not-self." This assumption is compatible with the finding that no histoincompatibility was found with regard to skin grafts from normal C3H mice to resistance-induced mice. Tumor antigens can be differentiated from normal tissue components, through whose deviations the tumor Ab is produced. Antigens should be recognized as "not-self" in a syngenic host, even if the grade of heterogeneity from normal tissue components might be subtle. In the course of breakdown of MM2 by rabbit Ab and C in syngenic host, a tumor antigen–rabbit Ab–C3H/He C1423 complex would be formed. The complex would be trapped more efficiently by macrophages. As postulated above, more extensive information from the macrophages would be expected to induce more efficient Ab production in lymphatic cells. Then, following the repeated challenges with fresh MM2 tumor acting as a booster and eliciting recycling of the process postulated above, syngenic antibody against MM2 tumor was demonstrated in the sera of syngenic mice (Takeuchi et al., 1969).

V. C1 Fixation and Transfer Reaction

A. Principle and Methods

As sensitive indicators for the presence of antigen-antibody complex on the cell surface, binding and activation of C1 have been utilized based

on the technique of C1 fixation and transfer as described by Borsos and
Rapp (1965a). The principle of this test comprises three steps. According
to Borsos *et al.* (1968), this test is capable of measuring antigen, antibody, or C1 concentration on an absolute molecular basis based on a
"one-hit" process of Mayer (1961b). First, antigen-antibody complex
was reacted with excess amount of CĪ (activated form of the first component of C) at i.s. 0.065. Second, CĪ reacted and bound to the antigen-
antibody complex was transfered to sensitized sheep erythrocytes carrying
C4 on their surface (EAC4) at ionic strength (i.s.) 0.150 to generate
EACĪ4. Third, the EACĪ4 thus formed was lysed by the addition of C2
and the remainder of C components in excess. Thus there are the three
stages:

1. Fixation stage Ag-Ab + excess C1 → AgAbCĪ at i.s. 0.065
2. Transfer stage Ag-Ab-CĪ + EAC4 → EACĪ4 + Ag-Ab at i.s. 0.150
3. Lysis stage EACĪ4 + C2 + C in EDTA → hemolysis.

Finally from the degree of lysis, the number of CĪ bound by the antigen-
antibody complex was calculated. Detection of cell surface antigens of
virus-induced mouse leukemia was reported after the leukemia cells were
reacted with corresponding antiserum. Employing Forssman IgM antibody on sheep erythrocytes 30 to 50% of the CĪ measured by this
technique was detected by direct cytolysis and only 0.03% of the
CĪ sites on sensitized mouse leukemia cells measured by this test were
detectable by direct cytolysis. In the latter case, the immune cytolysis of
mouse leukemia cells proved to be a one-hit reaction. CĪ fixation transfer
test also gives a very high sensitivity, to detect or quantitate cell surface
antigen or antibody (Borsos *et al.*, 1968).

This method is applicable for the analysis of antibody-complement
interactions which lead to a variety of manifestations of immunological
reaction. Borsos and Rapp (1965b) demonstrated that a single molecule
of IgM antibody in combination with antigen at the cell surface fixed one
molecule of CĪ, while two molecules of IgG in proximity on the cell surface are required to fix one molecule of C1; but recently a unique type of
IgG which fixes CĪ by a single molecule was found in the New Zealand
white rabbit immunized by boiled sheep erythrocyte stromata in Freund's
adjuvant (Frank and Gaither, 1970). Problems such as heterogeneity of
IgM antibodies, avidity of anti-Forssman antibodies, and difference
among immunoglobulin classes in complement fixation abilities have been
widely examined employing this technique (T. Ishizaka *et al.*, 1966;
Hoyer *et al.*, 1968; Linscott, 1969a).

Although the CĪ fixation and transfer test has made it possible to
quantitate interactions between antigen, antibody, and complement on a

moleclular basis, it needs some modification when more quantitative analysis is required in various experimental conditions. It was demonstrated at physiological i.s. (0.147), that the formation of EAC1, using sheep erythrocytes sensitized with purified IgG, was greater at 0°C. than at 37°C.; in contrast, the formation of EAC1 with IgM proceeded more efficiently at 37°C. than at 0°C. (Tamura and Nelson, 1968). The ionic strength 0.115 was found to be optimal for $C\bar{I}$ transfer to EAC4; and at 30°C., transfer of $C\bar{I}$ from the IgG sensitized cells was much better than at 0°C. but with IgM antibody it was the converse (Linscott, 1969b). Furthermore, the amount of IgG (and to a lesser extent IgM) which is used to make antigen-antibody C1 complex has a dramatic effect on the transferability to EAC4 (Linscott, 1969c). According to his experiments, Linscott suggested that C1 bound to IgG dimers transfers readily at i.s. = 0.0063, while C1 bound to IgG trimers transfers readily only at i.s. = 0.14; and $C\bar{I}$ bound to IgG tetramers may fail to transfer altogether. It is also necessary, to minimize reutilization of C1 by reduction of site to site transfer of $C\bar{I}$ not to overestimate $C\bar{I}$ molecules. For this reason, EAC4 prepared from rabbit IgG antibody was not suitable for the assay of $C\bar{I}$ and it is preferred to employ EAC4 prepared from rabbit IgM antibody (Colten et al., 1969). Furthermore, the physicochemical heterogeneity of C1 molecules might interfere with the quantitative measurement by these immune hemolytic assays (M. Takahashi et al., 1965; Tachibana, 1967; Hoffmann, 1968; Nagaki and Stroud, 1969).

B. Detection of in Vivo Immune Response against Tumor Cells

Despite the problems of the measurement of C1 on an absolute molecular basis which remains for solution, the measurement of C1 bound on tumor cells taken directly from experimental animals or clinical material, would give definitive information on whether the autochthonous host may react immunologically against its own tumor. Our experiments based on these points will be described (Nishioka et al., 1968).

1. Measurement of C1 Attached on Heterografted, Homografted, and Isografted Tumors

Ascites rat hepatoma AH-13, Ehrlich ascites tumor, and transplantable mouse mammary tumor MM2 were employed as heterograft, homograft, and isograft tumors. AH-13 and MM2 tumor were transplanted intraperitoneally into two groups of C3H/He mice and Ehrlich ascites tumor was transplanted in dd mice. Four, 6, 8, 10, and 12 days after the transplantation, the tumor cells were collected from three mice in each group, and the number of C1 attached to the cells was determined.

In the case of heterograft AH-13 in C3H/He mice, the number of C1/cell was 60 after 4 days. It increased to 120 and 176 on 6 and 8 days, respectively. These values reflected the immune responses in C3H/He mice to AH-13 and resulted in disappearance of tumor cells from the peritoneal cavity after 10–12 days. The cell populations collected at this stage were composed of nonmalignant C3H/He cells and the number of C1 attached to these cells was only 22–25. Serum antibody against AH-13 tumor cells was detected by the direct agglutination test at this stage.

In the case of Ehrlich ascites tumor homografted to dd mice, the number of C1 attached to tumor cells was 88 in the inoculum itself. It increased to 176 on the fourth day, probably as a result of sensitization by natural allogenic antibody and suddenly decreased to 36 on the sixth day. This might reflect the competitive relationship between tumor growth and immunological sensitization of the allogenic host. The value increased again after 8 to 10 days and simultaneously showed a prolongation of survival time. In such a situation MM2 tumor can be harvested after 30 to 45 days. As shown in Table VII, a much higher amount of C1 was present on tumor cells. These tumor cells showed regression later.

These preliminary C1 transfer tests may reflect the immune responses of the heterografted, homografted, and isografted host. According to all experience, the strength of the immune response increases with increasing genetic distance. The present results are in line with this. It is of particular interest that an immune response is even present in the syngenic host against the MM2 tumor, as indicated by the C1 transfer test. This system has been characterized previously with regard to the antibody and the immunochemical nature of the antigenic substance carried out by the target cell (Nishioka et al., 1969a,b; Takeuchi et al., 1969; Irie et al., 1969). These findings support the view that tumor-

TABLE VII

NUMBER OF C1 BOUND TO TUMOR CELLS IN HETEROGRAFTED, HOMOGRAFTED, AND ISOGRAFTED TUMOR CELLS IN C3H/HE MICE

Tumor	Origin	Host mouse strain	Days after transplantation							
			0	4	6	8	10	12	30	45
AH-13	Rat	C3H/He	0.3	60	120	176	25[a]	22[a]		
Ehrlich ascites tumor	dd mice	dd	88	176	36	110	341	454		
MM2	C3H/He mice	C3H/He	45	25	35	63	57	62	149[b]	163[b]

[a] Nonmalignant cells in peritoneal cavity of C3H/He mice.
[b] These mice were inoculated with AH-13 simultaneously.

specific antibody reacted against the surface antigen of the MM2 tumor cell and this was followed by the fixation of C1 on the antigen-antibody complex on the cell.

2. *Measurement of C1 Attached to Burkitt Lymphoma Cells*

Based on the above observations, a search was made for evidence of an immune reaction in an autochthnous tumor-host system by measurement of C1 bound to human tumor cells. Membrane fluorescence staining was performed in parallel on the same biopsy material and the results are compared.

Table VIII lists the results with biopsy cells from the Burkitt lymphoma patients, Daudi [Kenya Cancer Council (KCC) number 750], Opasa (KCC 766), and Isaac (KCC 788). C1/cell of 32.6 and 52.3 were demonstrated on the biopsy cells of Daudi, sampled on May 23 and 30, 1967 respectively, while a very small amount of C1 was found on the cells of Opasa and Isaac. Membrane fluorescence tests showed that a high percentage of Daudi cells were positive with anti-IgG, anti-IgM, and conjugates, and the kappa + lambda anti-light chain conjugate as well. Only a very low percentage of the Opasa or Isaac cells were positive. These data showed good correlation with the C1 measurement. It was shown, however, that the IgM coating on the surface of the Daudi cell is due to the surface-accumulating production of IgM by the Daudi cell, and not the coating from the outside (E. Klein *et al.*, 1968). Membrane IgM reactivity was maintained in the derived, established lines during prolonged cultivation *in vitro* in contrast to the IgG coating which was promptly lost. Therefore, the Daudi cells stained by the IgM reagent should not be considered as the cells sensitized by IgM antibody *in vivo*. This was confirmed in the present experiment with Daudi cells in tissue culture. The cell line started from the biopsy taken on May 23, 1967, and subcultured for 12 passages *in vitro* showed 100% membrane positivity with the anti-IgM and anti-kappa reagents but was negative with anti-IgG. Tissue culture cells derived from the May 30 sample, the first biopsy taken after massive tumor necrosis had been induced by cytosin arabinoside therapy, were, however, completely negative with both the IgM and IgG reagents. This fact indicates that the IgG coating of both the May 23 and 30 biopsies may reflect an immune response *in vivo*.

The number of C1 attached to the surface of tissue-cultured Daudi cells still showed values between 6.7 and 7.5. These C1 units can be removed by the addition of fetal calf serum employed in tissue culture medium. Therefore, the small amount of fixed C1 on the cultured cell may be attributed to the occurence of natural antibody and C1 in the fetal calf serum.

Table IX shows the results from 7 biopsy specimens. Three serial

TABLE VIII

Number of C1 Bound to Tumor Cells and Percentage of Cells with Membrane Fluorescence After Exposure to Fluorescein-Conjugated Anti-Human Immunoglobulin Reagents

Anti-Ig reagent	Biopsy						Derived tissue culture Daudi			
	Daudi (KCC[a] 750)				Opasa (KCC 766)	Isaac (KCC 788)				
	0502[b]	0509	0523	0530			0502(6)[c]	0509(4)	0523(12)	0530(8)
IgG	24	17	75	82	0	7	0	0	0	0
IgM	100	100	97	20	4	10	100	96	100	0
IgA	24	20	24	60	0	7	0	0	17	4
Kappa + lambda	100	100	100	25	4	2	100	100	96	—
Kappa									100	11
Lambda									11	
C1 cell			32.6	52.3	3.7	2.4			6.3	7.5

[a] Kenya Cancer Council number.
[b] Date of biopsy.
[c] No. of subcultures *in vitro*.

TABLE IX

NUMBER OF C1 BOUND TO TUMOR CELLS AND PERCENTAGE OF CELLS WITH
FLUORESCENCE AFTER EXPOSURE TO FLUORESCEIN-CONJUGATED ANTI-HUMAN
IMMUNOGLOBULIN REAGENTS

Anti-Ig reagent	Biopsy material						
	Isaac (KCC 788)			Katana (KCC 801)	Abwao (KCC 812)	Kibe (KCC 813)	Ekesa (KCC 816)
IgG	7	3	0	29	26	0	24
IgM	3	13	0	32	59	4	88
IgA	15	0	3	3	6	0	13
Lambda	3	6	5	18	22	29	20
Kappa	4	4	34	44	53	100	61
C1/cell	2.5	5.0	2.9	14.2	12.2	442	46

biopsies taken from the same patient (Isaacs) gave low values for both Ig-binding by the membrane fluorescence test and bound C1 per cell. Biopsy materials from three other patients (Katana, Abwao, and Ekesa) showed moderately positive membrane staining with the anti-IgG and IgM reagents. The value of bound C1/cell was also moderately elevated. An exceptional result was obtained with the Kibe cell. Only slight positivity was observed by IgM or IgG staining whereas anti-kappa staining was 100% positive. A very high value (442/cell) was obtained for C1 binding. In this case, two explanations could be postulated regarding this interesting result. Some unknown immunoglobulin which has K chain but lacks μ or γ might be present on the cell, or C1 attached on the cell surface might interfere in the staining with anti-μ or anti-γ reagent.

These observations indicate that a certain relationship may exist between percentage of cells that show stainability with anti-IgG or IgM reagent and C1 attachment. This indicates that the IgG and/or IgM stained by membrane fluorescence carries antibody activity directed against cell surface antigens and is capable of fixing C1. More detailed and accumulated observations were carried out by Tachibana and G. Klein (1970). Correlation was found between the value of bound C1 and IgM or IgG staining on the Burkitt tumor cell surface but not IgA, noncomplement fixing immunoglobulin staining. Depletion of C4 by tumor cells carrying C1 on their surface was also demonstrated by Chang (1967).

These initial observations are in agreement with the postulate that the autochthonous tumor host may react immunologically against his own tumor. It is very important to clarify why tumor cells sensitized by autochthonous antibody and C1 did not undergo cytolysis. Unfruitful site generation through to immune cytolysis, participation of complement component inhibitors, blocking by noncomplement-fixing antibody, target cell resistance to complement-induced lysis (immunoresistance), and quantitative insufficiency of the immune response in relation to tumor growth may be considered.

VI. Complement Fixation Test

A. Principle and Methods

Depending on the two properties of the complement system, (a) the fixation of complement by antigen-antibody aggregates and (b) the lysis of sheep red cells sensitized by rabbit antibody, complement fixation has long been employed for detection of subcellular antigens, soluble antigens, and even intact cellular antigens. It has given a potential tool especially for the analysis of viral carcinogenesis by measuring type-specific or group-specific virion antigen or a variety of nonvirion antigens. The most adequate standard method was described by Mayer (1961a) based on fundamental work on the complement system. The principle of the complement fixation test (CFT) is represented as follows.

$Ag + Ab + C \rightarrow$ (fixation of C) $+$ sensitized cell (EA) $\rightarrow$ no hemolysis $=$ positive CFT

Ag or Ab alone $+ C \rightarrow$ (no fixation of C) $+ EA \rightarrow$ hemolysis $=$ negative CFT

Therefore, the essential key point in CFT is to employ a limited and carefully regulated quantity of complement in the reaction mixture, and factors influencing complement activity should be controlled throughout the experiment. Standardization of complement dose should be done in terms of the 50% hemolytic unit (CH50). Five CH50 should be employed in a total fixation volume of 1.3 ml. in GVB^{2+} at 2 to 4°C. for 20 hours followed by incubation at 37°C. for 30 minutes. Sensitized erythrocytes, 0.2 ml. of 5×10^8/ml. cell suspension in GVB^{2+} is added and reacted at 37°C. for 60 minutes. The reading was given as degree of hemolysis, $0 =$ no lysis, $1 =$ approximately 25% lysis, $2 =$ approximately 50% lysis, $3 =$ approximately 75% lysis, and $4 =$ complete lysis. If the antigen-antibody fixes 5CH50, there is no hemolysis. When the antigen-antibody fixes 4CH50 out of 5CH50 added, the remaining 1CH50 will produce 50% lysis of indicator sensitized sheep erythrocytes and usually this is taken as an end point of CFT. By these procedures, false positive reactions can be minimized.

Since a limited amount of complement is employed, the anti-complementary activity of test reagents, especially present in the antigen or antibody source separately, should be eliminated as far as possible. When separately tested at twice the concentration as in the test proper, antigen or antibody alone should not display anticomplementary action. Another useful control is to set up the antigen or antibody control with 3CH50 to exclude participation of even slightly anticomplementary activity (Mayer, 1961a). There also exists an optimal ratio in regard to antigen or antibody concentrations in the reaction mixture. It is necessary to determine the level of antigen concentration yielding the highest antibody titer by box titration for each antigen-antibody system. To save reagents, CFT with a small volume (0.7 ml.) was devised by Wasserman and Levine (1961). Recently microtiter technique has been employed widely (Sever, 1962). A total volume of 100 μl. in this test can economize on antigen or antibody as well as time. Using a V type microplate, 25-μl. aliquots of antigen, 5CH50 of complement, and antibody in GVB^{2+} were added in each well and sealed and incubated at 37°C. for 1 hour. The sensitized sheep erythrocytes, 25 μl. of 1×10^8/ml. cell suspension in GVB^{2+} were added and the plates were sealed and incubated for an additional hour at 37°C. The plates were then centrifuged at 1800g for 7 minutes and the degree of hemolysis in each well recorded as 0 to 4 according to the criteria of the complement fixation test. Each test should include a control for anticomplementary activity of serum or antigen as well as a back titration of complement employed in the test proper.

B. Interaction between Complement and Immunoglobulins

The limitation of techniques to measure the antigen-antibody reaction through complement-mediated immune reactions is to be considered in regard to the nature of antibodies or antigens. These limitations also should be considered in the immune adherence, $C\bar{1}$ fixation and transfer tests, and the immune cytotoxicity reaction. Of five human immunoglobulin classes, IgG and IgM are mainly concerned with complement-mediated reactions while A is not. This was clearly demonstrated on a molecular level by $C\bar{1}$ fixation and transfer tests (T. Ishizaka et al., 1966) with human anti-A isoantibodies.

Complement-fixing ability of these different immunoglobulin classes was also demonstrated by complement-dependent hemolysis of sheep erythrocytes coupled with nonantibody human IgG and IgM by means of Cr treatment but there was no hemolysis of the cells coupled with IgA (Inai and Tsuyuguchi, 1969). Hiramatsu et al. (1969) observed no complement hemolysis of sheep erythrocytes coupled with λ type IgD myeloma immunoglobulin for which antibody activity has been unknown.

Employing their original method, T. Ishizaka et al. (1970) found no complement fixation of nonspecifically aggregated IgE and IgD while aggregated IgG or IgM showed fixation of C and aggregated IgA failed as described before (K. Ishizaka and Ishizaka, 1960; T. Ishizaka et al., 1967). Although such nonimmunologically induced molecular assembly showed low efficiency in the manifestation of biological activities as compared with immunological specific molecular assembly of antigen-antibody complex, all these findings suggested that IgG and IgM are more likely to participate in complement-mediated reactions, while IgA, IgD, and IgE are not.

More detailed information concerning complement-fixing activity of IgG and IgM has been accumulated recently and will be briefly reviewed. Among horse antidiphtheria toxin antibodies belonging to the IgG class, Nakamura and Katsura (1964) separated noncomplement-fixing T-globulin and complement-fixing γ-globulin. These corresponded well with the ability to induce passive cutaneous anaphylaxis in the guinea pig (Nishioka et al., 1967b). As for guinea pig immunoglobulins belonging to the IgG class, Benacerraf et al. (1963) separated two different types of antibody, showing that the fast-moving $7S\gamma 1$-globulin did not fix complement while the slow-moving $7S\gamma 2$ did. In this case, the skin sensitizing activities of two immunoglobulins showed the reverse of complement fixation. However, a more precise examination was made of the complement-fixing ability of $7S\gamma 1$-immunoglobulin. Sandberg et al. (1970) showed that $7S\gamma 1$-globulins diminish the hemolytic activity in fresh serum when added as preformed antigen-antibody precipitates, although a profile of complement component fixation by $7S\gamma 1$ differs from $7S\gamma 2$. $7S\gamma 1$ immune complex reacted with C3 and the later components despite little, if any, utilization of C1, C4, and C2.

Within the IgG globulin class of human immunoglobulin, the presence of four distinct subgroups was recognized. Employing aggregation and fixation of C or C1 or interaction with C1q, which is the subcomponent of C1 which interacts directly with antibody, IgG1, IgG3, and IgG2 showed interaction with C1 or C1q while IgG4 protein did not (T. Ishizaka et al., 1967; Müller-Eberhard, 1968a). These aggregates were not formed by specific antigen-antibody reaction but the result suggests that not all human IgG immunoglobulins are inhomogeneous in regard to their interaction with complement.

IgM antibodies against erythrocytes have been known to have much higher hemolytic activity than IgG antibody (Talmage et al., 1956) and single IgM antibody molecules could establish one $C\bar{1}$ site; in contrast, at least two IgG antibody molecules as a doublet are required for formation of the site (Borsos and Rapp, 1965b). This does not seem to be a generalized principle; rabbit IgG hemolysin which could induce one single C1 site on the cell was reported (Frank and Gaither, 1970). Moreover, it has been suggested that all IgM antibody molecules of rabbit hemolysin or human isoagglutinin could fix C1 (T. Ishizaka *et al.*, 1966; Rapp and Borsos, 1966b), but actually only 21% of rabbit IgM benzenearsonate antibody, which showed different electrophoretic mobility, has the C1-fixing properties (Hoyer *et al.*, 1968). In addition, the existence of a noncomplement-fixing subpopulation of IgM molecules was found in mice (Plotz *et al.*, 1968) and in guinea pigs (Linscott and Hansen, 1969). As for complement-fixing ability of IgM antibody, the efficiency was quite different depending on the number and distribution of antigenic determinants on the antigen while this phenomenon was not observed with IgG (Cunniff and Stollar, 1968). As in C1 site generation or in the immune adherence reaction, IgG antibody showed more effective complement fixation at 4°C. than at 37°C. while IgM antibody did not (Cunniff and Stollar, 1968).

At present, complement-fixing activities of IgG and IgM have been demonstrated while those of IgA, D, and E have not yet been demonstrated. IgG and IgM globulins have much heterogeneity concerned with interaction with complement, depending on the subclasses or experimental conditions, or the nature of antigens.

VII. Immune Cytotoxicity

Taking viability of the nucleated cells as indicator, the immune cytotoxicity test has been employed most widely for detection of antigen and antibody in the presence of complement. This test has features of simplicity and seems likely to have most obvious relevance to the rejection mechanism *in vivo*. As the first step in immune cytotoxicity concerns the damage of the cell membrane caused by antibody and complement on the cell surface antigens, most information has come from prototype experiment on immune hemolysis of sheep erythrocytes and much information on immunochemical analysis of cytolytic phenomena has accumulated. Recently, a unique experimental model with a chemically constructed artificial synthetic membrane (liposome) has been developed (Haxby *et al.*, 1968; Kinsky *et al.*, 1969). Although the essential principle of immunocytolysis mediated by antibody and complement obtained from these experimental models might be applicable, in general the process observed in these experimental models sometimes does not fit the cytotoxicity phenomena of a variety of other nucleated cells, and other accessory factors should be analyzed for understanding the immunocytotoxic phenomenon occurring *in vivo*.

A. Principle and Methods

For the immune cytotoxicity test, various indicators have been employed. Leakage of intracellular contents is one of the indicators, such as oxyhemoglobin from erythrocytes as most widely employed for immune hemolysis, nucleoprotein (Green *et al.*, 1959), cellular ATP (Nungester *et al.*, 1969), or the electrolyte ^{86}Rb (Hingson *et al.*, 1969).

Wigzell (1965) developed a method using ^{51}Cr for labeling of target cells in the mouse H2 system and cytotoxicity is detected by the liberation from the cell of incorporated radioactivity. Kinetic assay of lymphoid cell lysis was performed by Sanderson (1965) employing this method and he showed that the reaction proceeded in an identical fashion with immune hemolysis of sheep erythrocytes. Thereafter this was employed more widely because of its high precision and reproducibility and applied to the characterization of histocompatibility antigens or antibody (Nathenson and Davies, 1966; Davies, 1968), and also to the tumor-specific transplantation antigen of Moloney virus-induced lymphoma cells (Haughton, 1965).

Metabolic impairments measured by cessation of glycolysis (Flax, 1956) or dehydrogenase activities (Yamamoto *et al.*, 1956; Nishioka *et al.*, 1956) also could be used as an indicator of cytotoxic effects. In the latter method, the capacity of living tumor cells to reduce a redox dye such as 2.6-dichlorophenol indophenol was taken as the indicator of the viability of the cells. This method was initially invented for the assay of antitumor antibiotics (Yamamoto *et al.*, 1959) but it has been successfully employed for detection of immune cytotoxicity of Ehrlich ascites tumor and Sarcoma 180 induced by rabbit antibody and guinea pig complement (Nishioka *et al.*, 1958). Any non-reduced 2.6 dichlorophenol indophenol remaining was transferred to a butanol layer and after extraction could be quantitated spectrophotometrically. When the reaction was carried out with target cells in soft agar, the blue color of the redox dye was decolorized by dehydrogenase activity of viable cells, whereas the color remained unchanged in the zone where the cells were killed. This was confirmed by the presence or absence of tumor-producing capacity after transplantation. The developed blue pattern corresponds to the hemolytic zone in complement-induced hemolysis in the agar.

Enzyme activity for hydrolysis of fluorescein diacetate of the viable cells in soft agarose could also be employed as an indicator of viability, as demonstrated by Rotman and Papermaster (1966). Fluorescein diacetate does not show fluorescence but fluorescein or its protein complex does. Therefore when the cell membrane is intact, fluorescein-diacetate incorporated in the cells was hydrolyzed to fluorescein, which complexes with a cellular component. The complex retained inside the cells showed fluorescence when observed with an ultraviolet microscope. When the cells died, they could not hydrolyze fluorescein diacetate; or, even if the enzyme activity was retained, the cell membrane was destroyed, the fluorescein-protein complex could not be retained, and these cells did not show fluorescence. The technique is not simple, but the sensitivity is high and economizes on cells, antibody, or complement. This is preferable when it is difficult to obtain a large number of target cells (Rotman and Papermaster, 1966; M. Inoue *et al.*, 1968).

The dye exclusion test with Trypan blue or eosin has been most widely employed as a convenient and rapid method This test consists in testing the permeability of cells after incubation with antibody and complement. When cytotoxic antibody is reacted with viable target cells, complement induces a permeability increase, leading to the death of target cells. The increased permeability is usually measured by addition of Trypan blue or eosin which penetrates into dead cells but leaves viable cells unstained. The original method of Gorer and O'Gorman (1956) has been most widely employed and an improved technique was reviewed by Boyse *et al.* (1964) and Batchelor (1967), and an improved 45-minute microcytotoxicity test was presented by Mittal *et al.* (1969). Technical details and evaluation of the results of the test were given in these reviews.

B. Mechanism of Immune Cytotoxicity

Depending on the differences of antigen-antibody systems, rabbit serum sometimes showed stronger cytotoxicity than guinea pig serum which has been known to be a most potent complement source for a sheep erythrocyte-antibody system. An example will be presented here. Immunocytotoxicity tests carried out with C3H/He mouse mammary tumor cells (MM102) and syngenic antibody were shown in Fig. 8. (Chang, 1970), employing three different sources of complement. The complement activity was measured by immune hemolysis according to Mayer (1961a), and cytotoxicity of tumor cells was measured after Gorer and O'Gorman (1956). At a dilution of 1:2 or 1:4 of mouse antiserum, inhibition was observed due to anticomplementary activity of mouse serum. At dilutions higher than 1:8, 1:9 CH50 units of rabbit complement are more strongly cytotoxic than 17.3 CH50 units of rat serum, and guinea pig complement showed the weakest cytotoxicity, even employing 82.7 CH50 units of hemolytic complement. High efficiency of rabbit complement was noticed in cytotoxicity tests of human (Amos, 1965), rat (Valentine *et al.*, 1967), and mouse nucleated cells (Haughton and McGehee, 1969). As a factor responsible for this high efficiency of rabbit serum in the cytotoxicity test, the enhancing effect of natural antibodies, which react either against target cells or against antibody globulin specifically combined with target cell surface, has been considered (Herberman, 1969; Haughton and McGehee, 1969). Actually, a

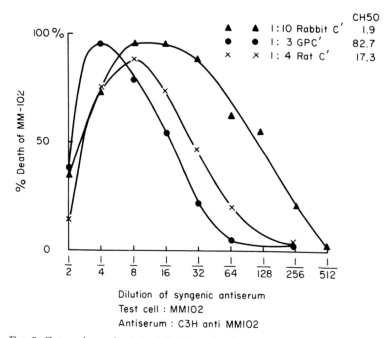

Fɪɢ. 8. Comparison of cytotoxicity test of ascites mouse mammary tumor cell by syngenic antibody reacting with rabbit, rat, and guinea pig complement. (From Chang, 1970.)

natural cytotoxic antibody was found and it is complement-dependent, heat-labile, and 7 S or 18 S in size (Herberman, 1969). This antibody reacted with an antigen on human nucleated cells but not with human or sheep erythrocytes. However, when the rabbit complement was absorbed off with target cells, still highly efficient cytotoxicity remained and it is not likely that natural antibody against target cells could play a significant role. On the other hand, the fact that addition of an optimal amount of antimouse globulin to guinea pig complement caused a modest increase in the cytotoxic efficiency of mouse antibody against alloantigen of mouse lymph node cells suggests the validity of the second possibility. However, they did not obtain the same effect of antimouse globulin on rabbit complement, and the dose-response curve also could not prove the existence of natural antiglobulin antibody in rabbit serum. It is difficult to explain why an extremely low unit of rabbit complement determined by the sheep erythrocyte system is stronger in cytotoxicity than rat serum which contains 9 times more CH50 or than guinea pig serum containing more than 40 times more CH50. Participation of an enhancing serum factor such as lysozyme, which accelerates bacteriolysis of gram-negative bacteria (Amano *et al.*, 1954; Glynn, 1969) might be plausible in this system. At this moment, more detailed information on the reaction mechanism of the complement component of rabbit or rat is required for understanding the entire mechanism of immune cytotoxicity of such nucleated cells. Some features may be pertinent. Rabbit serum requires extremely low concentrations of Ca^{2+} (Marney and Des Prez, 1969) and rat serum has a high efficiency of late-acting components (Miyakawa *et al.*, 1969). Some of the factors in target cells responsible for the different susceptibility of nucleated cells and erythrocytes, may be the difference in density of antigenic site on the cell surface, fragility of cellular membrane, distance of antigen site from the critical structure unit of membrane, and repair mechanism of nucleated cells against complement-induced damage. For practical purposes, rabbit serum showed great individual differences in complement activity and it is necessary to screen large numbers of individual rabbit sera to find suitable sources of complement for the immune cytotoxicity test in each system.

In accordance with the progress in measurement of complement-induced cytotoxicity by a quantitative technique, such as ^{51}Cr labeling (Wigzell, 1965) or electron microscopic observations (Humphrey and Dourmashkin, 1969), much more information has been accumulated on the mechanism of the immunocytotoxicity reaction as well as in a model experiment on immune hemolysis of sheep erythrocytes.

Requirement of doublet IgG mouse antibody and single IgM antibody directed against the H-2 system of mouse nucleated target cells in reaction with guinea pig complement was shown by Andersson *et al.* (1967) in a similar way to that of immune hemolysis of sheep or human erythrocytes.

Employing all nine components purified from guinea pig serum, Tamura *et al.* (1970) demonstrated that leukemia cells of the A strain mouse, RADA-1 sensitized with C57BL/6 antileukemia cell antibody and C1, C4, C2, C3, C5, C6, C7 were killed rapidly by a mixture of C8 and C9. Against leukemia cell antibody C1423567 cells, C9 without C8 did not show any significant immunocytotoxicity while C8 also produced a considerable cytotoxic effect. This experimental observation is in line with the idea that the action of guinea pig complement component on sensitized leukemia cells is essentially similar to its action on sensitized sheep erythrocytes. The heightened innate fragility of EAC1-8 cells was first described by Linscott and Nishioka (1963) and further investigated with guinea pig complement (Stolfi, 1968) and with human complement (Manni and Müller-Eberhard, 1969). A possibility that a trace of contaminated C9 causes the spontaneous lysis of EAC1-8 cells was excluded since monospecific anti-C9 antibody which functions as a specific inhibitor of hemolytic activity of C9 did not show any inhibition of the lysis of EAC1-8 (Tamura *et al.*, 1970). Although the evidence is good enough that EAC1-8 cells interact rapidly with 9, resulting in the prompt initiation of E* formation and the onset of lysis, one would prefer better cell stability in the absence of C9. In complement-mediated immune cytolysis in general, it appears as though interaction of SAC1423567 with C8 increases cell fragility by disrupting certain outer components of the cell wall, without effecting a complete breach of the integrity of this structure. The latter perhaps is then accomplished by subsequent interaction with C9.

Electron microscopic observation on complement-induced holes on the cell membrane were observed on a variety of erythrocytes as well as on ascites tumor cells by Humphrey and Dourmashkin (1965). They showed photographs of the membrane of tumor cells lysed by the action of rabbit 7 S antibody and rabbit or guinea pig complement in which multiple holes were present which were identical with those produced by similar complement in erythrocytes. The nature and characteristics of this complement-induced hole were fully described in their review (Humphrey and Dourmashkin, 1969) and it should be noted that essentially similar morphological changes were induced by complement and antibody on the membrane of erythrocytes, tumor cells, and bacterial or viral particles. As for a quantitative relationship of the number of holes to the molecular number of complement, Borsos *et al.* (1964) clearly demonstrated that the number of holes visualized correlated with the number of sites predicted by the one-hit theory, suggesting that each site produced one hole in the cell membrane. However, it is now known that the single site-single hole relationship is also observed when rabbit IgM antibody and guinea pig C were employed. In other cases, when rabbit IgG and guinea pig complement are used, or when fresh serum is used as a source of complement with both rabbit IgG and IgM antibody, the number of holes visualized was far greater than predicted, and thousands of holes may be formed at each predicted site. The results suggest that the multiple holes were produced at a step in the cytolytic sequence prior to the damage-producing step (Frank *et al.*, 1970).

C. Biological Implications

Complement-induced cytotoxic reaction has been considered to play an essential role in the humoral immune reaction in participation with all C1-C9 or C1-C8 components with complement-fixing IgG and IgM antibodies. With synergistic function of leukocytes, however, the first four or the first seven components of complement showed cytotoxic effects on target cells. Employing ^{51}Cr-labeled chicken erythrocytes with rabbit anti-Forssman antibody (A), isotope release from chicken E-EAC1-7 and E-AC1423 cells was described (Perlmann et al., 1969; Perlmann and Hölm, 1969). The first reaction proceeds more rapidly, within 4 hours and extensively with purified lymphocytes and a monocyte-rich leukocyte fraction, while the latter reaction occurred only with a monocyte-rich leukocyte fraction in 14 hours and purified lymphocytes could not cause the cytotoxic effect. Although these phenomena were described only with a single type of target cells and the background of lysis of chicken EAC1-7 cells was moderately high, these data indicate that complement is also of importance for induction of cell-mediated cytotoxicity. The lysis of chicken EAC1-3 cells with a monocyte-rich cell preparation is related to immune phagocytosis following a step of immune adherence. The destruction of chicken EAC1-7 with lymphocytes and C8 as mentioned above gave a general principle that cytotoxicity will be triggered by target cell-bound C7 and the buildup of lymphocytes or C8-susceptible sites on target cells should proceed in the sequence of reactions initiated by antibody and C1 to C7.

A possibility that the conventional sequence would be by-passed was demonstrated in the experiments of reactive lysis (Thompson and Lachmann, 1970; Lachmann and Thompson, 1970). Acute phase sera or normal sera treated with anti-C7 was mixed with zymosa, and $C\overline{56}$ complex was prepared first as "an activated reaction." The $C\overline{56}$, "an activated reactor" then combined with C7 as "indicator," resulting in formation of $C\overline{567}$ complex, which can attach itself to a normal unsensitized red cell membrane with a half-life of less than 1 minute. The E-$C\overline{567}$ complex thus formed without participation of antibody on the target cells was susceptible to the lytic action of C8 and C9. In this way, the reactive hemolysis described by Thompson and Rowe (1968) represents complement-mediated lysis of unsensitized cells initiated at the C5 stage by a stable complex ($C\overline{56}$) which was generated by complement activation at a distance. A mechanism by which complement activation at one site can lyse normal cells at a distance was demonstrated and a pathway to analyze the immunocytolysis caused by complement and lymphocyte on a molecular level was presented.

Another complement-mediated immune cytolysis without participation of antibody on the target cell was demonstrated by Inai and Tsuyuguchi (1969). Sheep erythrocytes nonspecifically coupled with human C1 by $CrCl_3$ could be lysed by sequential addition of the remaining components of complement without any antigen-antibody reaction. Analysis of immune cytolysis by such physically bound C1 or reactive lysis would give information on the mechanism of immune cytolysis on a molecular level, but the significance of such immune cytotoxic phenomena *in vivo* must await further investigation.

Immune reactions of tumors have been analyzed employing histocompatible hosts to avoid transplantation artefacts and for this purpose, inbred mice have been employed most widely in experimental tumor immunology. To analyze immunological phenomena of the tumor, it is most preferable to employ syngenic antibody and syngenic complement *in vitro* as the model most approximate to the immune reaction *in vivo*. From this point, studies on mouse complement have been considered to be important, but their low efficiency in hemolytic activity in general and the limited volume available from individual mice have made the situation for study of mouse complement difficult. By increasing the amount of hemolysin to sensitize sheep erythrocytes, mouse complement from some strains of C57 BL and C3H/He mice could be measured hemolytically (Rosenberg and Tachibana, 1963) and marked differences are found in hemolytic complement activity among inbred strains of mice. It was shown by Fujii *et al.* (1969) and Goto (1970) that rabbit anti-non-Forssman antibody could work efficiently in mouse complement-mediated immune hemolysis. By decreasing the ionicity of the reaction mixture to 0.07 and reducing the number of sheep erythrocytes to 5×10^7/ml., they increased the sensitivity of measuring the mouse complement. C3H/He, C57/BL/6, and BACB/C mice sera showed values of approximately 60 to 170 CH50/ml. Even in this condition, whole serum of A, AKR, DDD, DBA and 12 other strains of mice did not show immune hemolysis. It was shown that sheep erythrocytes with the first three components of mouse complement ($EAC1^m4^m2^m$) proceeded with non-Forssman antibody but not with Forssman antibody, and it was also demonstrated that mouse serum destroyed the SAC14 site prepared with Forssman antibody. These factors could explain the overall low reactivity of mouse complement, as has been suggested by the experiment of Borsos and Cooper (1961) employing CFW mice sera.

According to Terry *et al.* (1964), differences in serum complement activity among inbred strains of mice could be attributed to the differences of late-acting component. In the sera of males of complement-competent strains, male mice had significantly greater complement and late-acting complement component activity than did the sera of females of the same strains. This difference is due to the effect of androgen and estrogen which have greater effect on C6 activity and on C5 to some extent (Churchill *et al.*, 1967). Therefore, it seems that the level of mouse complement is controlled both genetically and hormonally. As for genetic markers associated with the complement level in inbred mice, Erickson *et al.* (1964) showed that complement activity and serum protein called hc' always segregated together and were determined by a single gene which has been named Hc. Cinader *et al.* (1964) also investigated a similar protein which they called MuBl which is supposed to be a genetically controlled component analogous to human C5 (Nilsson and Müller-Eberhard, 1967).

Such regulation mechanism of the complement level in inbred mice is of importance for analysis of immunological phenomena occurring *in vivo* and would give a proper tool for analysis of tumor-host relationships although many more difficulties might be encountered with *in vitro* assays.

VIII. Comments and Future Problems

During the past two decades, much attention has been paid to demonstration of immune reactions against experimental tumors in genetically compatible hosts in many laboratories, and it has been well documented that isograft or autograft reactions of varying intensities have been demonstrated against a large number of chemically and virally induced tumors in different species, including some spontaneous tumors. Complement research also has developed extensively during the last decade, resulting in characterization of each complement component and determination of sequences of reactions in immune cytolysis. At present, in accordance with purification of complement components, their biological activities participating in various immunological phenomena, and chemical characterization in terms of enzymes are making remarkable progress.

In conjunction with these two newly developing fields of medical science, a brief review is presented here. This has been mainly concerned with practical application and theoretical consideration of a variety of methods of characterization of the immunological cell marker of tumor cells, because this problem is considered to be most fundamental to analyze host-tumor relationships in future experiments.

What should be done to develop the next step in pursuing host-tumor relationships in the field of complement research? Although the biological implications of each immune reaction have been mentioned briefly, the significance of the biological activities of each complement component in the manifestation of body defense reactions or in immunopathological phenomena should be clarified more. This will be substantiated by recent progress in complement research. The complement system participating in the generation of a variety of mediators which seem to be involved in the induction of acute inflammatory response have been identified as molecular fragments or assemblies of complement components, such as anaphylatoxin (Cochrane and Müller-Eberhard, 1968), or chemotactic factors (Ward, 1970). The role of C3 in immune phagocytosis and antigen uptake was discussed above. Sequential reactions of complement components are now translated into biochemical terms of enzymology, and evidence for association of enzyme systems in each complement component is now accumulating (Müller-Eberhard, 1969; Mayer, 1970). This will contribute to the clarification of the biological activity of complement on the molecular level.

Since the recognition of neoplastic cells as antigens by autochthonous or syngenic host is well documented, it has been postulated that tumor antigen-antibody complex exists in the tumor-bearing host. This would be assumed to result in consumption of complement from circulating blood by immune complex present *in vivo*, as has been demonstrated in a variety of allergic diseases such as systemic lupus erythematosus (Morse *et al.*, 1962), glomerulonephritis (West *et al.*, 1964), or experimental serum sickness (Dixon *et al.*, 1958). In tumor-bearing hosts, however, no significant consumption of serum complement was observed. It might be due to weak antigenicity of tumor cells or weakened immunological responsiveness of the tumor-bearing host. Analysis of complement level in local tissue fluid such as in intraocular fluids (Shimada, 1970) or in synovial fluids (Sonozaki and Torisu, 1970) would give more information than measuring the level of complement in circulating blood. More direct demonstration of C1 or C3 bound on tumor cells as measured by C1 transfer test or immune adherence, or by fluorescence antibody technique would indicate a possibility of the existence of tumor cell antigen-antibody complexes *in vivo* as discussed earlier.

In many cases, elevated levels of whole complement activity or complement component activity was described in the sera of experimental tumor-bearing animals (Weimer *et al.*, 1964; Nishioka *et al.*, 1966; Yoshida and Ito, 1968) or in sera of patients with neoplastic diseases (Southam and Goldsmith, 1951; Baltch *et al.*, 1960; Zarco *et al.*, 1964; McKenzie *et al.*, 1967; Sakai, 1967; Yoshikawa *et al.*, 1969). A possibility of increased rate of release from reservoir or increased rate of production of complement after consumption by weak but repeated antigen-antibody reactions might have been postulated but much remains to be done in accordance with the progress of measurement of complement components.

In the field of tumor immunology or homograft rejection, much attention has been paid to cellular immunity. However, circulating antibody could be in a cell-bound state on the basis of immunochemical cross reactions, and show the reaction of so-called "cellular immunity." Such a possibility was strongly indicated by the experiments on cross-reactivity and transfer of antibody in Forssman-type antigen by Fujii and Nelson (1963) and antigen exchange in cross-reacting antigen-antibody complexes by M. Inoue (1966). Presence of such types of complement-requiring IgM antibody was demonstrated by Fujii *et al.* (1971) in homotransplantation experiments. If we emphasize the role of cellular immunity too much and do not pay much attention to detection of classical serum antibody, it is possible that important antigens or antibodies participating in tumor-host relationships might escape detection. In a weak antigen-antibody system such as tumor immunity, the immunological phenomena might have been misunderstood as "cellular immunity" simply because of the low sensitivity to measurement of antibody activity. Considering these possibilities, the author would like to mention again that immunological phenomena occurring in tumor-host relations especially in syngenic or autochthonous systems should be analyzed by a method with the highest possible sensitivity. As mentioned in the chapter on immunocytotoxicity, the synergistic action of cellular factor (lymphoid cells and/or macrophages) and complement-mediated antibody activity are of importance for analysis of tumor-host relationships on the basis of medical immunology.

ACKNOWLEDGMENTS

The work of our group described in this article was supported by grants from the Ministry of Health and Welfare, Ministry of Education, Princess Takamatsu Fund for Cancer Research and the Society for Promotion of Cancer Research. I am grateful to Dr. Waro Nakahara, Director of the National Cancer Center Research Institute, Dr. George Klein, Karolinska Institute and the late Dr. Masaru Kuru, former President of the National Cancer Center for their valuable discussions and encouragement throughout the work on tumor immunology. I wish to thank Drs. T. Tachibana, N. Tamura, S. Chang, T. Sekine, and T. Okuda for prepublication copies of their papers. The assistance of Miss H. Kato in the preparation of the manuscript and bibliography is gratefully acknowledged.

REFERENCES

Abelev, G. I. (1963). *Acta Unio Int. Cantra Cancrum* **19**, 80–82.

Abelev, G. I. (1968). *Cancer Res.* **28**, 1344–1350.

Adler, F. L. (1956). *J. Immunol.* **76**, 217–227.

Amano, T., Inai, S., Seki, T., Kashiba, S., Fujikawa, K., and Nishimura, S. (1954). *Med. J. Osaka Univ.* **4**, 401–427.

Amos, D. B. (1965). *In* "Histocompatibility Testing 1965" (H. Balner, F. J. Cleton, and J. G. Ernisse, eds.), p. 151, Munksgaard, Copenhagen.

Andersson, B., Wigzell, H., and Klein, G. (1967). *Transplantation* **5**, 11–20.

Aoki, T., Stück, B., Old, L. J., Hämmerling, U., and de Harven, E. (1970). *Cancer Res.* **30**, 244–251.

Ball, J. K. (1970). *J. Nat. Cancer Inst.* **44**, 1–10.

Baltch, A. L., Osborne, W., Bunn, P. A., Canarile, L., and Hassirdjian, A. (1960). *J. Lab. Clin. Med.* **56**, 594–606.

Barth, R. F., Espmark, J. A., and Gagraeus, A. (1967). *J. Immunol.* **98**, 888–892.

Batchelor, J. R. (1967). *In* "Handbook of Experimental Immunology" (D. M. Weir, ed.), pp. 988–1008. Blackwell, Oxford.

Benacerraf, B., Ovary, Z., Bloch, K. J., and Franklin, E. C. (1963). *J. Exp. Med.* **117**, 937–949.

Berken, A., and Benacerraf, B. (1966). *J. Exp. Med.* **123**, 119–144.

Blumberg, B. S., Harvey, J. A., and Visnich, S. (1965). *J. Amer. Med. Ass.* **191,** 541–546.

Blumberg, B. S., Sutnik, A. I., and London, W. T. (1968). *Bull. N. Y. Acad. Med.* **44,** 1566–1586.

Borsos, T., and Cooper, M. (1961). *Proc. Soc. Exp. Biol. Med.* **107,** 227–232.

Borsos, T., and Rapp, H. J. (1965a). *J. Immunol.* **95,** 559–566.

Borsos, T., and Rapp, H. J. (1965b). *Science* **150,** 505–506.

Borsos, T., Dourmashkin, R. R., and Humphrey, J. H. (1964). *Nature (London)* **202,** 251–252.

Borsos, T., Colten, H. R., Spalter, J. S., Rogentine, N., and Rapp, H. J. (1968). *J. Immunol.* **101,** 392–398.

Boyse, E. A., Old, L. J., and Churoulinkov, I. (1964). *Methods Med. Res.* **10,** 39–47.

Boyse, E. A., Old, L. J., Stockert, E., and Shigeno, N. (1968). *Cancer Res.* **28,** 1280–1287.

Bross, I. D. J. (1958). *Biometrics* **14,** 18–88.

Bungay, C., and Watkins, J. F. (1966). *Brit. J. Exp. Pathol.* **45,** 48–55.

Capra, J. D., Winchester, R. J., and Kunkel, H. G. (1969). *Arthritis Rheum.* **12,** 67–80.

Chang, S. (1967). *Jap. J. Exp. Med.* **37,** 97–106.

Chang, S. (1970). Personal communication.

Churchill, W. H., Weintraub, R. M., Borsos, T., and Rapp, H. J. (1967). *J. Exp. Med.* **125,** 657–672.

Cinader, B., Dubiski, S., and Wardlaw, A. C. (1964). *J. Exp. Med.* **120,** 897–924.

Coca, A. F. (1914). *Z. Immunitastsforsch.* **21,** 604–622.

Cochrane, C. G., and Müller-Eberhard, H. J. (1968). *J. Exp. Med.* **127,** 371–386.

Colten, H. R., Borsos, T., and Rapp, H. J. (1969). *Immunochemistry* **6,** 461–467.

Coombs, R. R. A., and Franks, D. (1969). *Progr. Allergy* **13,** 174–272.

Cooper, N., and Becker, E. L. (1967). *J. Immunol.* **98,** 119–131.

Cunniff, R. V., and Stollar, B. D. (1968). *J. Immunol.* **100,** 7–14.

da Silva, W. D., Eisele, J. V., and Lepow, I. H. (1967). *J. Exp. Med.* **126,** 1027–1048.

Davies, D. A. L. (1968). *Transplantation* **6,** 660–662.

Deichman, G. I. (1969). *Advan. Cancer Res.* **12,** 101–136.

de Planque, B., Williams, G. M., Siegel, A., and Alvarez, C. (1969). *Transplantation* **8,** 852–860.

de Thé, G., Ambrosion, J. C., Ho, H. C., and Kwan, H. C. (1969). *Nature (London)* **221,** 770–771.

Dixon, E. J., Vasquez, J. J., Weigle, W. O., and Cochrane, C. G. (1958). *AMA Arch. Pathol.* **65,** 18–28.

Epstein, M. A., Achong, B. G., and Barr, Y. M. (1964). *Lancet* **1,** 702–703.

Erickson, R. P., Tachibana, D. K., Herzenberg, L. A., and Rosenberg, L. T. (1964). *J. Immunol.* **92,** 611–615.

Fagraeus, A., Espmark, J. Å., and Jonsson, J. (1966). *Immunology* **10,** 161–175.

Ferrata, A. (1907). *Berlin. Klin. Wochenschr.* **44,** 366–368.

Flax, M. H. (1956). *Cancer Res.* **16,** 774–783.

Frank, M. M., and Gaither, T. A. (1970). *J. Immunol.* **104,** 1458–1466.

Frank, M. M., Dourmashkin, R. R., and Humphrey, J. A. (1970). *J. Immunol.* **104,** 1502–1510.

Fugmann, R. Personal communication.

Fujii, G., and Nelson, R. A., Jr. (1963). *J. Exp. Med.* **118,** 1037–1058.

Fujii, G., Goto, S., and Ishibashi, Y. (1969). *J. Immunol.* **102**, 1343.

Fujii, G., Hirose, Y., Goto, S., and Ishibashi, Y. (1971). *Jap. J. Exp. Med.* **41** (in press).

Gajl-Peczalska, K. J., Fish, A. J., Meuwissen, H. J., Frommel, D., and Good, R. A. (1969). *J. Exp. Med.* **130**, 1367–1393.

George, M., and Vaughan, J. H. (1962). *Proc. Soc. Exp. Biol. Med.* **111**, 514–521.

Gigli, I., and Nelson, R. A., Jr. (1968). *Exp. Cell Res.* **51**, 45–67.

Glynn, A. A. (1969). *Immunology* **16**, 463–471.

Gold, P., and Freedman, S. O. (1965). *J. Exp. Med.* **122**, 467–481.

Gordon, J., Whitehead, H. R., and Wormall, A. (1926). *Biochem. J.* **20**, 1028.

Gorer, P. A., and O'Gorman, P. (1956). *Transplant. Bull.* **3**, 142–143.

Goto, S. (1970). *Jap. J. Allergol.* **19**, 317–329.

Green, H., Fleischer, R. A., Barrow, P., and Goldberg, B. (1959). *J. Exp. Med.* **109**, 511–521.

Grünbaum, F. T. (1928). *Virchows Arch. Pathol. Anat. Physiol.* **267**, 126–143.

Habel, K. (1969). *Advan. Immunol.* **10**, 229–250.

Harris, H., Miller, O. J., Klein, G., Worst, P., and Tachibana, T. (1969). *Nature (London)* **223**, 363–368.

Haughton, G. (1965). *Science* **147**, 506–507.

Haughton, G., and McGehee, M. P. (1969). *Immunology* **16**, 447–461.

Hauschka, T. S. (1952). *Cancer Res.* **12**, 615–633.

Haxby, J. A., Kinsky, C. B., and Kinsky, S. C. (1968). *Proc. Nat. Acad. Sci. U. S.* **61**, 300–307.

Hayashi, K., Gotoh, A., and Nishioka, K. (1970). Unpublished observation.

Hellström, K. E., and Hellström, I. (1969). *Advan. Cancer Res.* **12**, 167–233.

Hellström, I., and Sjögren, H. O. (1967). *J. Exp. Med.* **125**, 1105–1118.

Henle, G., Henle, W., and Diehl, V. (1968). *Proc. Nat. Acad. Sci. U. S.* **59**, 94–101.

Henson, P. M. (1969). *Immunology* **16**, 107–121.

Henson, P. M., and Cochrane, C. G. (1969). *J. Exp. Med.* **129**, 167–183.

Herberman, R. B. (1969). *Transplantation* **8**, 813–820.

Hingson, D. J., Massengill, R. K., and Mayer, M. M. (1969). *Immunochemistry* **6**, 295–307.

Hinuma, Y., and Grace, J. (1967). *Proc. Soc. Exp. Biol. Med.* **124**, 107–111.

Hiramatsu, S., Tsuyuguchi, I., and Inai, S. (1969). *Biken J.* **12**, 43–44.

Hoffmann, L. G. (1968). *Science* **159**, 322–323.

Howard, J. G., and Benacerraf, B. (1966). *Brit. J. Exp. Pathol.* **47**, 193–200.

Hoy, W. E., and Nelson, D. S. (1969). *Nature (London)* **222**, 1001–1003.

Hoyer, L. W., Borsos, T., Rapp, H. J., and Vanier, W. E. (1968). *J. Exp. Med.* **127**, 589–603.

Huber, H., and Fudenberg, H. H. (1968). *Int. Arch. Allergy Appl. Immunol.* **34**, 18–31.

Huber, H., Polley, M. J., Linscott, W. D., Fudenberg, H., and Müller-Eberhard, H. J. (1968). *Science* **62**, 1281–1283.

Huber, H., Douglas, S. D., and Fudenberg, H. G. (1969). *Immunology* **17**, 7–12.

Humphrey, J. H., and Dourmashkin, R. R. (1965). *Complement, Ciba Found. Symp., 1964* pp. 175–186.

Humphrey, J. H., and Dourmashkin, R. R. (1969). *Advan. Immunol.* **11**, 75–115.

Inai, S., and Tsuyuguchi, I. (1969). *Biken J.* **12**, 1–7.

Inoue, K., and Nelson, R. A., Jr. (1965). *J. Immunol.* **95**, 355–367.

Inoue, K., and Nelson, R. A., Jr. (1966). *J. Immunol.* **96**, 386–400.

Inoue, M. (1966). *Jap. J. Exp. Med.* **36**, 423–434.
Inoue, M., Handa, B., and Nishioka, K. (1968). *Igaku No Ayumi* **66**, 592–596.
Irie, R. F., Nishioka, K., Tachibana, T., and Takeuchi, S. (1969). *Int. J. Cancer* **4**, 150–158.
Irie, R. F., Kataoka, T., and Mistui, H. (1970). *Int. J. Cancer* **6**, 304–313.
Ishizaka, K., and Ishizaka, T. (1960). *J. Immunol.* **85**, 163–171.
Ishizaka, T., Ishizaka, K., Borsos, T., and Rapp, H. (1966). *J. Immunol.* **97**, 716–726.
Ishizaka, T., Ishizaka, K., Salmon, S., and Fudenberg, H. (1967). *J. Immunol.* **99**, 82–91.
Ishizaka, T., Ishizaka, K., Bennich, H., and Johansson, S. G. O. (1970). *J. Immunol.* **104**, 854–862.
Ito, M., and Tagaya, I. (1966). *Jap. J. Med. Sci. Biol.* **19**, 109–126.
Ito, Y., Takahashi, T., Kawamura, A., Jr., and Tu, S-M. (1969). *Gann* **60**, 335–340.
Kaplan, M. E., and Tan, E. M. (1968). *Lancet* **1**, 561–563.
Kawamura, A., Jr., Hamajima, K., Murata, M., Gotoh, A., Takada, M., Nishioka, K., Tachibana, T., Hirayama, T., Yoshida, T. O., Imai, K., Tu, S-M., Liu, C-H., and Lin, T-M. (1971). *Ann. N. Y. Acad. Sci.* (in press).
Kinsky, S. C., Haxby, J. A., Zopf, D. A., Alving, C. R., and Kinsky, C. B. (1969). *Biochemistry* **8**, 4149–4158.
Klein, E., and Klein, G. (1964). *J. Nat. Cancer Inst.* **32**, 547–568.
Klein, E., Klein, G., Nadkarni, J. S., Madkarni, J. J., Wigzell, H., and Clifford, P. (1968). *Cancer Res.* **28**, 1300–1310.
Klein, G. (1966). *Annu. Rev. Microbiol.* **20**, 223–252.
Kojima, K., Okada, H., Yoshida, T. O., and Nishioka, K. (1971). *Jap. J. Allergol.* **19** (in press).
Koulirsky, R., Pieron, R., Koulirsky, S., Robineaux, R., and Voisin, G. (1955). *Ann. Inst. Pasteur, Paris* **89**, 273–279.
Kritschewsky, I. L., and Tscherikower, R. S. (1925). *Z. Immunitactsforsch.* **42**, 131–149.
Kronman, B. S., Wepsic, H. T., Churchill, W. H., Zbar, B., Borsos, T., and Rapp, H. J. (1969). *Science* **165**, 296–297.
Kronman, B. S., Wepsic, H. T., Churchill, W. H., Zbar, B., Borsos, T., and Rapp, H. J. (1970). *Science* **168**, 252–279.
Lachmann, P. J., and Müller-Eberhard, H. S. (1968). *J. Immunol.* **100**, 691–698.
Lachmann, P. J., and Thompson, R. A. (1970). *J. Exp. Med.* **131**, 643–657.
Lay, W. H., and Nussenzweig, V. (1968). *J. Exp. Med.* **128**, 991–1007.
Lay, W. H., and Nussenzweig, V. (1969). *J. Immunol.* **102**, 1172–1178.
Linscott, W. D. (1969a). *J. Immunol.* **102**, 986–992.
Linscott, W. D. (1969b). *J. Immunol.* **102**, 993–1001.
Linscott, W. D. (1969c). *J. Immunol.* **102**, 1322–1326.
Linscott, W. D., and Hansen, S. S. (1969). *J. Immunol.* **103**, 423–428.
Linscott, W. D., and Levinson, W. (1969). *Proc. Nat. Acad. Sci. U. S.* **64**, 520–527.
Linscott, W. D., and Nishioka, K. (1963). *J. Exp. Med.* **118**, 795–815.
Lo Buglio, A. F., Contran, R. S., and Jandl, J. H. (1967). *Science* **158**, 1582–1585.
McKenzie, D., Colsky, J., and Hetrick, D. L. (1967). *Cancer Res.* **27**, 2386–2394.
Manni, J. A., and Müller-Eberhard, H. J. (1969). *J. Exp. Med.* **130**, 1145–1160.
Marney, S. R., and Des Prez, R. M. (1969). *J. Immunol.* **103**, 1044–1049.
Mayer, M. M. (1961a). *In* "Experimental Immunolochemistry" (E. A. Kabat and M. M. Mayer, eds.), 2nd ed., pp. 133–240. Thomas, Springfield, Illinois.

Mayer, M. M. (1961b). *In* "Immunochemical Approaches to Problems in Microbiology" (M. Heidelberger and O. J. Plescia, eds.), pp. 268–279. Rutgers Univ. Press, New Brunswick, New Jersey.

Mayer, M. M. (1970). *Immunochemistry* 7, 485–496.

Mayumi, M. (1971). Personal communication.

Mayumi, M., Okochi, K., and Nishioka, K. (1971). *Vox Sang.* 20, 178–181.

Melief, C. J. M., van der Hart, M., Engelfriet, C. P., and van Loghen, J. J. (1967). *Vox Sang.* 12, 374–389.

Milgrom, F. (1962). *Proc. 9th Congr. Int. Soc. Blood Transfusion,* pp. 335–340.

Mittal, K. K., Mickey, M. R., and Terasaki, P. I. (1969). *Transplantation* 8, 801–805.

Miyakawa, Y., Sekine, T., Shimada, K., and Nishioka, K. (1969). *J. Immunol.* 103, 374–377.

Möller, G. (1961). *J. Exp. Med.* 114, 415–434.

Morrison, S. K., and Terres, G. (1966). *J. Immunol.* 96, 901–905.

Morse, J. H., Müller-Eberhard, H. J., and Kunkel, H. G. (1962). *Bull. N. Y. Acad. Med.* 38, 641–651.

Mukojima, T. (1970). *Bull. Tokyo Med. Dent. Univ.* 17, 75–88.

Müller-Eberhard, H. J. (1968a). *Advan. Immunol.* 8, 1–80.

Müller-Eberhard, H. J. (1968b.) *Cancer Res.* 28, 1357–1360.

Müller-Eberhard, H. J. (1969). *Annu. Rev. Biochem.* 38, 389–414.

Müller-Eberhard, H. J., Dalmasso, A. P., and Calcott, M. A. (1966). *J. Exp. Med.* 123, 33–54.

Nagaki, K., and Stroud, R. M. (1969). *J. Immunol.* 102, 421–430.

Nakamura, H., and Katsura, T. (1964). *Jap. J. Exp. Med.* 34, 167–196.

Nathenson, S. G., and Davies, D. A. L. (1966). *Proc. Nat. Acad. Sci. U. S.* 56, 476–483.

Nelson, D. S. (1963). *Advan. Immunol.* 3, 131–180.

Nelson, D. S., and Boyden, S. V. (1967). *Brit. Med. Bull.* 23, 15–20.

Nelson, D. S., and Nelson, R. A., Jr. (1959). *Yale J. Biol. Med.* 31, 185–200.

Nelson, D. S., and Uhlenbruck, G. (1967). *Vox Sang.* 12, 43–67.

Nelson, R. A., Jr. (1953). *Science* 118, 733–737.

Nelson, R. A., Jr. (1956). *Proc. Roy. Soc. Med.* 49, 55–58.

Nelson, R. A., Jr. (1962). *In* "Mechanism of Cell and Tissue Damage Produced by Immune Reaction" (P. Grabar and P. A. Miescher, eds.), pp. 245–248. Benno Schwabe, Basel.

Nelson, R. A., Jr. (1965). *In* "The Inflammatory Process" (B. W. Zweifach, R. T. McCluskey, and L. Grant, eds.), pp. 819–879. Academic Press, New York.

Nelson, R. A., Jr. (1968). *Cancer Res.* 28, 1361–1365.

Nelson, R. A., Jr., and Biro, C. (1968). *Immunology* 14, 527–540.

Nelson, R. A., Jr., Jensen, J., Gigli, I., and Tamura, N. (1966). *Immunochemistry* 3, 111–135.

Niederman, J. C., McCollum, R. W., Henle, G., and Henle, W. (1968). *J. Amer. Med. Ass.* 203, 205–209.

Nilsson, U. R., and Müller-Eberhard, H. J. (1967). *J. Exp. Med.* 125, 1–16.

Nishioka, K. (1963). *J. Immunol.* 90, 86–97.

Nishioka, K. (1965). *Jap. J. Exp. Med.* 35, 29–33.

Nishioka, K. (1966). *Immunochemistry* 3, 501.

Nishioka, K. (1971). *Proc. Int. Congr. Allergol. 7th, 1970* (in press).

Nishioka K., and Linscott, W. D. (1963). *J. Exp. Med.* **118**, 767–793.

Nishioka, K., Takeuchi, T., and Fujii, G. (1956). *Gann* **47**, 426–427.

Nishioka, K., Yoshida, T., Kinugawa, H., and Kasahara, T. (1958). *Gann* **49**, Suppl., 6–7.

Nishioka, K., Chang, S., and Sakamoto, M. (1966). *Jap. J. Allergol.* **15**, 927–928.

Nishioka, K., Tachibana, T., and Stock, C. C. (1967a). In "Subviral Carcinogenesis" (Y. Ito, ed.), pp. 253–264. Editorial Comm. First Intern. Symp. Tumor Viruses, Nagoya.

Nishioka, K., Tachibana, T., Doi, R., Nakamura, H., and Okada, H. (1967b). *Protides Biol. Fluids, Proc. Colloq.* **15**, 419–426.

Nishioka, K., Tachibana, T., Klein, G., and Clifford, P. (1968). *Gann Monogr.* **7**, 49–59.

Nishioka, K., Irie, R. F., Inoue, M., Chang, S., and Takeuchi, S. (1969a). *Int. J. Cancer* **4**, 121–129.

Nishioka, K., Irie, R. F., Kawana, T., and Takeuchi, S. (1969b). *Int. J. Cancer* **4**, 139–149.

Nishioka, K., Okada, H., and Yamanushi, K. (1971a). *Jap. J. Allergol.* **19** (in press).

Nishioka, K., Tachibana, T., Sekine, T., Inoue, M., Hirayama, T., Yoshida, T. O., Takada, M., Kawamura, A., Sugano, H., and Wang, C-H. (1971b). *Gann Monogr.* **10**, 265–282.

Nördenskjold, B. A., Klein, E., Tachibana, T., and Fenyö, E. M. (1970). *J. Nat. Cancer Inst.* **44**, 403–412.

Nungester, W. J., Paradise, L. J., and Adair, J. R. (1969). *Proc. Soc. Exp. Biol. Med.* **132**, 582–586.

Nuttal, G. (1888). *Z. Hyg.* **4**, 353–394.

Odaka, T., Ishii, H., Yamaura, K., and Yamamoto, T. (1966). *Jap. J. Exp. Med.* **36**, 277–290.

Oettgen, H. F., Old, L. J., McLean, E. P., and Carswell, E. A. (1968). *Nature* (*London*) **220**, 295–297.

Okada, H., Kawachi, S., and Nishioka, K. (1970a). *Jap. J. Exp. Med.* **39**, 527–531.

Okada, H., Kawachi, S., and Nishioka, K. (1970b). *Biochim. Biophys. Acta* **208**, 541–543.

Okada, H., Mayumi, M., Mukojima, T., Sekine, T., and Torisu, M. (1970c). *Immunology* **18**, 493–500.

Okochi, K., and Murakami, S. (1968). *Vox Sang.* **15**, 374–385.

Okuda, T., Tachibana, T., and Nishioka, K. (1971). To be published.

Old, L. J., and Boyse, E. A. (1964). *Annu. Rev. Med.* **15**, 167–186.

Old, L. J., Boyse, E. A., Clarke, D. A., and Carswell, E. A. (1962). *Annu. N. Y. Acad. Sci.* **101**, 80–106.

Old, L. J., Boyse, E. A., Oettgen, H. F., de Haven, H. E., Geering, G., Williamson, B., and Clifford, P. (1968). *Proc. Nat. Acad. Sci. U. S.* **56**, 1699–1704.

O'Neill, C. H. (1968). *J. Cell Sci.* **3**, 405–421.

Osler, A. G. (1961). *Advan. Immunol.* **1**, 132–210.

Pasternak, G. (1969). *Advan. Cancer Res.* **12**, 1–99.

Perlmann, P., and Hölm, G. (1969). *Advan. Immunol.* **11**, 117–193.

Perlmann, P., Perlmann, H., Müller-Eberhard, H. J., and Manni, J. A. (1969). *Science* **163**, 937–939.

Pinckard, R. N., and Weir, D. M. (1966). *Clin. Exp. Immunol.* **1**, 33–43.

Plotz, P. H., Cotten, H., and Talal, N. (1968). *J. Immunol.* **100**, 752–780.

Prehn, R. T. (1968). *Cancer Res.* **28**, 1326–1330.

Prince, A. M. (1968). *Proc. Nat. Acad. Sci. U. S.* **60**, 814–821.

Pulvertaft, T. J. V. (1964). *Lancet* **1**, 238–240.

Rapp, H. J., and Borsos, T. (1966a). *J. Amer. Med. Ass.* **198**, 1347–1354.

Rapp, H. J., and Borsos, T. (1966b). *J. Immunol.* **96**, 913–919.

Ritz, H. (1912). *Z. Immunitactsforsch.* **13**, 62–83.

Roitt, I. M., Ling, N. R., Doniach, D., and Couchman, K. G. (1964). *Immunology* **7**, 375–393.

Rosenberg, L. T., and Tachibana, D. K. (1963). *J. Immunol.* **89**, 861–867.

Rotman, B., and Papermaster, B. W. (1966). *Proc. Nat. Acad. Sci. U. S.* **55**, 134–141.

Rubin, D. J., Colten, H. R., Borsos, T., and Rapp, H. J. (1970). *J. Nat. Cancer Inst.* **44**, 975–979.

Sakai, K. (1967). *Jap. J. Allergol.* **16**, 635–657.

Sakamoto, M., Nishioka, K., Kawachi, S., Okada, H., and Chang, S. (1967). *Jap. J. Allergol.* **16**, 800–801.

Salaman, M. H., and Wedderburn, N. (1966). *Immunology* **10**, 445–458.

Sandberg, A. L., Osler, A. G., Shin, H. S., and Oliveira, B. (1970). *J. Immunol.* **104**, 329–334.

Sanderson, A. R. (1965). *Immunology* **9**, 287–300.

Sekine, T. (1970). Personal communication.

Sekine, T., Nishioka, K., Yoshida, T., and Imai, K. (1970). *Immunobiology* **3**, 34–38.

Sell, K. W., and Spooner, R. L. (1966). *Immunology* **11**, 533–546.

Sever, J. L. (1962). *J. Immunol.* **88**, 320–329.

Shimada, K. (1970). *Invest. Ophthalmol.* **9**, 307–315.

Shin, H. S., and Mayer, M. M. (1968). *Biochemistry* **1**, 2991–2996.

Siqueira, M., and Nelson, R. A., Jr. (1961). *J. Immunol.* **86**, 516–525.

Sjögren, H. O. (1965). *Progr. Exp. Tumor Res.* **6**, 289–322.

Smith, M. R., and Wood, W. B. (1969). *J. Exp. Med.* **130**, 1209–1227.

Sobernheim, G. (1902). *Berlin. Klin. Wochenschr.* **39**, 516–518.

Sobernheim, G. (1904). *Deut. Med. Wochenschr.* **30**, 948–988.

Sonozaki, H., and Torisu, M. (1970). *Ann. Rheum. Dis.* **29**, 164–172.

Southam, C. M., and Goldsmith, Y. (1951). *Proc. Soc. Exp. Biol. Med.* **76**, 430–432.

Spencer, R. R. (1942). *J. Nat. Cancer Inst.* **2**, 317–332.

Stolfi, R. L. (1968). *J. Immunol.* **100**, 46–54.

Sugano, H., Takada, M., Chen, H-C., and Tu, S-M. (1970). *Proc. Jap. Acad.* **46**, 453–457.

Sutnik, A. I., London, W. T., Blumberg, B. S., Yanbee, R. A., Gerstley, B. J. S., and Millman, I. (1970). *J. Nat. Cancer Inst.* **44**, 1241–1249.

Suzuki, I., Okada, H., Takahashi, S. K., Takahashi, M., and Nishioka, K. (1971). *Jap. J. Allergol.* (in press).

Tachibana, T. (1967). *Symp. Cell Chem.* **18**, 1–10.

Tachibana, T., and Klein, E. (1970). *Immunology* **19**, 771–782.

Tachibana, T., and Klein, G. (1970). Personal communication.

Tachibana, T., Worst, P., and Klein, E. (1970). *Immunology* **19**, 809–816.

Takada, M., Lin, Y-C., Shiratori, O., Sugano, H., Yang, C-S., Hsu, M-M., Lin, T-C., Tu, S-M., Chen, H-C., Hamajima, K., Murata, M., Gotoh, A., Kawamura, A., Jr., Yoshida, T. O., Osato, T., and Ito, Y. (1971). *Gann Monogr.* **10**, 149–162.

Takahashi, M., Kuroiwa, T., Tachibana, T., and Yoshida, T. (1965). *Igaku No Ayumi* **55**, 745 (abstr.).

Takahashi, S., Okada, H., and Nishioka, K. (1970). *Jap. J. Allergol.* **19**, 859–867.

Takahashi, T., Old, L. T., and Boyse, E. A. (1970). *J. Exp. Med.* **131**, 1325–1341.

Takeuchi, S., Irie, R. F., Inoue, M., Irie, K., Izumi, R., and Nishioka, K. (1969). *Int. J. Cancer* **4**, 130–138.

Talmage, D. W., Freter, G. G., and Taliaferro, W. H. (1956). *J. Infec. Dis.* **98**, 300–305.

Tamura, N., and Nelson, R. A., Jr. (1967). *J. Immunol.* **99**, 582–589.

Tamura, N., and Nelson, R. A., Jr. (1968). *J. Immunol.* **101**, 1333–1345.

Tamura, N., Shimada, A., and Chang, S. (1970). *Proc. Int. Congr. Microbiol. 10th, 1970* (in press).

Taniguchi, T., Joogetsu, M., and Kasahara, T. (1930). *Jap. J. Exp. Med.* **8**, 55–64.

Terres, G., and Wilson, W. (1961). *J. Immunol.* **86**, 361–368.

Terry, W. D., Borsos, T., and Rapp, H. J. (1964). *J. Immunol.* **89**, 576–578.

Thompson, R. A., and Lachmann, P. J. (1970). *J. Exp. Med.* **131**, 629–641.

Thompson, R. A., and Rowe, D. S. (1968). *Immunology* **14**, 745–762.

Thomson, D. M. P., Krupey, J., Freedman, S. O., and Gold, P. (1969). *Proc. Nat. Acad Sci. U. S.* **64**, 161–167.

Ueno, S. (1938). *Jap. J. Med. Sci. 7* **2**, 201–225.

Uriel, J., de Neuchan, B., Stanislawski-Birencwajg, M., Masseyeff, R., Leblanc, L., Quenum, C., Loisillier, F., and Grabar, P. (1967). *C. R. Acad. Sci.* **265**, 75–78.

Valentine, M. D., Bloch, K. J., and Austen, K. F. (1967). *J. Immunol.* **99**, 98–110.

van Loghen, J. J., and van der Hart, M. (1962). *Vox Sang.* **7**, 539–544.

von Kleist, S., and Burtin, P. (1969). *Cancer Res.* **29**, 1961–1964.

Vroom, D. H., Schultz, D. R., and Zarco, R. M. (1970). *Immunochemistry* **7**, 43–61.

Ward, P. A. (1967). *J. Exp. Med.* **126**, 189–206.

Ward, P. A. (1970). *Arthritis Rheum.* **13**, 181–186.

Wasserman, E., and Levine, L. (1961). *J. Immunol.* **87**, 290–295.

Watkins, J. F. (1964a). *Nature (London)* **202**, 1364–1365.

Watkins, J. F. (1964b). *Virology* **23**, 436–438.

Watkins, J. F. (1965). *Virology* **26**, 746–753.

Weimer, H. E., Miller, J. N., Meyers, R. L., Baxter, Robberts, D. M., Godfrey, J. F., and Carpenter, C. M. (1964). *Cancer Res.* **24**, 847–854.

Weir, D. M. (1967). *In* "Handbook of Experimental Immunology" (D. M. Weir, ed.), pp. 844–876. Blackwell, Oxford.

West, C. D., Northway, J. D., and Davis, N. C. (1964). *J. Clin. Invest.* **43**, 1507–1517.

Wigzell, H. (1965). *Transplantation* **3**, 423–431.

World Health Organization Immunology Unit. (1968). *Bull. W. H. O.* **39**, 935–938.

Yamamoto, T., Komeiji, T., Nishioka, K., Takeuchi, T., and Nitta, K. (1956). *Gann* **47**, 424–426.

Yamamoto, T., Nishioka, K., Oda, A., Sakurai, T., Yoshida, T., and Kinugawa, H. (1959). *Acta Unio Int. Contra Cancrum* **15**, 306–312.

Yasuda, J., and Milgrom, F. (1968). *Int. Arch. Allergy Appl. Immunol.* **33**, 151–170.

Yoshida, T. O. (1971). *Gann Monogr.* **10**, 283–290.

Yoshida, T. O., and Ito, Y. (1968). *Immunology* **14**, 879–887.

Yoshida, T. O., Imai, K., Ito, Y., Sekine, T., and Nishioka, K. (1970). *Jap. J. Allergol.* **19**, 71.

Yoshikawa, S., Yamada, K., and Yoshida, T. O. (1969). *Int. J. Cancer* **4**, 845–851.

Yoshino, K., and Taniguchi, S. (1969). *J. Immunol.* **102,** 1341–1342.

Zarco, R. M., Flores, E., and Rodriquez, F. (1964). *J. Philipp. Med. Ass.* **40,** 839–864.

Zbar, B., Wepsic, H. T., Borsos, T., and Rapp, H. J. (1970a). *J. Nat. Cancer Inst.* **44,** 473–481.

Zbar, B., Wepsic, H. T., Rapp, H. J., Stewart, L. C., and Borsos, T. (1970b). *J. Nat. Cancer Inst.* **44,** 701–717.

zur Hausen, H., and Schulte-Holthausen, H. (1970). *Nature (London)* **227,** 245–248.

ALPHA-FETOPROTEIN IN ONTOGENESIS AND ITS ASSOCIATION WITH MALIGNANT TUMORS

G. I. Abelev

Laboratory of Tumor Immunochemistry, N. F. Gamaleya Institute
for Epidemiology and Microbiology, Moscow, USSR

I. Introduction: Major Steps in Development of the Problem

Ontogenetic studies on the protein composition of the blood serum have revealed a group of the so-called embryo-specific proteins, i.e., proteins peculiar to fetal or newborn sera and not present in blood of adult individuals. The first identified protein of this group was fetuin, an embryo-specific protein of calf serum discovered by Pedersen (1944). Next, Bergstrand and Czar (1956, 1957) described an embryo-specific α-globulin in human fetal serum.

At present, embryo-specific serum proteins have been demonstrated in each mammalian species studied in this respect (Gitlin and Boesman, 1966, 1967a; Masopust et al., 1971). Several types of such proteins have been shown to exist, belonging to α- and β-globulin serum fractions. Most characteristic among them is alpha-fetoprotein (AFP) which is represented, probably, in all mammalian species and exhibits similar physicochemical properties as well as common dynamics in ontogenesis. It is relevant to emphasize here that AFP is different from the classical fetuin of Pedersen (Kithier et al., 1968a).

Although antigenic relations between tumor and embryonic tissues were repeatedly investigated (see Day, 1965), the embryo-specific serum proteins have not been studied early by oncologists. Interest in the problem developed after the demonstration that transplantable hepato-cellular carcinomas of the mouse were synthesizing and secreting into the blood an embryo-specific α-globulin subsequently identified as AFP (Abelev, 1963; Abelev et al., 1963a,b).

It was soon found that AFP appeared also with primary tumors of the liver and that its synthesis was characteristic not only of mouse but of rat hepatomas as well (Abelev, 1965a; Grabar et al., 1967).

In 1964 Tatarinov first detected AFP with human hepatocellular carcinoma and by 1966 he described six such cases (Tatarinov, 1964a; Tatarinov and Nogaller, 1966). The prospect appeared of an immuno-chemical diagnosis of liver cell cancer, based on AFP detection in the blood serum; this suggestion determined the main direction of subsequent studies.

Abelev et al. (1967a) and Uriel et al. (1967) confirmed and con-siderably extended observations of Tatarinov on the diagnosis of primary liver cancer in humans. Simultaneously, it was found by two independent groups that AFP appeared not only with liver cancer but also with malignant teratoblastomas of the testis and ovary, possessing elements of embryonic cancer (Assecritova et al., 1967; Abelev et al., 1967a; Masopust et al., 1967, 1968). AFP was not detected with tumors of other localization, including those metastatic to the liver, nor was it found with nonneoplastic liver diseases.

These early observations have been fully confirmed by subsequent studies, carried out in 1968–1970 on a large supply of clinical material which was obtained from countries with a high frequency of liver cancer—Senegal, Union of South Africa, Mozambique, Kenya, Uganda, Congo, and Indonesia—as well as from the USSR, England, France, USA, and Greece, where the disease rate is low. By these studies high specificity of the AFP test has been demonstrated as a means for differential diagnosis of hepatocellular cancer. The same conclusion was reached in the collaborative study undertaken by the International Agency for Research on Cancer in 1967–1969 (O'Conor et al., 1970). New practical problems became apparent; they were primarily those of early identification of AFP-producing tumors and of increasing the percentage of hepatocellular cancers and teratocarcinomas revealed by the AFP test.

In all the above-mentioned studies, AFP was detected by an agar-gel immunoprecipitation technique, which was, however, inferior to some other immunologic methods. It was natural to apply the most sensitive techniques of AFP determination for cancer diagnosis. The very first results with highly sensitive methods—aggregate hemagglutination (Olovnikov and Tsvetkov, 1969; Abelev et al., 1971), immunoradioautography (Abelev et al., 1971), and radioimmunoassay (Purves et al., 1970c)—showed that the specificity of the AFP test for liver cell cancer was far from being absolute. Low levels of AFP were found to occur during pregnancy and certain periods of noncancerous diseases of the liver. As a result, quantitative and dynamic aspects of the problem became important, especially in early cancer diagnosis.

Active studies on practical aspects of the problem have not been accompanied, however, with equally active basic investigations. And though the phenomenon itself—the synthesis of AFP in ontogenesis and by malignant tumors of the liver—has been described rather adequately, both in animals and man, its mechanism remains almost unstudied. Both the nature of control of AFP synthesis in ontogenesis and the reasons of resumption of its synthesis in tumors are to be determined.

In the present work, experimental and clinical evidence will be reviewed, the main attention being paid to approaches and prospects concerning research on the nature of the phenomenon and new aspects of its practical application.

II. Alpha-Fetoprotein Synthesis in Ontogenesis and Pathologic States. An Outline of the Phenomenon

Before detailed analyses of different aspects of the subject are given, we would like to present the general scheme of the phenomenon. It is given in Fig. 1 with its proved and assumed elements indicated. In the embryonic period of ontogenesis, AFP is synthesized and secreted into

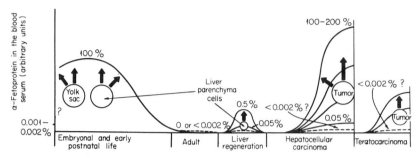

F<small>IG</small>. 1. Schematic representation of AFP synthesis in normal development and pathologic states. Solid line, serum AFP level, in arbitrary units. Broken line, expected AFP level. ?, not known.

the blood by cells of hepatic parenchyma and yolk sac. After birth, during the early postnatal period, AFP synthesis is carried out by liver cells only. In blood of healthy adult animals and humans AFP is not detectable by conventional methods. Some background serum level of this protein can, probably, exist in normal adult individuals, but it should not exceed 0.001% or 0.002% of its maximal level in fetal serum. AFP synthesis is resumed in animals during regeneration of the liver and seems to be carried out by cells of hepatic parenchyma. In this case, the synthesis has reversible character. Its intensity varies greatly in different species. It is not known whether liver regeneration can proceed without the AFP synthesis.

Synthesis of AFP is resumed during development of hepatocellular carcinomas or germinal tumors with elements of embryonic cancer, the production being permanent. In both neoplastic diseases, tumor itself is the site of synthesis, although additional proof may be required in case of teratocarcinomas, where cell elements responsible for AFP synthesis have not yet been identified. The level of the synthesis in "AFP-positive" tumors varies within very broad limits, more than 1000-fold. Some hepatomas and teratocarcinomas do not produce AFP, or rather produce it in undetectable amounts.

These are the main features of the phenomenon. As to its nature, which remains not yet elucidated, three possibilities have been discussed in the literature:

1. AFP synthesis may be an inducible process, similar to induction of certain enzymes in the liver by appropriate substrates or hormones. In tumor, a fortuitous and nonregular inactivation takes the place of a corresponding repressor (Grabar *et al.*, 1967).

2. AFP formation is believed to be a property of specialized cells of liver parenchyma. These cells are the final stage of the peculiar branch of liver stem cell differentiation. The alternative pathway results

in the formation of hepatocytes producing the "adult" serum proteins. The dynamics of AFP in ontogenesis and appearance in tumors, according to this view, is a reflection of the presence of the hypothetical AFP-forming cells and changes in their number (Abelev, 1968).

3. Only a certain stage in the hepatocyte development is considered to be endowed with the potential for AFP synthesis. Hepatocytes of earlier and later stages of differentiation do not synthesize AFP. In hepatomas a dedifferentiation of the hepatocyte ("retrodifferentiation") takes place, which results in an "AFP-positive" tumor if it corresponds to the "AFP-producing" stage (Uriel, 1969).

In subsequent discussions we shall consider individual aspects of the above points, with special attention to unsolved problems.

III. Alpha-Fetoprotein (AFP). Definition and Physicochemical Characteristics

A. DEFINITION AND IDENTIFICATION

To reveal and identify specific proteins in the embryonic serum, immunochemical methods are commonly used. An antiserum against fetal serum absorbed with a homologous adult serum serves as a specific reagent for embryo-specific antigens in immunoelectrophoresis or immunodiffusion. Depending on the animal species, such antisera reveal from one to three components in fetal sera. AFP is the most characteristic representative of this group and has been reported for 18 mammalian species examined in this way (Gitlin and Boesman, 1966, 1967a; Masopust *et al.*, 1971).

According to the definition proposed by WHO-IARC experts, AFP is the first α-globulin to appear in mammalian sera during development, and the dominant serum protein in early embryonic life. It reappears in the adult serum during certain pathologic states, primarily with hepatocellular carcinoma (Annual Report of International Agency for Research on Cancer, 1969).

AFP's from different animal species exhibit clear-cut cross-reactions. Taking advantage of this property, one can distinguish AFP from other embryo-specific proteins by demonstrating cross-reactivity with a reference AFP preparation, for instance that of rat or man.

Table I summarizes present knowledge of the physical, chemical, and immunological properties of AFP's, distinguishing this protein class from other embryo-specific proteins, and the unified terminology proposed for them. The corresponding table composed by the WHO-IARC expert group has been taken as a basis (Annual Report of International Agency for Research on Cancer, 1969). The table includes AFP of man and of most studied animals.

Additional information concerning other animals may be found in

TABLE I

Alpha-Fetoprotein and Other Embryospecific Serum Proteins. Terminology, Physico-Chemical and Immunochemical Properties[a]

Species	Unified term	Synonyms	Electrophoretic position	S_{20}	Molecular weight	Carbohydrates	Cross-reactions with α-fp or other species	Methods of detection	Isolation and purification techniques	Occurrence besides the embryo
Man	α-Feto-protein	x-component (1) ESA-globulin (2) F-protein (42) α₁-Fetoprotein (3) α₁-Feto-specific serum protein (4) Fetoprotein (5) Fetal α-globulin (6) αF-Globulin (7)	α₁-globulin (postalbumin)	4.5 S (8) 4.7 S (17)	64,000 (8)	± (5,9)	Dog and pig (10) Monkey Dog Cat Sheep Armadillo (11) Calf Mouse Rat (12)	1. Immunoelectrophoresis and gel precipitation 2. Electrophoresis on: (a) paper (1) (b) cellulose-acetate (11) (c) starch gel (13) (d) PAAG (14) (e) PAAG-agarose (4) 3. Aggregate-hemagglutination (15) 4. Immunoradioautography (16) 5. Radioimmunoassay (9)	1. Preparative electrophoresis in PAAG combined with anti-albumin antibodies (14) 2. Isolation from specific immune precipitate (8)	Found specific for hepatocellular carcinomas and germinal teratocarcinomas
		β-Fetoprotein (18) Embryo-specific β₁-Globulin (ESB₁)(19) β-Feto-specific serum protein (20)	β-globulin	~10 S (21)	>100,000 (21)		No cross-reaction with α-fp	Immunoelectrophoresis		Present in different diseases (19, 20)
		Embryo-specific β₂-globulin (ESB₂)(19)	β₂-globulin				No cross-reaction with α-fp	Immunoelectrophoresis		Present in different liver diseases (19)
Cattle	α-Feto-protein	Fetal α-globulin (22)	α₂-globulin (23)				No cross-reaction with α-fp Man (12) Goat Sheep (23)	Immunoelectrophoresis (22) PAAG electrophoresis (23)		Found in hepatocellular carcinomas (24)
	Fetuin	Fetuin (25)	α₁-globulin (26)	2.86 S (26) 3.47 S (27)	45,000 (26) 48,400 (27)	++ Glyco-protein (26,27)	No cross-reaction with α-fp (22)	Electrophoresis and immunoelectrophoresis (22,25)	Physicochemical (26, 27)	Present in low levels in adult bovine serum (22)

Species	Protein	Synonyms	Electrophoretic mobility	Sedimentation	Molecular weight	Cross-reaction	Cross-reacting species	Methods of demonstration	Methods of purification	Remarks
Rat	α-Feto-protein	Postalbumin (29) LA-antigen (31) Fetal-α_1-globulin (31) α_1-Feto-specific serum protein (4) α_1-Globulin (32)	α-Globulin (Postalbumin)	2.9 S[b] (30) 4.43 S (29) 4.7 S (17) 4.4 S (8)	30,000[b] (30) 64,800 (29) 65,000–70,000 (8)	± (30)	Mouse-man (12,43)	1. Immunoelectrophoresis and agar precipitation 2. Electrophoresis (a) in starch gel (33) (b) in PAAG (14) (c) in PAAG-agarose (4) 3. Immunofiltration (34) 4. Immunoradioautography (16)	1. Electrophoresis in pevicon block (29) 2. Electrophoresis in PAAG combined with antialbumin antibodies (14) 3. Purification by antibody immunosorbent against adult serum proteins (30)	Found specific for hepatocellular carcinoma
Rat	α-Macro-feto-protein	Slow-α_2 globulin (37) Abnormal serum component (35) α_2-Glycoprotein (30) α_2-Macroglobulin (28, 36) Acute phase protein (38) Embryonal α-globulin (43)	α_2-Globulin	17,8 S (28)		++ (30)	No cross-reaction with α-fp	1. Immunoelectrophoresis (3) 2. Starch-gel electrophoresis (37,36)		Appears in various injuries and pathologic states (30,35,43,44)
Mouse	α-Feto-protein	α_1-Globulin (39)	α_2-Globulin	4,4, S (17)			Rat, man (12)	1. Immunoelectrophoresis (39) 2. Electrophoresis in starch gel (40) 3. PAAG electrophoresis (14) 4. Immunoradioautography (16)	1. Immunofiltration (41,34) 2. Electrophoresis in PAAG (14)	Found specific for hepatocellular carcinoma

ᵃ Numbers in parentheses refer to the following references.

1. Bergstrand and Czar (1956, 1957).
2. Tatarinov (1964a).
3. Muralt and Roulet (1961).
4. Uriel (1969).
5. Masopust (1966).
6. Houstek et al. (1968).
7. Abelev et al. (1967a).
8. Nishi et al. (1971).
9. Purves et al. (1970).
10. Tatarinov and Afanassieva (1965).
11. Gitlin and Boesman (1966, 1967a).
12. Jazova and Gusev (1971).
13. Purves et al. (1969).
14. Gusev and Jazova (1970a).
15. Olovnikov and Tsvetkov (1969).
16. Elgort and Abelev (1971).
17. Gusev and Jazova (1971, unpublished).
18. Vasileysky and Yablokova (1964).
19. Tatarinov (1965a,b).
20. de Nechaud et al. (1969).
21. Vasileysky (1966).
22. Kithier et al. (1968a).
23. Masopust et al. (1971).
24. Kithier et al. (1968b).
25. Pedersen (1944).
26. Deutsch (1954).
27. Spiro (1960).
28. Boffa et al. (1965).
29. Kirsh et al. (1967).
30. Stanislawski-Birencwaig (1965, 1967).
31. Kithier and Prokes (1966).
32. Abelev (1965a).
33. Wise et al. (1963).
34. Abelev (1965b).
35. Lawford (1961).
36. Boffa et al. (1964).
37. Beaton et al. (1961).
38. Weimer and Benjamin (1965).
39. Abelev et al. (1963a,b).
40. Pantelouris and Hale (1962).
41. Abelev and Tsvetkov (1960).
42. Galdo et al. (1959).
43. Perova and Abelev (1967).
44. Van Gool and Ladiges (1969).

ᵇ Seems to be erroneous.

the reports of Tatarinov and Afanassieva (1965), Gitlin and Boesman (1966, 1967a), and Masopust et al. (1971).

B. Detection

Methods of AFP determination should be briefly discussed here, since the evaluation of experimental and clinical conclusions is essentially dependent on their specificity and sensitivity.

AFP in fetal and cancer patient sera can be assayed by a variety of analytical electrophoresis procedures: on paper, cellulose-acetate strips, and most clearly in starch and polyacrylamide [Table I; Fig. 2(a)]. Sensitivity of these methods is not high since they depend on zone densities detectable by staining. Their specificity is fair in the case of sera possessing characteristic patterns of component distribution, but it seems almost impossible to identify AFP in tissue extracts with these methods.

Much more sensitive and specific are the immunochemical methods—immunoelectrophoresis and agar-gel precipitation—especially when a specific anti-AFP serum is employed. The agar-gel precipitation test with single or double diffusion is a standard procedure of AFP determination providing for quantitative assay and possessing a sensitivity level of 1–3 μg./ml. AFP with absolute specificity (Khramkova and Abelev, 1961; Purves et al., 1968).

This level of sensitivity appears, however, not to be sufficient for some experimental and clinical investigations. New and highly sensitive tests for AFP determination have been suggested recently: aggregate-hemagglutination (Olovnikov, 1967; Olovnikov and Tsvetkov, 1969), indirect immunoradioautography (Rowe, 1969, 1970a; Abelev, 1971; Elgort and Abelev, 1971) and radioimmunoassay (Purves et al., 1970). In modifications used, the sensitivity limit of these tests is about 0.05 μg./ml. AFP, that is 25–50 times lower than with agar-gel precipitation.

The essence of these methods is as follows:

1. The aggregate-hemagglutination test may be considered as "reverse hemagglutination." The erythrocytes are conjugated with a pre-polycondensed anti-AFP-serum which renders them agglutinable with a corresponding antigen. Agglutination may be observed with as little antigen as thousandth portions of micrograms per milliliter, but since first dilutions of the antigen assayed are not taken into consideration (up to 1:10 or 1:15), the practical sensitivity limit is about 0.05 μg./ml. The reaction does not possess resolving power and its specificity depends on that of the antiserum used.

2. The radioimmunoassay is based on competition for corresponding antibody between the AFP in the assayed sample and reference [125]I-

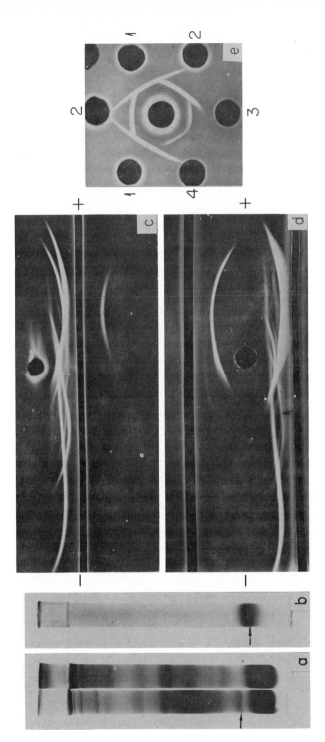

FIG. 2. Characteristics of human AFP. (a) PAAG electrophoresis pattern of fetal (left) and adult (right) human serum. AFP position is indicated by the arrow. (b) PAAG electrophoresis pattern of purified AFP. (c) Immunoelectrophoretic pattern of a fetal human serum (above) and of the purified AFP (below). Developed by antiserum to fetal human serum. (d) Immunoelectrophoretic pattern of a fetal human serum, developed by the antiserum to fetal human serum (bottom trench) and by unabsorbed anti-AFP serum (upper trench). (e) Cross-reactions of human AFP (wells 1) with that of calf (wells 2) mouse (well 3) and rat (well 4). In the central well rabbit antihuman AFP serum. (According to Gusev and Jazova, 1970a,b and Jazova and Gusev, 1971.)

labeled AFP preparation. The antigen-antibody complex is precipitated with antibodies against the immunoglobulin used in the reaction. From a displacement of ^{125}I-AFP in the test sample relative to the control, one can judge the presence of AFP in the examined sample.

Sensitivity of the method is extremely high (for some antigens to nanograms), while its specificity depends on the degree of purity of the reference AFP-anti-AFP system.

3. The indirect immunoradioautography test is a modified gel-precipitation reaction. Sensitivity of gel precipitation is known to increase directly with dilution of the antiserum and reference antigen comprising the test system. The precipitation zone formed by highly diluted reagents becomes invisible, however. In the modified test, visualization of the invisible precipitation band is accomplished with anti-γ-globulin antibodies labeled with ^{131}I or ^{125}I followed by autoradiography of agar plates. The method is about 15 to 30 times more sensitive than agar gel precipitation, and preliminary concentration of examined samples allows an additional 2- or 3-fold increase in sensitivity. As distinct from the above two methods, the immunoradioautography test is absolutely specific.

C. Isolation and Physicochemical Properties

Table I includes the available information on the purification methods and physicochemical characteristics of AFP's. The molecular weights of AFP's are approximately 65,000–70,000; they contain only traces of carbohydrate. The electrophoretic mobility differs depending on animal species: it is similar to that of albumin in man, monkey, or rat. Mouse AFP is located in the α_2-globulin fraction while dog AFP is in the α_3-fraction (Tatarinov and Afanassieva, 1965; Masopust et al., 1971).

Table I reflects certain progress in the study of different animal AFP, which has been obtained due to development of several effective methods for isolation and purification of this protein.

In physicochemical properties AFP is very close to serum albumin. AFP is almost inseparable from the albumin by agar-gel or paper electrophoresis of fetal sera of man, monkey, or rat. Even using polyacrylamide-gel electrophoresis, one cannot obtain complete preparative separation between the two proteins in human and rat sera. All the effective methods proposed for AFP purification employ a combination of physicochemical and immunochemical approaches. Thus, in the initial method of AFP purification, immunofiltration, the separation from electrophoretically inseparable impurities was obtained by a counterelectrophoresis of the antigen mixture through a "filter" composed of antibodies against the impurities (Abelev and Tsvetkov, 1960; Abelev, 1965a,b). Stanislawski-

Birencwajg (1967) purified AFP from fetal sera using adsorption of all "adult" antigens on an immunosorbent prepared from polycondensed antiserum against adult rat serum. Nishi (1970) and Nishi et al. (1971) obtained pure AFP from its precipitate with a corresponding antibody.

The most simple and effective method of purification seems to be that proposed by Gusev and Jazova (1970a), which combines preparative separation in polyacrylamide gel (PAAG) with a final purification step employing antibody. According to this procedure, AFP is first isolated from fetal serum by two cycles of preparative PAAG electrophoresis. The AFP fraction contains some serum albumin, and by addition of the equivalent amount of antialbumin antibody, followed by PAAG electrophoresis, a highly purified AFP preparation is obtained [Fig. 2(b,c)].

The method has been successfully used for isolation of human, rat, and mouse AFP. Pure AFP preparations have enabled us to find out the reliable physical and chemical characteristics and particularly to demonstrate the similarity of AFP from experimental animals and man.

Of no less importance is the use of pure AFP for the preparation of potent, strictly specific antisera. Thus, using immunization of rabbits into lymph nodes with purified AFP, very potent AFP antisera have been obtained (Gusev and Jazova, 1970b). Serum antibody titers reached 1:500 in immunodiffusion, with the immunizing antigen dose as little as 0.5 mg [Fig. 2(d)]. Potent AFP antisera clearly reveal cross-reactions between AFP's from distant species, such as man, cow, mouse, and rat [Fig. 2(e)]. The occurrence of cross-reactivity is good evidence in favor of the assumption that AFP's of the experimental animals and man are indeed homologous proteins, as are their serum albumins and immunoglobulins.

D. FURTHER STUDIES

Basic information on physical, chemical, and structural peculiarities of AFP presents more interest as an approach to understanding control of its synthesis. The available evidence does not provide a basis so far for any suggestions regarding the control mechanism of AFP production. It would be very helpful to have information on the submolecular structure of AFP.

First of all, one can expect that AFP is replaced during development by some "adult" protein with a similar function in the organism. Since in physicochemical properties AFP is close to serum albumin and seems to replace it (at least on electrophoreograms) at the earliest stages of development when the albumin is present only in trace amounts, it can be suggested that serum albumin is the counterpart of AFP, just as "adult" hemoglobin displaces the embryonic type of hemoglobin.

It would not be unreasonable to suppose that these proteins are close in function and homologous in origin. On this basis, similarity in their primary structure can be expected. It would be quite desirable, therefore, to know the primary structure of the polypeptides constituting both proteins or, at least, to compare their peptide maps (fingerprints).

Second, by comparing replacement of embryonic hemoglobin with the adult type protein, one might think of partial alterations in the submolecular structure of AFP rather than of total discontinuation of its synthesis in the adult organism. In this respect it is necessary to know first of all, whether AFP consists of one or more peptide chains. No studies of this kind have been reported so far.

Both of the above questions can be answered in the near future, since availability of simple and effective isolation and purification methods provides full opportunity for such studies.

Detection of genetic variants of AFP would be of indisputable interest for elucidating mechanisms controlling the synthesis of this protein. It would provide approaches for determining the number of genes controlling the synthesis, their localization and expression at cellular and organism levels. Very important in this respect are the reports of Purves *et al.* (1969) and Portugal *et al.* (1970) who detected by electrophoresis a rare "slow" variant of human AFP, significantly different in mobility from the usual type. Genetic analysis would undoubtedly be interesting in this case, as would establishment of the biochemical basis of this property— whether it results from a deviation in primary structure of the protein or from some secondary aggregation defect, or from complex formation with other compounds.

From the point of view of genetic analysis, detailed physicochemical and immunochemical investigation of AFP's from various mouse and rat lines is also promising. Interline and interspecies immunization might reveal line-specific determinants similar to allotypes in immunoglobulins. That would provide the basis for genetic analysis.

It is known that lost or greatly reduced ability to form certain proteins can also be a genetic trait. Analyzing composition of sera from individual human fetuses, Tatarinov (1965b, 1968) found that about 2% of the fetal sera contained no AFP. The age of the fetuses was 24 and 27 weeks and it is possible to think of changed dynamics of AFP formation, namely, of its premature disappearance from serum. Be that as it may, these observations require confirmation and a more detailed analysis.

Finally, one can mention the problem of similarity or difference between the embryonic AFP and that of tumor origin and of AFP's produced by various tumors. Detailed analysis of the protein from individual patients and individual fetuses might reveal possible "abnormalities" or at least heterogeneity in AFP. The latter is an important indication in the analysis of control of protein synthesis, as it has been shown, for example, in immunoglobulin studies.

Human and mouse AFP's behave as single proteins both in electrophoretic and sedimentation analysis. AFP of the rat, however, reveals a definite double zone in starch gel (Wise *et al.*, 1963; Kirsh *et al.*, 1967; Gusev and Jazova, 1970a; Nishi *et al.*, 1971). It is not known what this "bifurcation" is related to and whether or not it is developed by AFP synthesized by rat hepatomas.

Considerable material has accumulated on electrophoretic behavior of AFP's from individual patients (Purves *et al.*, 1969; Portugal *et al.*, 1970). No significant differences have been observed in their electrophoretic patterns. The above-mentioned "slow" variant was detected in less than 2% of cases. This seems to indicate that human AFP possesses no important heterogeneity.

Comparison of AFP's from sera of individual fetuses and patients showed very small differences between the groups in electrophoretic mobility in agar gel and PAAG. Fetal AFP's possessed a mobility which was only ∼5% higher than that of patient AFP's (Gusev *et al.*, 1971a). In this particular study, fetal sera of Europeans and patient sera of Africans were used. The possibility that the above differences were race-determined is not excluded.

Summarizing this section, we may conclude that AFP of different mammals is similar in physicochemical properties and contains common antigenic determinants. Its physicochemical study is fairly satisfactory, but characteristics which could be used in investigation of mechanisms controlling its synthesis are still lacking. Search for such characters is the significant task in studying properties of this protein.

IV. Site of AFP Synthesis in Ontogenesis

It may be considered established at present that during the embryonic period of ontogenesis, AFP is synthesized by the liver parenchyma cells and yolk sac cells. Two kinds of evidence support this statement: *in vitro* synthesis of AFP by the embryonic liver and yolk sac, and specific localization of AFP in cells of liver parenchyma and yolk sac.

A. LIVER

The synthesis of AFP by embryonic liver *in vitro* has been demonstrated by immunoradioautography technique according to Hochwald *et al.* (1961). Surviving pieces of embryonic or newborn liver of mice, rats, and man actively incorporated ^{14}C-amino acids into AFP. The labeled protein was determined by autoradiography in the precipitation band obtained in immunoelectrophoresis or agar double diffusion with a mono-specific anti-AFP serum. The incorporation was specific, since no ^{14}C-amino acids were found included in precipitates of proteins, not synthe-sized but present in the system, and no incorporation of the label resulted in AFP following incubation of other embryonic organs: spleen, kidney, lung, placenta,[1] intestine, stomach, heart, and brain (Abelev, 1965a; Wise and Oliver, 1966; Abelev and Bakirov, 1967; Gitlin and Boesman, 1967b; Van Furth and Adinolfi, 1969; Uriel, 1969).

Further support of the above statement has been obtained from experiments with organ cultures of mouse embryonic liver. Such cultures actively synthesized AFP, albumin, and transferrin and secreted them into the medium in the course of 2 or 3 weeks of cultivation (Luria et al., 1969).

Accumulation of AFP went on with multiple renewals of the medium, so that the total amount of AFP greatly exceeded that introduced with the explant. Besides, the occurrence of AFP synthesis was confirmed by incorporation of ^{14}C-amino acids into the protein.

Thus, AFP formation by the liver of the embryo has been sufficiently well documented. But embryonic liver is not homogeneous in cell com-position; moreover, it is a place of active hematopoiesis, and it remained unknown which liver cells were responsible for AFP synthesis and whether or not the hematopoietic tissue could be the site of its formation. Of course, the specific relation of AFP to hepatocellular cancer, when tumors themselves produced AFP, indicated, although indirectly, that the AFP formation in normal conditions was a function of liver parenchyma cells.

More directly, this was supported by immunofluorescence studies of AFP in sections of different embryonic organs and of cultured embryonic liver. Application of this method for AFP localization had encountered serious difficulties for a long time, since the usual cryostat technique, combined with various fixing reagents, either failed to reveal AFP in sections at all or produced obscure and poorly reproducible results. Only in one study, by Gitlin et al. (1967), was AFP shown rather definitely to be located in the embryonic liver parenchyma and yolk sac.

Much more reliable results were obtained when the paraffin technique of Sainte-Marie was used (Sainte-Marie, 1962; Hamashima et al., 1964). Engelhardt et al. (1969) using this method showed specific localization of AFP in the liver parenchyma cells of mouse and human embryos (Fig. 3)

---

[1] In experiments of Van Furth and Adinolfi (1969), AFP synthesis was reported for human placenta in 2 cases of 7. This was not noted in other studies (Wise and Oliver, 1966; Gitlin and Boesman, 1967b) and no explanation can be proposed at present for the discrepancy.

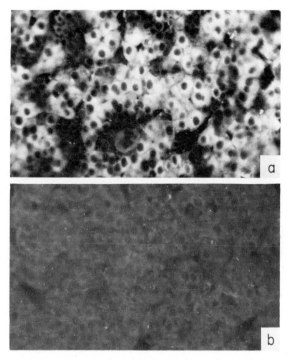

FIG. 3. Localization of AFP in human embryo liver by immunofluorescence. (a) A section of 6-weeks-old embryo liver, treated by antibodies to AFP, and then by fluorescein-conjugated antibody to rabbit γ-globulin. (b) The same as in (a) but anti-AFP serum was neutralized by an equivalent amount of purified AFP. ×40. (According to Engelhardt et al., 1969.)

with concurrent absence of this protein from the liver hematopoietic tissue cells, bile ducts, and Kupfer's cells.[2]

In organ cultures of the liver, also, the AFP-containing cells were identified, both in sections and in total preparations (Basteris et al., 1971). These were hepatocytes, which, as a rule, were distributed in the tissues as trabecules (Fig. 4).

Thus, the conclusion that the liver parenchyma cells are a site of AFP synthesis in normal ontogenesis seems to be well substantiated by the above evidence.

B. Yolk Sac

The yolk sac has been much less studied in this respect. Gitlin and Boesman (1967b) demonstrated that this organ of rats incorporates [14]C-

---

[2] Erythroblastic localization of AFP was observed by Dufour et al. (1969) in the cell suspension of embryonic rat liver. They reported no data about the AFP localization in hepatocytes.

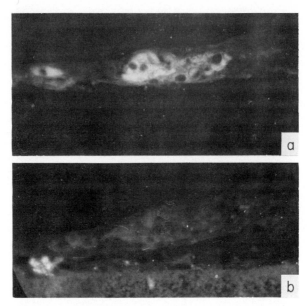

Fig. 4. Localization of AFP in organ cultures of the mouse embryo liver by immunofluorescence. (a) Culture section treated by rabbit antibodies to AFP and then by fluorescein-conjugated antibody to rabbit γ-globulin. (b) Serial section treated as in (a) but anti-AFP was neutralized by purified AFP. ×40. The membrane filter supporting the cultures is seen in (b). (According to Basteris *et al.*, 1971.)

amino acids into AFP during short-term cultivations *in vitro*. Besides, these authors have detected AFP in cryostat sections of the yolk sac (Gitlin *et al.*, 1967).

More detailed investigation of the yolk sac would be desirable.

V. The Dynamics of AFP in Ontogenesis

Detailed investigation of AFP dynamics in ontogenesis is of principal interest. It may throw light on still-unknown functions of the protein and on mechanisms controlling its synthesis.

Thus far the problem has been studied rather irregularly. Most information pertains to the middle and terminal periods of pregnancy or to the time when AFP synthesis is being stopped, while the period when the synthesis is established, early in ontogenesis, has been studied very little.

Conclusions about the dynamics of AFP and other serum proteins are exclusively based on data from electrophoretic and immunodiffusion analysis. No attempts have been made to measure the rate of AFP synthesis in comparison with other serum proteins. Neither were any correlations found between AFP production and other features of the developing organism. Studies on the cellular basis of AMP formation have just been started. All that still purely phenomenological information is absolutely necessary to proceed to the analytical stage of research concerning the function of AFP and regulation of its synthesis.

A. THE EARLY EMBRYONIC PERIOD

There are no data so far about the exact time in ontogenesis when AFP first appears, nor about the initial site of its production.

Some idea of serum composition in the early embryonic period may be obtained from data relating to its termination, that is to the sixth or eighth week of development in man and to ~2 weeks in rats. The protein composition of sera at that time is very distinct from the adult serum, or even from sera of more advanced fetuses.

AFP is the dominating protein in sera of mice and rats, while albumin and transferrin—the main components of adult sera—are present in trace amounts (Fig. 5a), (Pantelouris and Hale, 1962; Wise *et al.*, 1963; Abelev, 1965a,b; Kirsh *et al.*, 1967; Perova, 1969). In human 8-week-old embryos, although albumin prevails over AFP, both proteins are present in comparable concentrations (Fig. 5b) (Galdo *et al.*, 1959; Andreoli and Robbins, 1962).

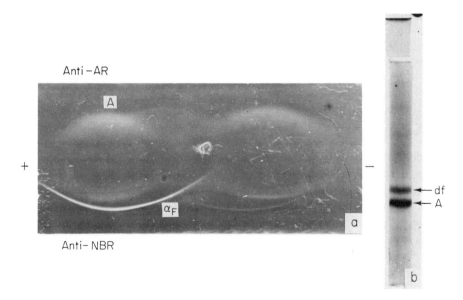

FIG. 5. AFP in early embryonal sera. (a) Immunoelectrophoresis of a rat embryo serum. (The weight of the embryo was about 0.15 gm.) Anti-AR, rabbit antiserum to adult rat serum; Anti-NBR, rabbit antiserum to newborn rat serum; α_F-AFP, A-albumin. (b) PAAG electrophoresis of human 8-week-old embryo serum. α_F-AFP, A-albumin.

Engelhardt[3] (1970) detected AFP in fluids of a 4-week-old human embryo, its concentration being much higher than that of the serum albumin.[4] It seems therefore, that AFP in humans, like that in mice and rats, is also the dominating protein during the earliest stages of development.

It is possible that true proportions between AFP, albumin, and transferrin in the "early" sera are masked by penetration into the fetal blood of mother serum proteins, already when in small amounts. In this respect, measurements of serum protein synthesis, accomplished by the embryo during this period, according to incorporation of ^{14}C-amino acids, would be extremely important, as would determinations of labeled proteins penetrating from the blood flow of the mother. The use of autoradiography of PAAG electrophoreograms (Herrich and Lawrence, 1965) would permit exact answers to these points.

By comparing the "early" sera with those from later stages, it is clearly indicated that an appearance of new components, peculiar to adult serum, is continuously taking place in the embryo, as well as an increase in albumin and transferrin concentrations (see Wise et al., 1963). It is obvious that the most "early" sera studied do not correspond to the first stage of the process, and it would not be unexpected if the initial "primary" sera contained AFP not only as principal but as the only protein component synthesized by the embryo.

It is possible that initially AFP is selectively synthesized in the yolk sac, which provides for its high concentration in embryonic sera with only trace amounts of the albumin. As soon as hepatocytes begin functioning, a rapid accumulation of the albumin would begin, along with a further increase in AFP. To test this possibility, AFP- and albumin-forming cells in the yolk sac and liver should be studied by immunofluorescence techniques during the earliest stages of embryonic development.

Should the "early" embryonic AFP be formed only by the yolk sac, it would be interesting to compare its properties with that of liver-produced AFP which can be obtained in early postnatal life or in animals with regenerating liver.

B. FROM THE MIDDLE OF PREGNANCY TO ITS TERMINATION

This period has been more completely investigated in man and animals (Bergstrand and Czar, 1957; Galdo et al., 1959; Muralt and

---

[3] Gamaleya Institute, Moscow.

[4] Van Furth and Adinolfi (1969) reported trace amounts of AFP in 6- or 7-week-old human fetuses (50 to 100 μg./ml.) with 1.6 to 3.0 mg./ml. for the albumin. It seems that the evidence on this point is not sufficient.

Roulet, 1961; Pantelouris and Hale, 1962; Andreoli and Robbins, 1962; Wise *et al.*, 1963; Tatarinov, 1965; Tatarinov *et al.*, 1967; Masopust, 1966; Masopust *et al.*, 1967; Van Furth and Adinolfi, 1969; Perova, 1969; de Nechaud and Uriel, 1971; Zizkovsky *et al.*, 1971). Figure 6 presents the AFP and albumin levels in sera of fetuses and newborns for man (a,b) and rat (c), the most studied species in this respect. In spite of the great difference in duration of the process and the different position of birth on the curves, the latter are of similar type. An initial rise of AFP level up to a maximum of about 4 mg./ml., some period of plateau, changing later into a period of AFP decline, until it completely disappears—are observed in both cases. It is not known what parameters of the developing embryo determine the character of the curve: its maximum turning point, and cessation of the AFP synthesis. It is certain, only, that neither the duration of development, so different in absolute values for man and rat, nor the time of birth constitute the determining factors for the curve of AFP dynamics.

Evidently, the curve type is dependent on some stage of maturation of the fetus, perhaps on that of its liver, which in man occurs before birth and in mice and rats, afterward (Zizkovsky *et al.*, 1971). It would be most important to identify this character of the developing embryo, equally positioned in relation to the AFP dynamics curve in different mammalian species. Possible correlations should be determined, for this purpose, between AFP synthesis and other principal functions of the liver or of other organs of the fetus. One of such correlations may be the obvious coincidence with the embryonic hematopoiesis. Both processes are successively taking place in the yolk sac and liver, and both terminate at about the same time. AFP might be one of the factors essential for the embryonic hematopoiesis, as Dr. Fridenstein[5] has suggested. The question may be clarified, perhaps, by comparison of the AFP dynamics curves with the period of hepatic hematopoiesis in various animals, significantly differing in time when the AFP synthesis is stopped (see Zizkovsky *et al.*, 1971). Of course, it is important to look for other characters, whose appearance and disappearance might correlate with the AFP dynamics.

Distribution of cells responsible for AFP production during the period of its maximal synthesis have not practically been studied. There is an indication that in the 6-week-old human embryo and in newborn mice, the overwhelming majority of liver parenchyma cells contain AFP (Engelhardt *et al.*, 1969). To investigate the cellular basis for the production of AFP, albumin, and transferrin in the developing embryo seems to be an exciting as well as quite feasible task. The paraffin technique of

[5] Gamaleya Institute, Moscow.

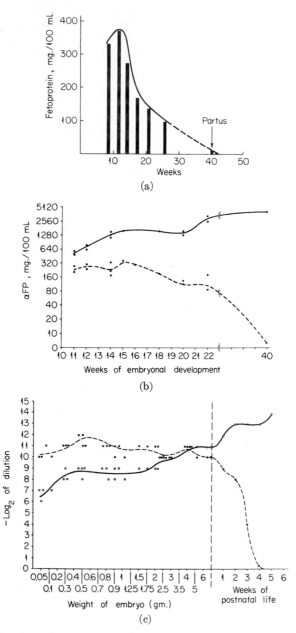

Fig. 6. The dynamics of AFP and serum albumin in the ontogenesis of man and rat. (a) AFP in human fetal sera. (From Masopust *et al.*, 1967.) (b) AFP and serum albumin in human fetal sera. (According to a report of Van Furth and Adinolfi, 1969.) Solid line, serum albumin. Broken line, AFP. (c) AFP and serum albumin in rat fetal sera. (According to Perova, 1969.) Solid line, serum albumin. Broken line, AFP.

Sainte-Marie, which is excellently suitable for cellular localization of serum proteins and permits use of serial sections, provides practical opportunities for detection of several proteins in the same tissue regions (Engelhardt *et al.*, 1971).

Such an investigation would answer the question whether the production of AFP and that of "adult" serum proteins takes place in the same hepatocytes, or if the liver may be considered as a mosaic of cells, specialized in the synthesis of one or another protein. It is absolutely necessary to know this for investigating the mechanisms which regulate serum protein synthesis during development.

C. The Early Postnatal Period

The termination of AFP synthesis is a stage of special interest since it is during this period that the controlling factors come into force. Nothing is known so far about their nature. It has been shown only that the intensity of proliferation of hepatic tissue does not correlate with AFP synthesis (Abelev *et al.*, 1967b). A temporary arrest of mitosis in the liver of 1- to 7-day-old rats (McKellar, 1949) was not accompanied by cessation of AFP synthesis, and on the other hand, termination of the synthesis (fourth week) took place during intensive proliferation of hepatocytes. Thus, the onset of division in hepatocytes or its decline does not seem to be a factor regulating AFP synthesis.

No answer can be given at present to even one of the principal questions, whether a gradual decline of ATP synthesis takes place in all hepatocytes or if only the number of AFP-forming cells decreases. In other words, is it the intensity which is controlled in the AFP synthesis taking place in all hepatocytes or, rather, is the number of cells involved the object of control?

We made an attempt to answer this question by determining AFP, using immunofluorescence, in sections of the mouse liver during the early postnatal period (Abelev, 1971; Shipova *et al.*, 1971). A notable heterogeneity in fluorescence was observed in newborn or 1- or 2-day-old mice.

The heterogeneity markedly increases, beginning from the third to the fifth day of postnatal life. It consisted in regular grouping around the central veins of brightly luminescent cells, clearly differing from the majority of cells in the lobe, which possessed a homogeneous unelevated level of fluorescence, exceeding, however, that of controls (Fig. 7). This may indicate either a difference in the level of ATP synthesis between different liver cells, or that the synthesis is accomplished by a limited number of cells regularly situated in the lobe. With fading of the synthesis, the number of brightly luminescent islets in the lobe diminished, together with the number of cells composing them. By the time AFP

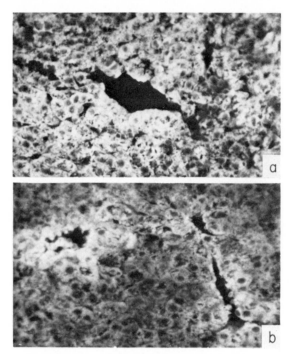

FIG. 7. Immunofluorescence of AFP in the liver of mice during early postnatal life. Sections are treated by rabbit antibody to AFP and then by fluorescein-conjugated antibody to rabbit γ-globulin. ×40. (a) The liver of a 1-day-old mouse. (b) The liver of 11-day-old mouse.

synthesis ceased—the fourth week of postnatal life—no luminescent cells in the liver were observed. We are inclined to think, therefore, that the decrease in AFP level is due to a smaller number of cells synthesizing AFP rather than to fading of a process taking place in all cells of the liver. The suggestion requires a further study with both *in vivo* systems and organ cultures of the liver.

Next, a no less important question is whether the hepatic AFP synthesis is completely discontinued in the adult organism, or if some background level of the protein is maintained. AFP has never been detected in adult animal and human sera by the agar precipitation technique. The sensitivity of the method is about 1 μg./ml., which constitutes 0.025% of the maximal AFP concentration in fetal blood. More sensitive methods—aggregate-hemagglutination and immunoradioautography (see Section III), with the sensitivity limit of 0.05 μg./ml.—in our experience likewise do not reveal AFP in human and rat sera, which brings its level below 0.001% of the maximal concentration.

However, in preliminary experiments, Rowe (1970b) has found trace amounts of AFP in some sera of normal donors by an immunoradio-autography test. Using a similar technique we[6] have demonstrated recently a regular presence of AFP in adult mouse sera, but not in that of rats or humans. The conclusive answer will probably be obtained from radioimmunoassay, but no corresponding studies have been reported up to now.

The problem of background level of AFP is important both for under-standing the nature of the phenomenon and in order to find out whether the tolerance to this antigen persists in adult animals and people. If AFP is completely absent from the adult organism, the tolerance may be lost. A possible immunologic response to AFP in patients with hepatomas might influence its blood level and must be considered in the evaluation of "seropositive" and "seronegative" hepatomas. No direct experiments have been reported, however, on immunization of adult animals or humans with the homologous AFP. Thus, the problem of tolerance to AFP, obviously important from the practical and theoretical points of view, still remains open.

Summarizing the available evidence on AFP dynamics during the embryonic and postnatal periods, it may be concluded that phenomeno-logical study of the problem is far from being completed. To obtain a fuller picture, the following directions of research seem to be necessary.

1. Detailed investigation of early embryonic sera: determination of time of AFP appearance relative to periods of functioning of the yolk sac and liver. Comparative studies on AFP from "albumin-less" sera and from sera of adult animals with regenerating liver.

2. Investigation of correlations between AFP production and other functions of the embryonic liver, particularly with the hepatic hematopoiesis.

3. Immunofluorescence study of the yolk sac and liver in ontogenesis, aimed at determining their contribution in the serum protein production during the early and later stages of embryonic development.

4. Analysis by immunofluorescence of the cellular basis for the syn-thesis of AFP and "adult" proteins: determination of mono- or multi-potency of the hepatocytes in the synthesis of different serum proteins, and of dynamics of the population of AFP-forming cells during ontogenesis.

5. Detection of a possible background level of AFP and of tolerance to it in the adult organism.

---

[6] In cooperation with Drs. D. Elgort and S. Perova.

VI. AFP Synthesis during Regeneration of the Liver

In the first study on AFP synthesis by mouse hepatomas (Abelev *et al.*, 1963a,b) it was established that a limited temporary "outbreak" of AFP synthesis occurred in normal adult animals after partial hepa-

TABLE II

ALPHA-FETOPROTEIN IN SERA OF PARTIALLY HEPATECTOMIZED RATS[a]
(IMMUNORADIOAUTOGRAPHY)

Treatment	No. of animal	Weight and sex	Results of IR-test[b]								
			Days after the operation								
			0	1	2	3	4	5	7	8	12
Hepatectomy	1	♂120	−	−	4+	3+	3+	.	.	.	.
	2	♂189	−	−	4+	3+	3+	.	.	.	.
	3	♀215	−	−	4+	3+	3+	.	.	.	.
	4	♂123	−	−	4+	2+	.	.	.	.	.
	5	♂148	−	−	4+	3+	.	.	.	.	.
	6	♂158	−	−	4+	3+	.	.	.	.	.
	7	♂155	−	−	4+	3+	.	.	.	.	.
	8	♂218	−	−	4+	3+	.	.	.	.	.
	9	♂204	−	−	4+	3+	.	.	.	.	.
	10	♀ 90	−	−	4+	3+	.	.	.	.	.
	11	♂140	−	−	4+	3+	3+	3+	.	.	.
	12	♂192	−	−	3+	3+	3+	2+	.	.	.
	13	♂183	−	−	4+	3+	3+	3+	.	.	.
	14	♂182	−	−	4+	3+	3+	3+	.	.	.
	15	♂170	−	−	4+	3+	3+	3+	.	.	.
	16	♂181	−	−	4+	3+	3+	3+	.	.	.
	17	♂181	−	−	4+	3+	3+	3+	.	.	.
	18	♂157	−	−	4+	3+	3+	3+	.	.	.
	19	♂181	−	−	4+	3+	3+	3+	.	.	.
	20	♂202	−	−	4+	3+	3+	3+	.	.	.
	21	♂153	−	−	4+	3+	3+	3+	.	.	.
	22	♂117	−	.	4+	.	.	.	2+	+	−
	23	♂155	−	.	4+	.	.	.	2+	+	−
	24	♀123	−	.	4+	.	.	.	+	+	−
	25	♂147	−	.	4+	.	.	.	2+	+	−
	26	♂146	−	.	4+	.	.	.	2+	+	−
	27	♂154	−	.	4+	.	.	.	2+	+	−
Laparotomy	28–	♂175–	−	.	−	−	−	.	.	.	.
	32	♂201									

[a] According to Perova *et al.* (1971).

[b] All serum samples were 3-fold concentrated before the analyses. From + to 4+ degree of positive reaction; − negative result; . not tested.

tectomy. These observations were repeatedly confirmed later, and the most efficient and reproducible method of AFP induction in mice was shown to be liver regeneration following inhalation of CCl_4 vapor (Bakirov, 1968). The response in mice was rather uniform with relatively high secretion of AFP into the blood. AFP appeared 2 days after the animals were poisoned reached a maximum (about 1% of the fetal blood level) on the third day, and then disappeared from the circulation in the course of 8 to 10 days. Laparotomy, inhalation of ether, and other "nonspecific" treatments did not result in resumption of AFP synthesis.

In rats with regenerating liver, an outwardly different picture was recorded. With adult animals, neither partial hepatectomy nor CCl_4 vapor inhalation resulted in AFP detectable by the agar-gel precipitation method (Grabar et al., 1967; Stanislawski-Birencwajg et al., 1967; Perova and Abelev, 1967; de Nechaud and Uriel, 1971).

At the age of 5 weeks, "induction" was observed only in some animals after partial hepatectomy (Perova and Abelev, 1967) or administration of CCl_4 (de Nechaud and Uriel, 1971). The distinctions between mice and rats could be either quantitative or qualitative, and in order to decide on this point, sera of partially hepatectomized rats were analyzed for AFP by the indirect immunoradioautography test. The result was regular detection of AFP on the second day after the operation with gradual decrease by the ninth to twelfth day (Table II) (Perova et al., 1971).

Thus, the dynamics of AFP in rats with regenerating liver has recapitulated that of hepatectomized or CCl_4-treated mice, although the absolute values were 10 to 30 times lower.

The experiments allowed one to think that AFP synthesis during regeneration of the liver occurs with general regularity.

Whether AFP appears during regeneration of the liver in humans was of interest not only from the point of view of the scope of the phenomenon, but as a possible source of complications in the diagnosis of hepatic tumors. Immunoprecipitation in agar gel, as a rule, did not reveal AFP in sera of patients with acute hepatitis and cirrhosis, the diseases commonly accompanied by more or less active liver regeneration (see Section VII). It was not until recently that AFP was reported, with this method, in 3 of 375 examined cases of Botkin disease and in 2 of 324 patients suffering from cirrhosis (Tatarinov, 1970; Massiukevitch, 1970).[7] The AFP concentration was just above the threshold level and the appearance was of

[7] One case of AFP appearance with acute hepatitis and one with cirrhosis were reported earlier by Alpert et al. (1968). See also a case described by Geffroy et al. (1970a).

TABLE III

ALPHA-FETOPROTEIN IN PATIENTS WITH LIVER DISEASES
(IMMUNORADIOAUTOGRAPHY)[a]

| | AFP in blood serum[b] | | |
Diagnosis	Number of AFP-positive cases	% of AFP-positive cases	Comments
Infectious and serum hepatitis	23/176	13%	2 cases were strongly positive in agar-precipitation
Cirrhosis	0/54	0%	
Chronic hepatitis	0/33	0%	
Other liver diseases	1/21	4.7%	"AFP+" case — mechanic jaundice

[a] According to Abelev et al. (1971).
[b] All serum samples were concentrated 2- or 3-fold.

short duration. In view of the above instance with rats, the matter had to be reinvestigated with more sensitive methods of AFP detection. No materials were available to us from patients with mechanical injury of the liver, the closest analogy of hepatectomy. But with other liver diseases, the investigation gave quite definite results, when indirect immunoradioautography was used (Table III) (Abelev, 1971; Abelev et al., 1971). Infectious and serum hepatitis were prominent among the liver diseases: in ~13% of the patients the test revealed AFP in concentrations from 0.05 to 0.5 μg./ml.; 2 patients from the total number of 176 possessed AFP levels considerably higher than the sensitivity limit of agar-gel precipitation.

Sixteen of the patients with AFP in their blood had been followed during the course of disease (Table IV). In all the cases, AFP disappeared from the serum after convalescence. Some of the patients were examined at 7- to 10-day intervals. The results suggested that in viral hepatitis the appearance and disappearance of AFP occurred within a period of 2 months or less. However, the available data are not sufficient for a final conclusion on this point.

The suggestion about liver regeneration as a cause of AFP formation in viral hepatitis is founded on principal similarity of the AFP dynamics during this disease and that of mice and rats with regenerating liver. No direct evidence is available, however, which could be obtained, for instance, from detailed comparison of the clinical course with the AFP dynamics. The need in such studies is obvious. There is no doubt, also, of the necessity to compare regenerative processes in the liver of patients

TABLE IV

ALPHA-FETOPROTEIN DYNAMICS IN ACUTE VIRAL HEPATITIS
AS REVEALED BY IMMUNORADIOAUTOGRAPHY TEST[a]

Patient	Results of IR test								
	Weeks from the onset of disease								
	1	2	3	4	5	6	7	8	More than 8 weeks
1. G-n	·	·	4+	·	·	·	·	·	— (14th week)
2. U-v	·	—	+	·	·	·	·	·	— (18th week)
3. S-v	>4+[b]	·	·	·	·	—	·	·	
4. P-r	—	·	4+	4+	·	·	·	·	
5. P-v	·	+	·	·	—	—	·	·	
6. Ch-v	—	·	4+	4+	·	·	·	2+	
7. B-va	·	·	4+	2+	+	—	·	·	
8. R-ja	·	—	·	·	3+	·	·	·	— (26th week)
9. Z-v	·	·	—	·	·	2+	2+	2+	
10. O-y	—	·	+	—	·	·	·	·	
11. T-n	·	·	>4+	·	·	·	—	·	
12. R-n	·	·	·	2+	·	—	·	·	
13. K-v	·	·	·	·	·	·	+	·	— (15th week)
14. Sh-y	·	·	·	·	·	·	·	·	>4+ on 20th week,[b] — on 32th week
15. L-v	? + after 6 weeks —								
16. G-k	? + after 1 week —								

[a] According to Abelev et al. (1971).

[b] Positive in agar precipitation test. · -not tested; — negative; + to 4+ degrees of positive reaction; ? -the onset of the disease not known; □ -period of jaundice.

who possess or lack AFP in their blood, although such studies in man are not easy to perform.

The patient group with cirrhosis has been sufficiently large, and the fully negative result is unexpected. To explain the contradiction between the absence of AFP in cirrhosis and its presence in infectious hepatitis— both diseases being attended by regeneration of the liver—the following suggestions can be offered: first, that a definite minimal regeneration rate is necessary for AFP "induction" to occur and, second, that the ability to synthesize AFP might become "exhausted" during long-lasting regeneration or with successive cycles of regeneration. The suggestions can be tested readily in experimental models. In this respect, of great interest is the experimental cirrhosis in rats induced by CCl_4 (Reuber and Glover, 1970), in which case AFP could be followed during all stages of disease. Repeated induction of the regenerative process in mice by CCl_4 vapor may also serve as a good model. Based on the above suggestions, it may be expected, also, that a low level of AFP will be found eventually in patients with active cirrhosis of the liver, especially during the acute stage.

Thus, it may be considered proved that regeneration of the liver results in temporary AFP synthesis in mice and rats, and seems to do so in man. The level of synthesis varies within broad limits in different species. Diagnostic implications of the phenomenon will be discussed in Section VIII.

A. AFP Synthesis during Regeneration of the Liver
   as a Model for Studying the Nature
   of the Phenomenon

The early negative findings encountered in detection of AFP during regeneration of the liver in rats and in clinical material have lessened interest in and even cast doubt on the correlation as such. Hence, the "induction" of AFP synthesis under these conditions has received undeservedly little study. The mechanism of "induction" is not known, although the system is probably most suitable for studying this aspect of the phenomenon as a whole. Indeed, AFP synthesis in this case can be induced deliberately under strictly controlled conditions and in adult animals. The response is pronounced and develops without undue variation in individual animals.

1. Cellular Aspects of AFP Synthesis

The first question arising in the analysis of AFP "induction" is whether all the hepatocytes resume synthesis or only some liver cells become "activated." Preliminary evidence, obtained by immunofluorescence on regenerating mouse liver, clearly indicates that AFP is observed only in certain cells distributed in small and rare groups.

The cells become detectable on the second day and are most pronounced on the third day after poisoning animals with CCl_4, which corresponds to the maximal level of AFP in the blood serum (Engelhardt et al., 1969). The majority of hepatocytes did not contain AFP.

Studies of this kind should also be made with hepatectomized mice, which contain no zones of necrosis in their liver, confusing the ordinary picture of that organ. It would be particularly significant to find out whether or not "AFP-positive" cells are revealed around central veins, the areas where AFP synthesis seems to persist longest in the postnatal period.

The next major question is whether the "inducible" cells of the liver are preexisting or appear always as a result of division of precursor cells, cambial cells, or differentiated hepatocytes. This problem can be solved, probably, by combining ^{3}H-thymidine autoradiography with immunofluorescent detection of AFP in the same sections. An occurrence of even a portion of AFP-containing cells which have not undergone division would indicate preexistence of hepatocytes capable of being induced to synthesize AFP. That would mean that AFP "induction" is dependent on some external factors, inducers or inhibitors which activate or switch off the synthesis. On the other hand, if it is found that all the "AFP-positive" cells belong to the proliferative pool of the regenerating liver and appear only as a result of division of precursor cells, the latter can be either the division of a mature hepatocyte, attended by dedifferentiation, or that of a cambial liver cell, leading to its differentiation into an AFP-producing hepatocyte.

2. Genetic Aspects in the "Induction" of AFP

For elucidating factors involved in AFP "induction" it is of interest to use line distinctions in this character, found in mice of C3HA[8] and C57BL/6 strains (Bakirov and Abelev, 1968). The distinctions are of quantitative nature, but quite significant: on the average, the AFP levels in the strains differ by a factor of 10. Hybridological analysis could show the number of genes determining this trait. It seems feasible also to derive coisogenic pairs, different only in AFP formation levels. The availability of such a specific pair, with distinction only in the studied character, would be of undoubted interest for determining factors which control AFP synthesis and understanding species differences in activity of the synthesis during regeneration of the liver.

In this connection, the existence in mice of a detectable background level of AFP, as distinct from the rat and man, is of primary importance. It seems most likely that the degree of "induction" of AFP during regeneration is in positive correlation with the background level of AFP. A quantitative investigation of this suggestion in "inducible" and "low-inducible" lines and their hybrids might give a definite answer to the question.

[8] The C3HA response is typical for most mouse strains tested.

VII. AFP in Hepatocellular Cancer

The evidence obtained with experimental models and in the clinic may be considered together in view of the principal similarity of the phenomenon in animals and man. This is especially justified since each of the approaches has its advantages: with animal tumors, a more detailed analysis has been done while the clinical material examined has been by far more rich and diverse than that from experimental models. Naturally, one must always bear in mind the species differences as well as the differences in etiology of hepatomas in experiments and nature, which exclude direct transfer of empirical generalizations from experimental model systems to man. First, we shall consider the problem of localization of the AFP synthesis in cancer of the liver, upon which proper evaluation of both clinical and experimental evidence is dependent.

A. SITE OF AFP SYNTHESIS IN CANCER OF THE LIVER

When AFP appears in the blood of a tumor-bearing animal or patient, both the tumor itself and the affected liver could be the source of the embryonic protein. There is sufficient evidence to believe that tumor constitutes the main site of AFP synthesis in the organism of the host, but the possibility of the synthesis being resumed by the liver, even if in some exceptional cases, by no means can be excluded.

Most convincing evidence about the site of AFP synthesis was obtained in experimental model systems. In experiments with a transplantable hepatoma of mice we have demonstrated that the tumor continues to synthesize murine AFP following its heterotransplantation into cortisone-treated rats or explantation *in vitro* (Abelev *et al.*, 1963a,b). Subsequent studies with stable cultures of the same tumor showed that, at least during first generations they maintained the ability to synthesize AFP *in vitro* together with albumin and transferrin (Irlin *et al.*, 1966). Accumulation of AFP was observed also in primary cultures of Zaidela's hepatoma of the rat (Perova and Abelev, 1967). Experiments of Hull *et al.* (1969b,c) on cultivation of primary hepatomas of monkeys, induced by carcinogen, have showed that AFP, albumin, and transferrin are synthesized by them *in vitro*.

Thus, data obtained with hepatomas of mice, rats, and monkeys convincingly demonstrate AFP production by tumors themselves. It should be emphasized that the evidence in itself does not at all exclude possible participation of the liver in the production.

Naturally, it is a more difficult task to determine the site of AFP synthesis in humans suffering from liver cancer. Three groups of evidence testify in favor of AFP production by tumor itself, apart from the analogy with the situation in animals: the highly specific correlation of AFP with hepatocellular cancer, the disappearance of AFP after surgical removal of the tumor, and the detection of AFP in tumor cells by immunofluorescence. The first group of evidence will be especially considered in the next section, while two others are discussed here.

Surgery with hepatomas is extremely rare. We have observed only one case. In a patient who had a high blood level of AFP, there was a sharp decrease in AFP, at times its complete disappearance, when the liver lobe affected by tumor had been ablated (Morkhov and Sokolov, 1970).

More information on the AFP synthesis site in human cancer of the liver has been obtained recently by immunofluorescence. It has been mentioned that AFP can be readily localized in tissues by the technique of Sainte-Marie. A major complication in work with hepatomas, especially with the autopsy material from humans, is connected with secondary nonspecific uptake of AFP from the serum by dead cells and, in general, by cells with impaired permeability. These are necrotic cells in tumor and dead or dying cells in normal tissue, because, usually, the material is available only several (2–6) hours after clinical death. To differentiate AFP-forming cells from those passively acquiring it along with other proteins of the plasma, we used a special control: parallel examination of the same cells in serial sections for presence of human γ-globulin (Engelhardt et al., 1971).

γ-Globulin is known to be elaborated only by plasma cells and does not penetrate living cells of the liver or tumor, while penetrating freely into dead cells. Parallel study of the same areas in sections of the liver or tumor for presence in the cells of AFP and human γ-globulin, has indeed showed the existence for both antigens of completely coinciding areas, with identical localization, as well as of tissue regions where only AFP was localized. A typical appearance of the "overlapping" and "nonoverlapping" distribution is shown in Fig. 8. Specific localization of AFP has been observed only in tumor tissue. The liver, lung, and kidney of the patient exhibited no AFP distribution differing from that of γ-globulin (Gusev et al., 1971b).

The immunofluorescence evidence is quite convincing. But the conclusive proof of AFP synthesis by human hepatocellular tumors could be provided by evidence on AFP synthesis by cultured hepatomas. It should be supposed that such evidence will soon be available.

Thus, the combined findings from experimental model systems and clinical material indicate that AFP synthesis is resumed by cells of hepatocellular carcinomas themselves. On the other hand, the occurrence of AFP synthesis during regeneration of the liver must be taken into

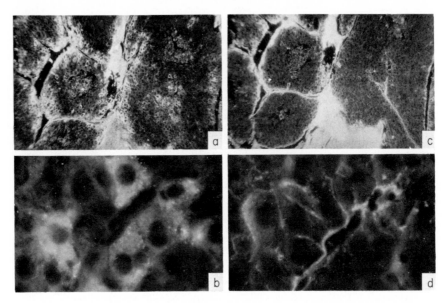

Fig. 8. Localization of AFP and γ-globulin in a human hepatocellular carcinoma. (a–b) A tumor section treated by rabbit antibody to AFP and then by fluorescein-conjugated antibody to rabbit γ-globulin. ×10 and ×90, respectively. (c–d) A parallel section treated by rabbit antibody to human γ-globulin and then by fluorescein-conjugated antibody to rabbit γ-globulin. ×10 and ×90, respectively. Note the γ-globulin-free cells containing AFP. (According to Engelhardt *et al.*, 1971.)

account as an additional possibility weakening the correlation of AFP with cancer of the liver.

B. Demonstration of AFP in the Blood in Cases of Liver Cancer and Other Diseases by the Method of Agar-Gel Precipitation

This section will be devoted to results of experimental and clinical studies on detection of AFP in cancer of the liver, other tumors, and noncancerous diseases of the liver. No consideration is given to AFP in embryonic tumors, since the problem requires special analysis, presented in Section IX.

Tables V and VI summarize published results on liver tumors in experimental animals together with appropriate control groups. Table VII presents clinical data available to us on more than 1000 cases of primary cancer of the liver and several thousand disease cases in the control group. It must be emphasized that the antisera used by different workers for AFP determination in humans, in the majority of cases, had been collated. All data presented in Tables V to VII were obtained by agar-gel precipitation.

TABLE V

ALPHA-FETOPROTEIN IN ANIMAL HEPATOMAS, ACCORDING TO THE
AGAR-GEL PRECIPITATION TEST

Species	Carcinogen	Primary or transplantable	Number of AFP-positive cases	References
Mouse	Spontaneous	Primary	1/25	Khramkova and Guelstein (1967); Abelev (1968)
	Ortoamino-azotoluene	Primary	7/29	Khramkova and Guelstein (1965)
	Ortoamino-azotoluene	Transplantable	6/8	Abelev (1965a, 1968)
Rat	3'-M DAB	Primary	78/94	Stanislawski-Birencwajg et al. (1967)
	DAB	Primary	22/28	Stanislawski-Birencwajg et al. (1967)
	N-dimetilnitrosoamine	Primary	1/2	Stanislawski-Birencwajg et al. (1967)
	Aflatoxin B	Primary	0/15	Stanislawski-Birencwajg et al. (1967)
	Aflatoxin B	Primary	0/60	Monjour and Mariage (1969)
	?	Transplantable strains	5/7	Stanislavski-Birencwajg et al. (1967)
	?	Transplantable strains	20/60	Nishi et al. (1971)
	DAB	Zaidela hepatoma	+	Perova and Abelev (1967); Dorfman (1967)
	DMBA	Transplantable strains	3/13[a]	Baldwin and Barker (1967)
Monkey	N-nitrosodiethylamine	Primary	33/37	Hull et al. (1969b,c)
Baboon	Pyridoxine deprived	Primary "preneo-plastic" lesions	5/10	Foy et al. (1970a,b)
Cattle	Spontaneous	Primary	2/4	Kithier et al. (1968b)

[a] The results of Baldwin and Barker (1967) are included in the table arbitrarily, since no identification of the embryonal antigen was made, either with AFP or with α-macro-fetoprotein.

TABLE VI

ALPHA-FETOPROTEIN IN NONHEPATIC TUMORS AND NONNEOPLASTIC CONDITIONS

Species	Tumor or treatment	Primary or transplantable	Number of AFP+ cases	References
Mouse	Carcinogen-induced sarcomas	Transplantable strains	0/9	Abelev et al. (1963a,b)
	Leukemia	Transplantable strains	0/5	Abelev et al. (1963a,b)
	Skin tumor	Transplantable strains	0/2	Abelev et al. (1963a,b)
	Mammary tumor	Transplantable strains	0/2	Abelev et al. (1963a,b)
	Krocer sarcoma	Transplantable strains	0/1	Abelev et al. (1963a,b)
	Ehrlich carcinoma	Transplantable strains	0/1	Abelev et al. (1963a,b)
Rat	M-1 and 45 sarcomas	Transplantable strains	0/2	Abelev (1965a)
	Renal blastoma	Primary	0/9	Stanislawski-Birencwajg et al. (1967)
	Renal myoneuroma	Primary	0/2	Stanislawski-Birencwajg et al. (1967)
	Adrenal epithelioma	Transplantable	0/1	Stanislawski-Birencwajg et al. (1967)
	Salivary gland epithelioma	Transplantable	0/1	Stanislawski-Birencwajg et al. (1967)
	Mammary tumor	Transplantable	0/1	Stanislawski-Birencwajg et al. (1967)
	Lymphosarcoma	Transplantable	0/1	Stanislawski-Birencwajg et al. (1967)
	Myeloma	Transplantable	0/1	Stanislawski-Birencwajg et al. (1967)
	Bile-duct carcinoma	Primary	0/30	Stanislawski-Birencwajg et al. (1967)
	Cirrhosis		0/7	Stanislawski-Birencwajg et al. (1967)
	Hepatitis		0/8	Stanislawski-Birencwajg et al. (1967)
	Nodular hyperplasia		0/3	Stanislawski-Birencwajg et al. (1967)
Monkey	N-Nitroso-diethylamine hepatitis		0/19	Hull et al. (1969b,c)
	Cycasin		0/16	Hull et al. (1969b,c)
	1 Nitroso-piperidine		0/7	Hull et al. (1969b,c)

TABLE VI (*Continued*)

Species	Tumor or treatment	Primary or transplantable	Number of AFP+ cases	References
	Aflatoxin B		0/15	Hull *et al.* (1969b,c)
	3′M-DAB		0/10	Hull *et al.* (1969b,c)
	2,7-FAA		0/13	Hull *et al.* (1969b,c)
Baboon	Riboflavin deprived		0/5	Foy *et al.* (1970a,b)
	Normal		0/8	Foy *et al.* (1970a,b)

It should be kept in mind that the total number of hepatoma patients in Table VII may be somewhat overestimated, because some authors included the same data in several publications. In known instances, the corresponding data in Table VII have been marked. From the reported results a few quite significant general conclusions can be drawn.

1. The appearance of AFP in the blood of adult animals and humans is highly specific for hepatocellular cancer and for mixed hepato- and cholangiocellular cancer of the liver. On the average, AFP has been found in about 70% of histologically confirmed hepatocellular cancers in humans.

2. The cholangiocellular cancer of the liver is not associated with AFP production.

3. Metastatic tumors of the liver, as a rule, are not associated with appearance of AFP, nor are malignant tumors of nonhepatic origin.

4. Liver diseases of noncancerous nature are usually not accompanied by AFP formation.

5. There is a significant group of histologically confirmed hepatocellular carcinomas in which AFP has not been detected (about 30% in humans).

6. A small portion of clinical cases constitute a histologically confirmed group of "false positives."

The material presented in the tables seems to be quite sufficient for a general conclusion about the practical value of the AFP test for differential diagnosis of hepatocellular cancer.

However, both the analysis of the nature of the phenomenon and further improvement of the test require additional evidence, primarily from studies of the differences between "AFP-positive" ("AFP+") and "AFP-negative" ("AFP−") hepatomas and of cases in which AFP appears in the absence of hepatocellular cancer.

The first problem which should be considered in comparing "AFP+"

TABLE VII
ALPHA-FETOPROTEIN IN HEPATOCELLULAR CANCER AND OTHER DISEASES OF MAN,

Country	Group	Hepatocellular and mixed type of primary liver cancer			Cholangio-cellular carcinoma		Metastatic liver cancer		Nonneoplastic liver diseases	
		AFP+ total	% of AFP+	Type of diagnosis	AFP+ total	% of AFP+	AFP+ total	% of AFP+	AFP+ total	% of AFP+
USSR	I Astrakhan	29/30	96%	Histological	0/8	0%	0/58	0%	5/1356	0.36%
	II Moscow	35/53	64%	Histological	0/16	0%	0/93	0%	2/374	0.55%
	III Siberia	22/29 includes 20/24	75.8% 83%	Clinical or histological Histological	1/21	4.7%	1/64	1.5%	0/410	0%
USSR (total)	I-III	86/112 84/107	76.8% 78.5%	Clinical or histological Histological	1/45	2.2%	1/215	0.4%	7/2140	0.33%
France	I	12/21	55%	Clinical or histological	0/1	0%	0/25	0%	0/114	0%
	II	18/30	60%	Clinical or histological	0/2	0%	0/25	0%	0/127	0%
	III						1/1			
France (total)	II-III	18/30	60%	Clinical or histological	0/2	0%	1/26	0.38%	0/127	0%
Greece	I	18/35	51%	Clinical or histological	0/4	0%	0/37	0%	0/203	0%
USA	I	8/28 for Caucasian 6/8 for Africans	28% 75%	Histological	.	.	.	.	0/250	0%
	II	15/39 includes 9/19	38% 47% 31% AFP+ caucasians, 71% AFP+ Africans	Clinical or histological Histological	0/12	0%	0/34	0%	0/45	0%
	III	7/12	58%	Histological	.	.	.	.	0/156	0%
USA (total)	I-III	36/87 30/67	41% 44.7%	Clinical or histological Histological	0/12	0%	0/34	0%	0/451	0%
England	I	14/35 includes	40%	Histological	0/10	0%	0/14	0%	0/185	0%

According to Gel Precipitation Method[a]

Nonhepatic neoplasmas		Nonneoplastic and nonliver diseases		Pregnancy		Normal donors		Comments on nonhepatoma group	References
AFP+ total	% of AFP+	AFP+ total	% of AFP+	AFP+ total	% of AFP+	AFP+ total	% of AFP+		
.	.	.	.	6/1049	0.5%	0/462	0%	(a) 2AFP+ from 324 in cirrhosis; 3 AFP+ out of 378 in viral hepatitis (b) Included part of hepatoma cases from group II	Tatarinov (1970); Massiukevitch (1970)
0/142	0%	.	.	.	.	.	.	(a) 2AFP+ out of 176 of viral hepatitis	Assecritova et al. (1967); Abelev et al. (1967a); Abelev (1968); Perova (1969)
.	.	.	.	.	.	0/11340	0%	(a) 1AFP+ —carcinoma of unknown origin with liver metastases	Babinov and Shain (1971)
0/142	0%	.	.	6/1049	0.5%	0/11862	0%		
.	.	0/9	0%	.	.	.	.		de Nechaud et al. (1969)
.	.	0/15	0%	.	.	.	.	Group II includes partly (?) the group I	Economopuolos et al. (1970)
.	.	.	.	.	.	.	.	Histologically confirmed case	Boureille et al. (1970)
.	.	0/15	0%	.	.	.	.	According to group II and III	
0/5 (liver sarcomas)	0%	0/168	0%	.	.	.	.		Economopuolos et al. (1970)
.	.	.	.	.	.	.	.		Alpert (1969)
0/143	0%	0/19	0%	.	.	.	.		Hull et al. (1969b,c, 1970)
.	.	0/25	0%	.	.	0/300	0%	Control group includes all kind of disease	Smith and Blumberg (1969); Smith and Todd (1968)
0/143	0%	0/44	0%	.	.	0/300	0%		
.	.	.	.	.	.	.	.		Foli et al. (1969)

(continued)

TABLE VII

Country	Group	Hepatocellular and mixed type of primary liver cancer			Cholangio-cellular carcinoma		Metastatic liver cancer		Nonneoplastic liver diseases	
		AFP+ total	% of AFP+	Type of diagnosis	AFP+ total	% of AFP+	AFP+ total	% of AFP+	AFP+ total	% of AFP+
England	II	9/27	33% for non-Africans							
		5/8	62% for Africans							
		4/9	44%	Clinical or histological						
	III	4/6	66% includes 2/2 Africans, 2/4 non-Africans	Histological						
England (total)	I-III	22/50	44%	Clinical or histological	0/10	0%	0/14	0%	0/185	0%
		18/41	43%	Histological						
Czechoslovakia	I	1/3	33%	Histological						
South Africa (Bantu)	I	76/93	82%	Histological					0/2119	0%
	II	102/130	78%	Clinical or histological						
South Africa (total)	I-II	76/93	82%	Histological					0/1219	0%
		178/223	79.8%	Clinical or histological						
Mozambique	I	29/56 includes	51.7% histological	Clinical or histological						
		25/37	67.6%	Histological						
Senegal	I	219/304 includes	72%	Clinical or histological					0/1248	0%
	II	35/44	79.6%	Histological					5/81[b]	
Kenya	I	13/28 includes	46.4%	Clinical or histological					0/83[b]	0%
		10/14	71.4%	Histological						
Nigeria	I	11/15 includes	73%	Clinical or histological					1/23[b]	4%
		10/14	71%	Histological						
Uganda	I	20/40	50%	Clinical or histological			0/8	0%	2/111	1.8%
	II	11/18 includes	61%	Clinical or histological						

(*Continued*)

Nonhepatic neoplasmas		Nonneoplastic and nonliver diseases		Pregnancy		Normal donors		Comments on nonhepatoma group	References
AFP+ total	% of AFP+	AFP+ total	% of AFP+	AFP+ tòtal	% of AFP+	AFP+ total	% of AFP+		
.	.	.	.	.	.	.	.		Clark (1970)
.	.	.	.	.	.	.	.		Kohn and Muller (1970)
.	.	.	.	.	.	.	.		
0/213	0%	.	.	.	.	.	.		Masopust *et al.* (1968) Kithier *et al.* (1966)
.	.	.	.	.	.	0/1384	0%	8 AFP+ in newborns are excluded from the control group	Purves *et al.* (1968, 1970c)
.	.	.	.	.	.	0/1384	0%		
.	.	1/300	0.3%	.	.	0/200	0%	(a) 1 AFP+ in control group-hepatoblastoma in 1-year child (b) Control group includes all nonhepatoma patients	Portugal *et al.* (1970)
3/106	2.9%	0/2485	0%	.	.	0/2025	0%	(a) Nonhepatic tumors include those with liver metastases	Uriel *et al.* (1967); Masseyeff *et al.* (1968)
								(b) 3 AFP+ cases—gastro-intestinal tumors with liver metastases; 2 AFP+ metastatic liver cancer; 2 AFP+ cirrhosis and 1 AFP+ —trypanosomiasis	O'Conor *et al.* (1970)
.	.	.	.	7/20	35%	.	.	7 AFP+ in pregnancy more than 30 weeks	O'Conor *et al.* (1970) Foy *et al.* (1970d)
.	.	.	.	.	.	.	.	AFP+ —hepatosplenomegaly (Clinical)	O'Conor *et al.* (1970)
.	.	0/50	0%	.	.	.	.	(a) AFP+ in histologically confirmed viral hepatitis (1 case) and cirrhosis (1 case)	Alpert *et al.* (1968)

(*continued*)

TABLE VII

Country	Group	Hepatocellular and mixed type of primary liver cancer			Cholangio-cellular carcinoma		Metastatic liver cancer		Nonneoplastic liver diseases	
		AFP+ total	% of AFP+	Type of diagnosis	AFP+ total	% of AFP+	AFP+ total	% of AFP+	AFP+ total	% of AFP+
	II	9/14	64%	Histological	.	.	.	.	0/108[b]	0%
Uganda (total)	I-II	31/58 includes	53%	Clinical or histological	.	.	0/8	0%	2/219	0.9%
		9/14	64%	Histological						
Congo	I	20/28 includes	71.4%	Clinical or histological	.	.	.	.	3/61[b]	4.9%
		17/22	77.3%	Histological						
Indonesia	I	87/100	87%	Clinical or histological	.	.	.	.	2/74	2.7%
Singapore	I	24/32 includes	75%	Clinical or histological	.	.	.	.	0/84[b]	0%
		21/29	72%	Histological						
Hong Kong	I	27/42	64%	Histological	.	.	.	.	0/14	0%
Jamaica	I	4/6 includes	66.7%	Clinical or histological	.	.	.	.	1/113[b]	0.9%
		3/3	100%	Histological						
Total		824/1209	68.2%	Clinical or histological	1/73	1.37%	2/334[c]	0.6%	15/5984	0.25%
		366/530	69.1%	Histological						

[a] Embryonal tumors not included; Data for Japan: see Addendum.
[b] Included different disease cases, namely: Liver diseases 212
                 Nonliver cancer—126
                 Nonliver and nonhepatoma diseases—217 (O'Conor et al., 1970).
[c] This group is significantly diminished since part of the patients are included in the group with nonliver tumors.
[d] All AFP+ cases—nonliver tumors with liver metastases.

and "AFP—" hepatomas is whether they have qualitative or only quantitative differences between them. The corresponding data are discussed below.

C. Quantitative Aspects of AFP Production by Liver Tumors

In connection with data considered in the previous section, it has been mentioned that all of them were obtained by a method possessing a definite sensitivity limit which, in the end, is of arbitrary value. Until quite recently, we did not know events occurring in the "subthreshold" area, or the degree in which the specificity of the phenomenon and, respectively, of the diagnostic test is maintained, when more sensitive methods of AFP detection are employed.

Blood levels of AFP with hepatomas in animals and man vary

(*Continued*)

Nonhepatic neoplasmas		Nonneoplastic and nonliver diseases		Pregnancy		Normal donors		Comments on nonhepatoma group	References
AFP+ total	% of AFP+	AFP+ total	% of AFP+	AFP+ total	% of AFP+	AFP+ total	% of AFP+		
.	.	.	.	.	.	.	.		O'Conor *et al.* (1970)
.	.	0/50	0%	.	.	.	.		
.	.	.	.	.	.	.	.	2 AFP+ in control group— metastatic liver cancer primary localization unknown. 1 AFP+— post-necrotic cirrhosis	O'Conor *et al.* (1970)
.	.	.	.	.	.	.	.	Only clinical diagnosis in control group	Kresno *et al.* (1970)
.	.	.	.	.	.	.	.		O'Conor *et al.* (1970)
.	.	0/94	0%	.	.	0/100	0%		Smith and Todd (1968) Smith and Blumberg (1969)
.	.	.	.	.	.	.	.	AFP+ in control group —gastric cancer with liver metastases (no histological)	O'Conor *et al.* (1970)
7/735[d]	0.9%	2/3373	0.06%	13/1069	1.2%	0/15731	0%		

within very broad limits, in man no less than 1000-fold, from 1 or 3 μg./ml.[9] up to 5 or 7 mg./ml. (Masseyeff *et al.*, 1968; Purves *et al.*, 1968, 1970). There is no doubt that some "AFP—" hepatomas elaborate subthreshold quantities of AFP and would be in the "AFP+" group with highly sensitive methods.

Some impression of the size of the "subthreshold" group of hepatomas can be gained from the analysis of hepatoma distribution curves based on their AFP production. By extrapolation of the curves beyond the sensitivity limit of the immunodiffusion method, the theoretically expected gain for the group can be obtained. Unfortunately, quantitative data are not given in the overwhelming majority of reports. Besides,

[9] Sensitivity threshold of immunodiffusion methods.

the distribution picture is distorted by cases of erroneous diagnosis which, naturally, accumulate in the "AFP—" group.

The distribution curves have been presented in only two publications: by Purves *et al.* (1968, 1970c) for the Union of South Africa and Masseyeff *et al.* (1968) for patients from Senegal. According to Purves, extrapolation of the distribution curve below the sensitivity limit of the agar-gel precipitation method, indeed, suggests existence of "AFP+" hepatomas in that range. As their preliminary results indicate with the radioimmunoassay, about one-third of "AFP—" cases are transferred into the "AFP+" group, resulting in about 90% of "AFP+" hepatomas, on the whole, for Bantu of South Africa (Purves *et al.*, 1970c).

The distribution curve for Senegal (Masseyeff *et al.*, 1968) is rather peculiar: it has a distinct maximum in the range of ~50 μg./ml. with symmetric slopes in both directions. But, near the sensitivity limit of the method, there is a noticeable increase, so that it is difficult to predict the ultimate direction of the curve (Fig. 9a). Of similar appearance is the distribution curve plotted using our data with the International Experiment materials for seven countries (O'Conor *et al.*, 1970). Again, there is a maximum in the range of 50 to 70 μg./ml., slopes on both sides, and a rise in the region of threshold values (Fig. 9b).

It appears therefore, that although the distribution curves clearly suggest the possibility of occurrence of hepatocellular cancers with sub-threshold levels of AFP, it may not be decided from their appearance, whether the particular range contains a "fading" branch of the curve or a new maximum.

The above-mentioned distribution curves are related to countries where a high percentage of "AFP+" hepatomas is observed. It would be very important to have similar curves for those countries which have considerably lower incidence of such tumors. It is not impossible that the corresponding curves would be "cut off" by the sensitivity limit of the method.

Experimental analysis of the quantitative aspects of AFP production by hepatomas has just been started. According to our data (Abelev, 1971, Abelev *et al.*, 1971), the indirect immunoradioautography test has revealed 22 positive cases in a group of 48 "AFP—" hepatomas studied (46%). The examined collection included 36 sera from Dakar[10] and 12 from the USSR. The percentage of "AFP+" findings in the former group was considerably lower (37%) than in the latter (75%). The material was not large and not homogeneous with respect to diagnosis. It is quite possible that the disagreement between the groups was due to unequal

[10] Courtesy of Prof. Masseyeff and Dr. Leblanc (Dakar University, Senegal).

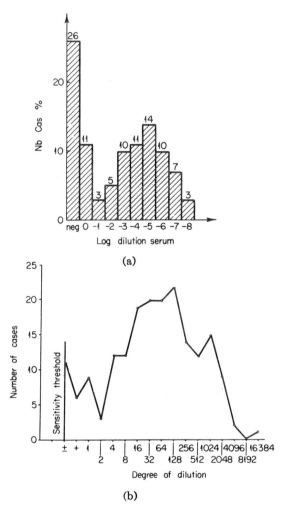

FIG. 9. The distribution of serum AFP levels in patients with cancer of the liver. (a) The distribution curve for Senegal. (From Masseyeff *et al.*, 1968.) (b) The distribution curve for seven countries, which includes all "AFP+" cases. (According to O'Conor *et al.*, 1970.)

accuracy of diagnosis. It is only natural that cases of misdiagnosis would accumulate in the "AFP—" group, bringing down the relative gain in "AFP+" cases. For the most part, the Moscow collection (11 cases) had histological confirmation while that from Dakar was confirmed in only half of the cases (Masseyeff *et al.*, 1968).

The available material is not sufficient for definite conclusions, but it clearly indicates the prospects for employing highly sensitive AFP determination tests for further progress in the diagnosis of liver cancer. Such development entails, however, the inevitable lowering of the specificity of the AFP test. This point is additionally discussed in Section VIII.

The pronounced increase in the "AFP+" group with higher sensitivity of the detection method also permits the suggestion that two kinds of hepatoma cases may exist, one corresponding to the maximum of 50 to 70 μg. AFP/ml. in the distribution curve, and the other to a maximum in the subthreshold range. It may be that the different incidence of "AFP+" hepatomas in various countries is due only to different occurrence of these two kinds of cases. This hypothesis requires quantitative determinations of AFP by usual and highly sensitive methods in groups of patients from countries with high and low incidence of "AFP+" hepatocarcinomas, as well as quantitative studies on experimental "models."

D. AFP Production by Hepatomas as Influenced by Etiologic and Pathogenic Factors

In order to get a deeper insight into the mechanism by which the AFP synthesis is resumed in hepatomas, as well as for practical purposes, it is necessary to know conditions under which the phenomenon takes place and correlations, if any, of this trait with other characters of hepatomas. It seems more accurate in this respect to speak of correlations between the tumor characters and the level of AFP synthesis, but until the group of "AFP—" hepatomas is sufficiently well analyzed, we have to deal with "AFP+" and "AFP—" groups, bearing in mind the provisional character of this division.

1. The Dependence of the Proportion of "Seropositive" Hepatomas on Areas of the World

In analyzing the frequency of occurrence of "AFP+" hepatomas in various parts of the world, considerable differences have been noted by all investigators engaged in this field. Moreover, as Hull *et al.* (1970) concluded, there is a positive correlation between the proportion of "AFP+" hepatomas and the incidence of liver cancer in a particular area of the world. Indeed, the highest percentages of "seropositive" hepatomas have been observed for areas endemic for primary cancer of the liver: the South African Union (82%), Senegal (79%), Congo (77%), Mozambique (67%), Indonesia (87%). The proportion of "seropositive" hepatomas among the native population in the USA, England, France, and Greece is considerably less—from 50 to 60%—but it approaches maximal values in those who come from Africa. Values for the USSR (Moscow) and Uganda are intermediate (64%). Unexplainably high are the figures for Astrakhan (96%) and Siberia (82%) (see Table VII).

Of course, not all of these data are equally comparable since they differ by exactness of diagnosis (the proportion of clinically and histologically confirmed cases in each of the groups), by selection of patients (a tendency to follow each "AFP+" case and loss of some "AFP—" cases), and by modifications of the AFP test used by different laboratories. But, even with all these reservations taken into account, the regularity seems to be evident: the incidence of "AFP+" hepatomas is higher in areas endemic for hepatocellular cancer.

This conclusion raises a number of problems, including those of dependence of the "serological type" of the tumor on the etiological agent, chemical nature of carcinogen, dose and route by which it penetrates the organism, on genetic and physiologic peculiarities of a particular population, and on characteristics of the tumors arising in different populations.

2. Dependence on Carcinogen

Among the hepatomas of rats, mice, and monkeys which are characterized in Table V above, there are tumors induced by various carcinogens—OAAT, 3'-Me-DAB, DAB, nitrosoamine and aflatoxin, as well as spontaneous hepatomas and preneoplastic nodules resulting from pyridoxine deficiency. As can be seen, "AFP+" tumors are present in all groups of hepatomas, both spontaneous and induced, with one notable exception. Aflatoxin, a most probable carcinogen for man, has induced hepatomas in rats, which formed no AFP. It seems to us that these observations indicate the need of further studies. They include results of two series of experiments with primarily induced tumors, which malignancy has not been proved by transplantation. For definite conclusions, it is necessary to study transplantable alfatoxin-induced hepatomas with application, if required, of highly sensitive tests for AFP detection.

In the rest of the groups, no correlations can be found between the carcinogen used, on the one hand, and the frequency of "AFP+" hepatomas, or the AFP level, on the other. Moreover, one carcinogen (3'-Me-DAB) acting on the same animals under similar conditions of application exhibited rather significantly differing results: 52% and 100% of "AFP+" hepatomas (Stanislawski-Birencwajg et al., 1967). It has been noted in all studies that with hepatomas induced by the same carcinogen there are great differences in the levels of AFP.

In spite of the fact that the above material is small, episodic, not always studied under comparable conditions, and clearly requires confirmation, we are inclined to believe that AFP production is determined rather by the character of the induced tumor than by etiologic factors.

3. *The Dependence of AFP Production on Biological Characteristics of the Tumor*

In our initial study on AFP formation by mouse hepatomas, it was noted that the degree of malignancy positively correlated with the level of AFP production by the tumors (Abelev, 1965a, 1968). This is shown in Table VIII together with more recent data which have supported and extended the observation. As can be seen, trace amounts of AFP, detectable only by the immunoradioautography test were associated with growth of hepatomas, which type may be defined as "minimally deviated from normal." Threshold levels (by agar-gel precipitation) were observed with slowly growing strains while three fast-growing anaplastic hepatomas produced the greatest amounts of AFP. Similar correlation between AFP formation and degree of malignancy was noted also when primary OAAT-induced hepatomas were compared with their first generations and transplantable stable strains (Abelev, 1965a, 1968; Khramkova and Guelstein, 1965; Guelstein and Khramkova, 1965).

The above observations and conclusions strongly disagree with those of other authors who studied primary tumors in rats, monkeys, and man. Thus, no regularity was found when AFP production was analyzed with respect to histological type of primary tumors of rats (Stanislawski-Birencwajg *et al.*, 1967) and monkeys (Hull *et al.*, 1969b,c).

TABLE VIII
ALPHA-FETOPROTEIN IN MICE BEARING HEPATOMAS OF DIFFERENT GROWTH RATE

Hepatoma strain	Latent period of growth[a]	AFP in agar precipitation test	AFP in IR test
22 a	5–7	++++	.
22 a ascitic	5–7	++++	.
56	7–10	++++	
22	21–28	+	.
38	23–30	+	.
60	19–36	±	++++
61	28–116	+	++++
46	30–90	−	+++
48	55–90	−	+++
Normal adult C3HA	−	−	+[b]

[a] According to Guelstein (1966).
[b] Approximately 8 times lower than in the hepatoma-bearing mice.

Also unsuccessful were attempts to reveal any correlations for human tumors between the occurrence or level of AFP in the blood and the degree of malignancy or histological type of the tumor. In all groups analyzed in this respect no correlation was found (Masseyeff et al., 1968; Abelev et al., 1967a; Purves et al., 1970c; Foli et al., 1969; O'Conor et al., 1970). Only in the study of Purves et al. (1970c) was a slight tendency noted: the percentage of "AFP+" hepatomas was lower in patients with highly differentiated tumors than in those with less differentiated ones, and became lower again in a group with anaplastic cancer of the liver.

It is difficult at present to find explanations for the existing contradictions. It is possible that the regularity noted in mice is an occasional observation, which will not be corroborated with larger material. It seems to us, however, that the reason for the discrepancy may lie with the fact that tumors studied in the former case were mostly transplantable, while those in the latter case were primary. It is natural to expect that any correlations between AFP production and some other character of the tumor should be more pronounced in comparing relatively homogeneous transplantable tumors which have undergone extended selection. Primary tumors, especially in man, are large and heterogeneous. Individual nodules may differ in the degree of malignancy and differentiation. To look for a correlation there, obviously, is more difficult.

It seems to us that the problem can be adequately solved by measuring AFP in a series of transplantable Morris hepatomas of rats which present a complete spectrum of tumors discretely differing in the degree of malignancy, as well as in separate biological and biochemical characters (Morris et al., 1964).

It is necessary, also, to elaborate quantitative criteria for the evaluation of AFP production by an individual tumor, perhaps on the basis of incorporation of ^{14}C-amino acids in this protein in vivo, taking into account the weight of the tumor. It is also extremely desirable in this type of study to use the high-sensitivity tests.

As for primary tumors, especially those of man, another approach seems to be promising: a study of specific features of AFP-producing cells and of regularities determining their appearance within tumors of various structure. The method of detecting AFP by immunofluorescence (see Section VII,A) provides opportunities for such investigations. Initial results obtained with this method in human hepatomas indicate that only few cells of the tumor specifically contain AFP, and that these cells always form groups "gravitating" to vessels in the tumor (Gusev et al., 1971b). The latter evidence strongly suggests that the resumption of AFP synthesis in cells of the tumor is probably not a random process, and that there is some regularity in appearance of such cells, which can be revealed, possibly, by combining methods of immunofluorescence, histochemistry, and autoradiography.

Demonstration in human and animal hepatomas of the isozyme spectrum peculiar to the embryonic liver (Schapira et al., 1963, 1970; Nordmann and Schapira, 1967; Uriel, 1969) is of undoubted interest for determining correlations between AFP production and other biochemical characters of hepatomas. It is especially important that the shift toward embryonic type is differently expressed in individual human tumors and in various strains of transplantable hepatomas of the rat. In the latter case, aldolases of the embryonic type were detected only in fast-growing tumors, whereas slowly growing tumors possessed the isozyme typical of the adult liver (Schapira et al., 1970).

Parallel investigations of AFP formation by hepatomas, possessing the adult or embryonic aldolase spectra, would be of great interest. Also important would be parallel immunofluorescence studies on localization of AFP and embryonic type aldolase in the tumor tissue, especially with human primary tumors.

4. *The Dependence of AFP Synthesis on Stage of Cancerogenesis and Tumor Progression*

This aspect is important both for understanding the nature of the phenomenon and the evaluation of feasibility of early diagnosis of hepatomas. Practically no experiments have been made in this direction in simple mouse and rat "models," but there are studies in monkeys and single observations in the clinic. Foy et al. (1966), working with baboons deprived of pyridoxine in their diet, have shown that such animals develop lesions in their liver which resemble hepatocellular carcinoma in structure.

The lesions were not malignant tumors, but are considered by the authors as preneoplastic formations. Monkeys fed pyridoxine-less diets contained AFP in their blood, its level being not transitory, but maintained in the course of several months (Foy et al., 1970a,b). These observations indicate the possibility of AFP appearance in monkeys during the process of cancerogenesis.

Investigations of Hull et al. (1969b,c) on monkey hepatomas induced by nitrosoamine showed that AFP may appear in the blood before the tumor is detectable by palpation and before any clinical signs appear. Besides, the authors noted that a high level of AFP can be observed with a very small tumor. These observations, although not fixing a definite stage in cancerogenesis, clearly show that AFP in AFP-producing tumors is detected during early clinical stages of development of the tumor.

Clinical evidence which bears on this problem is episodic. It is of special interest, for determining the clinical stage at which AFP may appear, to examine cases for which the initial time of AFP detection has been registered. We have had only two observations of this kind among studied patients (Khasanov *et al.*, 1971). Patient S., suffering from cirrhosis and severe pancreatitis, gave a negative AFP test. Two months after the first examination a weakly positive reaction for AFP developed. No clinical symptoms of primary cancer of the liver were observed. Following AFP detection, the patient was twice examined by scanning of the liver and selective angiography, but it was not possible to localize exactly the suspected tumor. During the following months, the AFP level increased continuously. In 7 months after the initial detection of AFP, some increase in dimensions of the left liver lobe was noted. Clinical signs of progressing liver cancer became evident only 1 year after the appearance of AFP. The lethal outcome from another cause confirmed the presence of primary cancer of the liver. This case clearly shows that with "seropositive" hepatomas AFP may appear at sufficiently early stages of disease, prior to its clinical symptoms. But there is no doubt that opposite cases may exist, when AFP appears after the clinical symptoms (Hull *et al.*, 1969a; Khasanov *et al.*, 1971).

Obviously, the problem cannot be solved empirically, and thorough experimental analysis is required. Studies on chemically induced cancerogenesis in mice and rats, using highly sensitive tests for AFP detection and immunofluorescence, seem to be quite expedient.

5. The Dependence of the Incidence of "Seropositive" Hepatomas on Age of the Patients

This problem has not been studied at all in experimental models. In the analysis of a large amount of material from Senegal (Masseyeff, 1971), a slight tendency was revealed toward lower percentage of "AFP+" hepatomas with increasing age of the patients. However, it should be noted that the material examined was from Africa, where a relatively young population group is affected by cancer of the liver, and where the percentage of "AFP+" hepatomas is rather high ($\sim$75%). A greater incidence of "AFP+" hepatomas in males has also been noted (O'Conor *et al.*, 1970).

Mawas *et al.* (1970, 1971) demonstrated a definite correlation between the age and the incidence of "AFP+" hepatomas in a group of patients from France. In children not older than 11 years of age, ∼ 90% of hepatomas (21 cases of 24) appeared to be "AFP+", which greatly exceeds the average incidence of such hepatomas for France (60%), and even the corresponding indexes for countries of Africa and Southeast Asia.

The work of Mawas and his associates has been corroborated by Bagshawe and Parker (1970) on a group of patients from Kenya. Nine patients with hepatocellular cancer, whose age was from 10 to 30 years, were 100% "AFP+"; in the patient group aged 31 to 40 years, the proportion of "AFP+" cases was 66% (4 cases out of 6), while at ages over 40 years there were only 22% of "AFP+" patients (2 out of 9). These extremely remarkable observations could throw light on the reason why there are geographical differences in the incidence of "AFP+" hepatomas. It is well known that the age of hepatoma patients from Africa is, on the average, some three decades less than that of patients from Europe and America.

The problem of dependence of the incidence of "AFP+" cases upon the age merits a most thorough investigation and accumulation of greater material. This may help to elucidate whether hepatomas developing at a young age possess any specific features, or whether there is some other determining factor which is extraneous to the tumor and changes with the age of the organism.

The age dependence strongly suggests the existence of an external factor ("inducer"), which influences the rate of AFP synthesis in tumor tissue, and which diminishes with age. It may be supposed that a certain part of hepatomas, belonging to the "subthreshold" group according to their AFP formation, are competent to respond to the "inducer" by elevated AFP production, and that the same phenomenon underlies AFP "induction" during regeneration of the liver. If it is so, we can expect that in younger patients, possessing a greater level of the "inducer" than the older group, an increase in AFP production by low-productive ("AFP−" in the standard test) hepatomas will take place and that they will appear in the "AFP+" group.

This supposition can be tested experimentally. First, there must be a deviation from the symmetric shape in patient distribution curves, based on AFP level, in the group of young patients, as compared with elderly patients, with an increase in the range of low AFP concentrations.

Second, according to the above suggestion, an exposure to higher concentration of the "inducer" should result in increased AFP synthesis on the part of highly differentiated mouse hepatomas which produce little AFP. Higher levels of the "inducer" may be expected either in the early postnatal period or during regeneration of the liver. A tumor growing in such conditions should produce more AFP than that in normal adult mice. This can be checked, for example, by the immunofluorescence method, which allows one to calculate "AFP+" cells directly in the tissue studied.

Age dependence may alternatively be explained from quite a different position. If it is assumed that tolerance to AFP in humans is lost with age, then it will follow that AFP elimination from the blood would take place in adult patients much more frequently than in younger patients, creating a seeming impression of dependence between the hepatoma "serotype" and the age of the host.

Thus, in the consideration of possible correlations between AFP production and etiologic and pathogenic factors, a number of remarkable regularities and contradictions are revealed. This character of hepatomas has been shown to depend on "endemicity" of the area and age of the patients. The evidence on AFP production as related to degree of malignancy appears to be contradictory, while the role of the carcinogen and of the stage of cancerogenesis has been studied very little. The available evidence does not permit one to present any general picture concerning the resumption of AFP synthesis in tumors. But there are approaches and still unused opportunities for analyzing the problem.

VIII. Clinical Aspects of the Diagnosis of Liver Cancer

In this chapter, we should like to discuss the use of the AFP test for differential diagnosis of hepatocellular cancer and for its early diagnosis.

The differential diagnosis based on the standard AFP test may be considered, on the whole, a solved problem. The summary of the corresponding studies, presented in Table VII, testifies for very high specificity of the AFP test when working with the agar-gel precipitation methods.

It should be noted that the percentage of "AFP+" cases was, as a rule, significantly higher in the groups with histologically confirmed hepatocellular cancer in comparison with those which include both types of diagnosis. This indicates that the AFP test give less false positive results than diagnoses based on clinical data only.

False positive reactions can also be observed here, most likely with cases of infectious and serum hepatitis and of stomach cancer metastatic to the liver. In the former cases, to obtain a differential diagnosis, the reversible character of AFP dynamics with noncancerous diseases of the liver may be taken into account, besides the clinical symptoms. Repetition of the analysis in the course of 2–4 weeks will indicate whether the production of AFP is transient or an increase in its level takes place.

In case of metastases to the liver, the situation is more complicated, as the reason for AFP production is not clear. Tumor itself is unlikely to be the source of AFP. More probable is another mechanism, namely, via necrosis and regeneration of the liver parenchyma.[11] In this case we also have a right to expect transient appearance of AFP and its very low levels.

Another, more "ponderable" problem is that of "false negative" reactions, especially for America and Europe where they amount to 50% of hepatoma cases. We consider it quite substantiated here to use highly sensitive tests, first of all the immunoradioautography. In our experience, 75% of "false-negative" hepatomas from the USSR (9 out of 12 cases) appeared to be clearly positive with this test. The reaction itself, being absolutely specific for AFP, is not much more difficult to perform than the agar-gel precipitation test and thus is quite feasible in hospital laboratories.

However, when dealing with AFP levels of the order of 0.05 to 0.5 μg./ml., much more frequent are "false positive" reactions due to pregnancy, viral hepatitis, metastases to the liver and other liver diseases (Table IX).

Thus, using the immunoradioautography test, we may expect to have about 90% of serologically revealed hepatomas (together with those diagnosed by agar-gel precipitation) and about 15% of "false positives" in groups with metastatic liver cancer and viral hepatitis. As was already mentioned above, the basis for differential diagnosis in case of Botkin disease can be obtained by following the AFP dynamics, together with clinical symptoms (Table IV). It is well established that with primary cancer of the liver there is either a stable or a slowly growing AFP level (Purves et al., 1970c; Masseyeff et al., 1968). Detailed studies on AFP dynamics in metastatic liver cancer are urgently required.

Can the AFP test provide any additional information on the clinical state of a patient? Thorough investigations in this direction, carried out by Masseyeff et al. (1968) and Purves et al. (1970c) on large groups of patients in Senegal and South Africa, permit only a negative answer to this question. No correlation is apparent between the AFP level in a patient and the stage or gravity of the disease. Observation of AFP levels may serve, apparently, as a control of success of surgical treatment, judging from disappearance of AFP after resection of the tumor, or an indication of a relapse or metastases if AFP reappears.

---

[11] For instance: liver regeneration due to biliary obstruction (Cameron, 1935; Fahan et al., 1966).

TABLE IX

ALPHA-FETOPROTEIN IN NONHEPATOMA PATIENTS ACCORDING TO
IMMUNORADIOAUTOGRAPHY TEST[a]

Diagnosis	AFP-positive/ Number of cases	% of AFP positives	Comments
Healthy donors	0/47	0%	
Pregnancy Before 15 weeks	2/19	10%	
Pregnancy After 15 weeks	45/46	98%	
Cholangiocellular carcinoma	0/6	0%	
Metastatic liver cancer	3/21	14%	2 "AFP+" gastric cancer with liver metastases. 1 "AFP+"—Wilms tumor with liver metastases
Malignant disease of blood	0/15	0%	
Other malignant tumors[b]	1/26	3.9%	AFP+ carcinomatosis of the peritoneum, original site unknown
Acute viral hepatitis	23/176	13%	Two cases positive in agar precipitation
Other liver diseases (cirrhosis, chronic hepatitis, echinococcosis and others)	1/108	0.9%	AFP+ case-mechanic jaundice
Noncancer and nonliver diseases	0/39	0%	

[a] After Abelev et al. (1971).
[b] Embryonal tumors not included.

As far as early diagnosis of hepatocellular cancer is concerned, we have already discussed what evidence there is on the time of AFP appearance during development of liver cancer. Experiments in monkeys and single observations in the clinic permit an optimistic view of prospects of an early diagnosis in some cases of hepatocellullar cancer. But a direct answer may be obtained only from broad epidemiological examination of the population in areas of the world endemic for liver cancer.

Such investigations, employing the standard AFP test, were being conducted by the International Agency for Research on Cancer in the Ivory Coast, at the time the present review was written (Annual Report of International Agency for Research on Cancer, 1969). It is very tempting to introduce highly sensitive tests in studies of this kind. In spite of the inevitable increase in the percentage of false positive reactions, these methods provide a considerably better chance of detecting clinically unapparent forms of liver cancer. It is essential for such work to follow AFP dynamics in detected positive cases.

Broad examinations of certain population groups by the high-sensitivity tests have some technical difficulties. To perform the radioimmunoassay or immunoradioautography with samples from tens of thousand people is a complicated, time-consuming, and expensive undertaking. Here, it may be extremely helpful to apply the aggregate-hemagglutination reaction.

In a comparative trial of the aggregate-hemagglutination reaction and immunoradioautography, performed on the same collection of sera, it has been found that the former reaction gives considerably more positive results than the latter, mostly with low dilutions of sera (1:8 and 1:16) (Abelev *et al.*, 1971). This disagreement was not due to sensitivity of the methods, which was comparable.

It was found recently that the disagreement between two tests could be sharply diminished, if not completely excluded, by the use of additional control—erythrocytes sensitized by nonimmune serum. The "false positive" samples were equally active in agglutination of both types of erythrocytes—conjugated with immune as well as with normal serum. The absorption of such serum samples by erythrocytes loaded with nonimmune serum inhibited their reactivity against the control erythrocytes. The same treatment did not influence the specific activity of AFP-containing samples.

According to our data, however, the aggregate-hemagglutination test gives almost no "false negative" reactions, i.e., it has not, practically, been negative with samples obviously positive for AFP in the immunoradioautography test. The only group in which such results were registered was that of pregnant women (76% positives by the aggregate-hemagglutination reaction and 98% positives according to the immunoradioautography test). No false negative reactions were observed in patient groups with primary liver cancer, embryonal tumors, infectious hepatitis, etc., provided the aggregate-hemagglutination titer of a serum equal to 1:8 was recorded as a positive reaction.

It is clear, therefore, that the aggregate-hemagglutination test can be used for preliminary screening, with subsequent verification of selected sera by the immunoradioautography test. The simplicity and speed of performance of the aggregate-hemagglutination reaction allows its application in broad epidemiological surveys. One operator is capable of testing several hundred sera a day.

Summarizing the discussion on the clinical aspects of the phenomenon, the following three statements can be made.

1. The differential diagnosis of hepatocellular cancer on the basis of the AFP test, carried out by the agar-gel precipitation method, is highly specific, but always gives a definite percentage of false negative results.

2. The proportion of diagnosed hepatomas can be significantly increased with application of highly sensitive tests for detecting AFP. False positives may be obtained in pregnant women and a part of patients with metastases to the liver and viral hepatitis. To obtain a differential diagnosis in the above cases, it is necessary to follow the AFP level in dynamics.

3. For the prospect of an early diagnosis of liver cancer, it is expedient to undertake a broad-scale study of the population in the "endemic" areas, with application of highly sensitive tests for AFP detection and regularly following the dynamics of positive reactions.

IX. Alpha-Fetoprotein with Teratocarcinomas

This problem has been much less studied than that of AFP with liver cancer, although its practical importance for countries of Europe and America is, probably, not less than in liver cancer. First of all, it should be emphasized that studies in experimental models are completely lacking in this case, which, naturally, deprives the problem of a basis for theoretical exploration. This is the more a pity, as tetratocarcinomas of mice are known and well-studied tumors (Kleinschmit and Pierce, 1964; Kahan and Ephrussi, 1970; Rosenthal et al., 1970).

AFP has been reported to occur in blood of patients with malignant teratoblastomas of the testis and ovary, as well as in those rare cases when this tumor has retroperitoneal localization. Published evidence, obtained with the agar-gel precipitation method, is summarized in Table X. It follows from these data that:

1. The occurrence of AFP is specific for malignant testicular and ovarian teratocarcinomas with elements of embryonal cancer.

2. Tumors of this type are associated with AFP in about 50% of cases.

3. Other embryonal tumors—seminomas, chorionepiteliomas, neuro- and nephroblastomas and Wilms' tumors are not accompanied by AFP in patients' blood.

Thus, AFP may be of quite definite significance in the differential diagnosis of the germinal cancers. Besides, in the case of "AFP+" teratoblastomas, the AFP level reflects the effectiveness of surgery and chemotherapy (Mawas et al., 1969a,b).

An important observation was made by Mawas et al. (1971) who noted a correlation between the incidence of "AFP+" teratoblastomas and the degree of their malignancy. Of 29 cases which they studied,

TABLE X
ALPHA-FETOPROTEIN IN PATIENTS WITH EMBRYONAL TUMORS AS REVEALED BY AGAR-GEL PRECIPITATION TEST

Group	Teratoblastoma of testis and ovary with elements of embryonal cancer		Teratoblastoma with elements of chorion epithelioma or seminoma		Stromal tumor of testicle		Seminoma		Chorion-epithelioma		Sympatho- and neuro-blastoma		Nephro-blastoma		Wilms tumor		References and comments
	AFP+ total	% of AFP+	AFP+ total	% of AFP+	AFP+ total	% of AFP+	AFP+ total	% of AFP+	AFP+ total	% of AFP+	AFP+ total	% of AFP+	AFP+ total	% of AFP+	AFP+ total	% of AFP+	
I	17/34	50%	3/12	25%	0/7	0%	0/27	0%	0/11	0%	0/14	0%	.	.	0/9	0%	Abelev (1968); Perova (1969)
II	5/8	62%							0/1		0/14	0%	0/7	0%			Masopust et al. (1968)
III	15/29	51%					0/1				0/42	0%	0/43	0%			Mawas et al. (1969a,b)
IV	9/33	27%					0/11	0%	2/8	25%							Hull et al. (1969c, 1970) 1 AFP+ case retroperitoneal teratocarcinoma
Total	47/104	45.2%	3/12	25%	0/7	0%	0/39	0%	2/15	13%	0/70	0%	0/50	0%	0/9	0%	

AFP was found in 15, while from the remaining 14 "AFP—" cases, 13 tumors underwent complete regression. It is possible that with tumors of this type, the occurrence and level of AFP may characterize to some extent the character of the tumor and the course of the disease.

It was natural to examine patients with embryonal tumors using methods of higher sensitivity. The corresponding results, obtained with indirect immunoradioautography, are presented in Table XI. Considering these results, it should be borne in mind that only those patients were reexamined in the teratoblastoma group who failed to exhibit AFP in the standard test. The results make evident both a pronounced increase in serologically diagnosed teratoblastomas and some decline in the diagnostic specificity of the reaction. It should be recalled in this connection that teratoblastomas are most frequent in children, and that child hepatopathy is often associated with "false positive" reactions (Masopust *et al.*, 1971). This possibility should be taken into account when highly sensitive tests are applied for the diagnosis of child tumors.

Thus, the AFP test presents undoubted clinical interest with teratoblastomas, and an extension of studies in this direction is extremely desirable.

As far as the theoretical aspect of AFP formation with embryonal tumors is concerned, it remains completely unstudied. There is no adequate proof that AFP is formed by tumor itself, although it is most probable, taking into account the specificity of the phenomenon and the fact that the AFP formation is stopped by resection of the tumor. It

TABLE XI

ALPHA-FETOPROTEIN IN PATIENTS WITH EMBRYONAL TUMORS AS REVEALED
BY THE IMMUNORADIOAUTOGRAPHY TEST[a]

Diagnosis	AFP+ / Total number	% of AFP+	Comments
Teratoblastoma of testis and ovary with elements of embryonal tumor	15/20	75%	Only sera AFP-negative in agar precipitation are included
Chorion-epithelioma	0/11	0%	
Wilms tumor	1/9	11%	(a) 1 AFP+—Wilms tumor with liver metastases (b) 1 AFP+ case— Wilms tumor with acute viral hepatitis is not included

[a] After Abelev *et al.* (1971).

cannot be excluded, of course, that teratocarcinomas induce AFP synthesis in the liver. The finding of AFP in the cells of tumor by immunofluorescence technique (Mawas *et al.*, 1969a) is not quite convincing since passive uptake of AFP from the serum was not excluded (see Section VII,A).

Should the synthesis occur in the tumor, it is extremely interesting to identify the structures responsible for the tumor. As is known, teratocarcinomas are capable of forming differentiated tissues, including the development of a yolk sac and, less frequently, of hepatocytes (Kleinschmit, and Pierce, 1964; Berry *et al.*, 1969). It seems logical, therefore, that it is precisely these tumors, together with hepatomas, that are associated with the occurrence of AFP. We consider it most likely that the AFP synthesis with teratocarcinomas is determined by the formation of a yolk sac, i.e., a structure which is most typical of malignant teratocarcinomas and is able to produce AFP. The problem could be solved unequivocally using the immunofluorescence technique.

Thus, the phenomenon of association of AFP with teratocarcinomas obviously requires experimental studies with "models" and with clinical material, both for its adequate description and for evaluating the prospects of its clinical use.

X. Concluding Remarks

It was the central objective of this article to emphasize the importance of basic research on the alpha-fetoprotein phenomenon; such studies, aimed to decipher its nature, would contribute to understanding of both normal ontogenesis and pathogenesis of tumors. An essential task in this respect is to elucidate factors which control AFP production during the embryonic period of ontogenesis and resumption of its synthesis in tumors.

Analyzing specific aspects of the phenomenon, we made an attempt to formulate experimental approaches to some immediate problems:

1. Is there any external factor which could control AFP synthesis and determine its intensity?

2. Is the synthesis carried out by certain type of cells, specialized in AFP production, or is this function inherent in any hepatocyte?

3. Is the control of AFP synthesis accomplished by regulation of intensity of the process taking place in individual cells, or by involvement of varying numbers of cells with a constant level of AFP production?

4. Is the AFP synthesis in a tumor due to maintained ability of the stem tumor cell to differentiate, or is it the result of dedifferentiation of the mature hepatocyte?

Answers to these questions are essential, in our opinion, in order to bring the research up to a molecular level.

There is no doubt that elucidation of the AFP phenomenon is facilitated by progress in related fields, as it is not only with tumors of the liver and teratoblastomas that the resumption of the synthesis of embryo-specific proteins takes place. Well known are investigations on the carcino-embryonic antigens of the human digestive system (Gold and Freedman, 1965; Gold et al., 1968; Thomson et al., 1969; Kleist and Burtin, 1970), a phenomenon, which is principally similar to that discussed in the present article. It is not impossible that resumption of the synthesis of embryonic antigens in tumors is a general regularity (Brawn, 1970; Duff and Rapp, 1970; Coggin et al., 1970).

In the practical aspect, the development of a simple and accessible test for AFP with high sensitivity and its trial in a broad epidemiological survey seem to be most important. This approach would help to determine the feasibility of early diagnosis of the liver cancer, at stages permitting surgical treatment.

Acknowledgments

Sincere gratitude is expressed to Dr. L. N. Mekhedov for the English translation of the article, to Dr. N. V. Engelhardt, for the critical reading of the manuscript, to Dr. A. I. Gusev and Miss A. K. Jazova for providing illustrations, and to Dr. S. D. Perova for assistance in the preparation of the manuscript.

XI. Addendum

Since the manuscript was written, several important publications have appeared. A new purification procedure for human AFP has been suggested by Purves et al. (1970a), which includes physiochemical and immunochemical treatments. The AFP preparations obtained were found homogeneous in neutral and alkaline pH ranges, but revealed distinct heterogeneity at pH 4.5. Nishi (1970) has described in detail a method of isolation of human AFP from its precepitate with specific antibody. The purified AFP had $S_{20} = 4.50$ S and a molecular weight of 64,000. This is in good agreement with data presented in Table I.

Clinical observations for Japan have been reported in the same paper. AFP was found in 23 patients with hepatocellular carcinoma out of 31 examined; from the histologically confirmed 20 cases there were 16 AFP—positive (80%). No positives were found among 500 patients with noncancerous liver diseases, but one case with AFP was observed among 100 patients with nonliver tumors. The "AFP+" serum belonged to a patient with gastric cancer complicated by massive liver metastases.

One more case of AFP appearance with gastric cancer metastatic to the liver has been reported by Geffroy *et al.* (1970b).

Purves *et al.* (1970b) have found that the blood levels of AFP in liver cancer patients reflect to some degree the effect of chemotherapy on the tumor size.

Gitlin and Pericelli (1970) have demonstrated, using the immunoautoradiography technique, the synthesis of AFP, transferrin, and albumin by human yolk sac.

A direct proof of AFP production by human hepatocellular carcinomas has been obtained by Rioche *et al.* (1970), who demonstrated AFP accumulation in a medium of cultured liver tumor cells.

References

Abelev, G. I. (1963). *Acta Unio Int. Contra. Cancrum* **19**, 80–82.

Abelev, G. I. (1965a). *Progr. Exp. Tumor Res.* **7**, 104–157.

Abelev, G. I. (1965b). *In* "Viruses, Cancer, Immunity" (N. Blokhin, ed.), pp. 327–351. Medicine, Moscow.

Abelev, G. I. (1968). *Cancer Res.* **28**, 1344–1350.

Abelev, G. I. (1971). *Protides Biol. Fluids, Proc. Colloq.* **18** (in press).

Abelev, G. I., and Bakirov, R. D. (1967). *Vopr. Med. Khim.* **13**, No. 4, 378–383.

Abelev, G. I., and Tsvetkov, V. S. (1960). *Vopr. Onkol.* **6**, No. 6, 62–72.

Abelev, G. I., Perova, S. D., Khramkova, N. I., Postnikova, Z. A., and Irlin, I. S. (1963a). *Transplantation* **1**, 174–180.

Abelev, G. I., Perova, S. D., Khramkova, N. I., Postnikova, Z. A., and Irlin, I. S. (1963b). *Biokhimiya* **28**, 625–634.

Abelev, G. I., Assecritova, V., Kraevsky, N. A., Perova, S. D., and Perevodchikova, N. I. (1967a). *Int. J. Cancer* **2**, 551–558.

Abelev, G. I., Perova, S. D., Bakirov, R. D., and Irlin, I. S. (1967b). *In* "Specific Tumor Antigens" (R. J. G. Harris, ed.), UICC Monograph Series, Vol. 2, pp. 32–33. Munksgaard, Copenhagen.

Abelev, G. I., Tsvetkov, V. S., Biryulina, T. I., Elgort, D. A., Olovnikov, A. M., Gusev, A. I., Jazova, A. K., Perova, S. D., Rubzov, I. V., Kantorovich, B. A., Tur, V., Khasanov, A. I., and Levina, D. M. (1971). *Byull. Eksp. Biol. Med.* No. 4, 75–81.

Alpert, M. (1969). *Clin. Res.* **17**, 461.

Alpert, M., Uriel, J., and de Nechaud, B. (1968). *N. Engl. J. Med.* **278**, 984–986.

Andreoli, M., and Robbins, J. (1962). *J. Clin. Invest.* **41**, 1070–1077.

Annual Report of International Agency for Research on Cancer. (1969). pp. 58–59. IARC, Lyon.

Assecritova, I. V., Abelev, G. I., Kraevsky, N. A., Perova, S. D., and Perevodchikova, N. I. (1967). *Vestn. Akad. Med. Nauk SSSR* **22**, No. 5, 75–81.

Babinov, B. A., and Shain, A. A. (1971). *Vopr. Onkol.* (in press).

Bagshawe, A., and Parker, A. (1970). *Lancet* **2**, 268.

Bakirov, R. D. (1968). *Byull. Eksp. Biol. Med.* No. 2, 45–47.

Bakirov, R. D., and Abelev, G. I. (1968). Unpublished experiments.

Baldwin, R. W., and Barker, C. R. (1967). *Brit. J. Cancer* **21**, 338–345.

Basteris, B., Engelhardt, N. V., Gusev, A. I., Prussevich, T., and Luria, E. A. (1971). In preparation.

Beaton, G. H., Selby, A. E., Veen, M. J., and Wright, A. M. (1961). *J. Biol. Chem.* **236,** 2005.

Bergstrand, C., and Czar, B. (1956). *Scand. J. Clin. Lab. Invest.* **8,** 174.

Bergstrand, C., and Czar, B. (1957). *Scand. J. Clin. Lab. Invest.* **9,** 277–283.

Berry, C. L., Keeling, J., and Hilton, C. (1969). *J. Pathol.* **98,** 241–252.

Boffa, G. A., Nadal, C., Zajdela, F., and Fine, J. M. (1964). *Nature (London)* **203,** 1182–1184.

Boffa, G. A., Jagout-Armand, J., Candin-Harding, F., Susbielle, H., and Fine, J. (1965). *C. R. Acad. Sci.* **159,** 1307–1312.

Bourreille, J., Metayer, P., Sanger, F., Matray, F., and Fondimare, A. (1970). *Presse Med.* **78,** 1277.

Brawn, R. I. (1970). *Int. J. Cancer* **6,** 245–249.

Cameron, G. R. (1935). *Pathol. Bacteriol.* **41,** 283–288.

Clark, J. V. (1970). *Lancet* **1,** 88.

Coggin, J., Ambrose, K., and Anderson, N. (1970). *J. Immunol.* **105,** 524–526.

Day, E. (1965). "Immunochemistry of Cancer." Thomas, Springfield, Illinois.

de Nechaud, B., and Uriel, K. (1971). *Protides. Biol. Fluids, Proc. Colloq.* **18** (in press).

de Nechaud, B., Economopoulos, P., and Uriel, J. (1969). *Presse. Med.* **77,** 1945–1947.

Deutsch, H. F. (1954). *J. Biol. Chem.* **208,** 669–678.

Dorfman, N. A. (1967). *Vopr. Med. Khim.* **13,** 267–272.

Duff, A., and Rapp, F. (1970). *J. Immunol.* **103,** 521–523.

Dufour, D., Barrett, D., and Tremblay, A. (1969). *Rev. Immunol. Ther. Antimicrob.* **33,** 315–321.

Economopoulos, P., Theodoropoulus, G., and Sakellaropoulos, N. (1970). *Lancet* **1,** 1337.

Elgort, D. A., and Abelev, G. I. (1971). *Byull. Eksp. Biol. Med.* No. 2, 118–120.

Endo, Y. *et al.* (1969). *Naika Hokan* **14,** 24–28.

Engelhardt, N. V. (1970). Unpublished experiments.

Engelhardt, N. V., Shipova, L. Ja., Gusev, A. I., Jazova, A. K., and Ter-Grigorova, E. N. (1969). *Byull. Eksp. Biol. Med.* No. 12, 62–64.

Engelhardt, N. V., Gusev, A. I., Shipova, L. Ja., and Abelev, G. I. (1971). *Int. J. Cancer* **7,** 198–206.

Fahan, F., Kropackova, L., Sirlova, A., and Magrot, T. (1966). *Naturwissenschaften* **53,** 555–556.

Foli, A., Sherlock, S., and Adinolfi, M. (1969). *Lancet* **2,** 1267–1269.

Foy, H., Gillman, T., Kondi, A., and Preston, J. (1966). *Nature (London)* **212,** 150.

Foy, H., Kondi, A., Linsell, C., Parker, A., and Sizaret, P. (1970a). *Nature (London)* **225,** 952–953.

Foy, H., Kondi, A., and Linsell, C. (1970b). *Lancet* **1,** 411.

Foy, H., Kondi, A., Parker, A., Stenley, R., and Venning, C. (1970c). *Lancet* **1,** 1336.

Foy, H., Kondi, A., and Linsell, C. (1970d). *Lancet* **2,** 663.

Galdo, A., Casado, J., and Talavera, R. (1959). *Arch. Fr. Pediat.* **16,** 954–962.

Geffroy, Y., Denis, P., Colin, R., Sanger, F., Matray, F., and Fondimare, A. (1970a). *Presse Med.* **78,** 1107–1108.

Geffroy, Y., Metayer, P., Denis, P., Phillip, J., Matray, F., Sanger, F., Laumonier, R., and Duval, C. (1970b). *Presse Med.* **78**, 1896.

Gitlin, D., and Boesman, M. (1966). *J. Clin. Invest.* **45**, 1826–1838.

Gitlin, D., and Boesman, M. (1967a). *Comp. Biochem. Physiol.* **21**, 327–336.

Gitlin, D., and Boesman, M. (1967b). *J. Clin. Invest.* **46**, 1010–1016.

Gitlin, D., and Pericelli, A. (1970). *Nature* **228**, 996–997.

Gitlin, D., Kitzes, J., and Boesman, M. (1967). *Nature* (*London*) **215**, 534.

Gold, P., and Freedman, S. (1965). *J. Exp. Med.* **122**, 464–481.

Gold, P., Gold, M., and Freedman, S. (1968). *Cancer Res.* **28**, 1331–1334.

Grabar, P., Stanislawski-Birencwajg, M., Oisgold, S., and Uriel, J. (1967). *In* "Specific Tumor Antigens" (R. J. C. Harris, ed.), UICC Monograph Series, Vol. 2, pp. 20–32. Munksgaard, Copenhagen.

Guelstein, V. I. (1966). Dissertation Thesis, Moscow.

Guelstein, V. I., and Khramkova, N. I. (1965). *Neoplasma* **12**, 251–260.

Gusev, A. I., and Jazova, A. K. (1970a). *Biokhimiya* **35**, 172–181.

Gusev, A. I., and Jazova, A. K. (1970b). *Byull. Eksp. Biol. Med.* No. 4, 120–122.

Gusev, A. I., Jazova, A. K., and Poljakova, E. (1971a). *Byull. Eksp. Biol. Med.* No. 3, 69–72.

Gusev, A. I., Engelhardt, N. V., Masseyeff, R., Camain, R., and Basteris, B. (1971b). *Int. J. Cancer* **7**, 207–217.

Hamashima, J., Harter, J., and Coons, A. (1964). *J. Cell Biol.* **20**, 271–279.

Herrich, H., and Lawrence, J. (1965). *Anal. Biochem.* **12**, 400–402.

Hochwald, G., Thorbecke, G., and Asofsky, R. (1961). *J. Exp. Med.* **114**, 459.

Houstek, J., Masopust, J., Kithier, K., and Radl, J. (1968). *J. Pediat.* **72**, 186–193.

Hull, E., Moertel, C., and Carbone, P. (1969a). *Clin. Res.* **17**, 403.

Hull, E., Carbone, P., Gitlin, D., O'Gara, R., and Kelly, M. (1969b). *J. Nat. Cancer Inst.* **42**, 1035–1044.

Hull, E., Carbone, P., O'Gara, R., Moertel, C., O'Conor, G., and Smith, C. (1969c). *IARC Conf. Primary Liver Cancer, London* (unpublished).

Hull, E., Carbone, P., Moertel, C., and O'Conor, G. (1970). *Lancet* **1**, 779.

Irlin, I. S., Perova, S. D., and Abelev, G. I. (1966). *Int. J. Cancer* **1**, 337–347.

Jazova, A. K., and Gusev, A. I. (1971). *Byull. Eksp. Biol. Med.* (in press).

Kahan, B., and Ephrussi, B. (1970). *J. Nat. Cancer Inst.* **44**, 1015–1036.

Khasanov, A. I., Abelev, G. I., Perova, S. D., Polenko, V. K., Ryaposova, U. K., and Shirenkova, O. (1971). *Vopr. Onkol.* (in press).

Khramkova, N. I., and Abelev, G. I. (1961). *Byull. Eksp. Biol. Med.* No. 12, 107–111.

Khramkova, N. I., and Guelstein, V. I. (1965). *Neoplasma* **12**, 239–250.

Khramkova, N. I., and Guelstein, V. I. (1967). Unpublished data.

Kirsh. I., Wise, R., and Oliver, I. (1967). *Biochem. J.* **102**, 763–766.

Kithier, K., and Prokes, J. (1966). *Biochim. Biophys. Acta* **127**, 390–399.

Kithier, K., Houstek, J., Masopust, J., and Radl, J. (1966). *Nature* (*London*) **212**, 414.

Kithier, K., Masopust, J., and Radl, J. (1968a). *Biochim. Biophys. Acta* **160**, 135–137.

Kithier, K., Valenta, Z., and Zizkovsky, V. (1968b). Conference on Veterinary Pathology, Brno (unpublished).

Kleinschmit, L., and Pierce, B. (1964). *Cancer Res.* **24**, 1544–1552.

Kleist, S., and Burtin, P. (1970). *In* "Immunity and Tolerance in Oncogenesis" (L. Severi, ed.), pp. 286–296. Perugia.

Kohn, J., and Muller, U. (1970). *Lancet* **1**, 142.

Kresno, S., Gandasoebrata, K., and Rumke, P. (1970). *Lancet* **1**, 1178.

Lawford, P. J. (1961). *Biochem. Pharmacol.* **7**, 109.

Luria, E. A., Bakirov, R. D., Yeliseyeva, T. A., Abelev, G. I., and Fridenstein, A. I. (1969). *Exp. Cell Res.* **54**, 111–117.

McKellar, M. (1949). *Amer. J. Anat.* **85**, 263.

Masopust, J. (1966). "Ontogeny of Human Serum Proteins," Vol. 45. Babakova Sbirka, Prague.

Masopust, J., Kithier, K., Fuchs, V., Kotal, L., and Radl, J. (1967). *In* "Intra-uterine Dangers to the Foetus" (J. Horsky and Z. Stembera, eds.), pp. 30–35. Excerpta Med. Found., Amsterdam.

Masopust, J., Kithier, K., Radl, J., Koutecky, J., and Kotal, L. (1968). *Int. J. Cancer* **3**, 364–373.

Masopust, J., Zizkovsky, V., and Kithier, K. (1971). *Protides Biol. Fluids, Proc. Colloq.* **18** (in press).

Masseyeff, R. (1971). *Protides Biol. Fluids, Proc. Colloq.* **18** (in press).

Masseyeff, R., Sankale, M., Onde, M., Menye, A., Camain, R., Quenum, C., Magdat, L., Mattern, P., Ancelle, I., and Leblanc, L. (1968). *Bull. Soc. Med. Afr. Noire Langue Fr.* **13**, 537–548.

Massiukevitch, V. (1970). Dissertation Thesis, Astrakhan (USSR).

Mawas, C., Buffe, D., Lemerle, J., Schweisguth, O., and Burtin, P. (1969a). *Arch. Fr. Pediat.* **26**, 779.

Mawas, C., Kohen, M., Lemerle, J., Buffe, D., Schweisguth, O., and Burtin, P. (1969b). *Int. J. Cancer* **4**, 76–79.

Mawas, C., Buffe, D., and Burtin, P. (1970). *Lancet* **1**, 1291.

Mawas, C., Buffe, D., Schweisguth, O., and Burtin, P. (1971). *Protides Biol. Fluids., Proc. Colloq.* **18** (in press).

Monjour, L., and Mariage, C. (1969). *C. R. Soc. Biol.* **163**, 1288–1290.

Morkhov, J. K., and Sokolov, J. N. (1970). *Khirurgia (Moscow)* No. 2, 133–136.

Morris, H., Dyer, H., Wagner, B., Myah, H., and Rechigl, M. (1964). *Advan. Enzyme Regul.* **2**, 321–333.

Muralt, P., and Roulet, D. (1961). *Helv. Paediat. Acta.* **16**, 517–533.

Nishi, S. (1970). *Cancer Res.* **30**, 2507–2513.

Nishi, S., Watanabe, H., Tsukada, J., and Hirai, H. (1971). *Protides Biol. Fluids, Proc. Colloq.* **18** (in press).

Nordmann, Y., and Shapira, F. (1967). *Eur. J. Cancer* **3**, 247–250.

O'Conor, G. T., Tatarinov, Ju. S., Abelev, G. I., and Uriel, J. (1970). *Cancer* **25**, 1091–1098.

Olovnikov, A. M. (1967). *Immunochemistry* **4**, 77–80.

Olovnikov, A. M., and Tsvetkov, V. S. (1969). *Byull. Eksp. Biol. Med.* No. 12, 102–104.

Pantelouris, E., and Hale, P. (1962). *Nature (London)* **195**, 79.

Pedersen, K. (1944). *Nature (London)* **154**, 575.

Perova, S. D. (1969). Dissertation Thesis, Moscow.

Perova, S. D., and Abelev, G. I. (1967). *Vopr. Med. Khim.* **13**, 369–377.

Perova, S. D., Elgort, D. A., and Abelev, G. I. (1971). *Byull. Eksp. Biol. Med.* No. 3, 45–47.

Portugal, M. L., Azevedo, M. S., and Manso, C. (1970). *Int. J. Cancer* **6**, 383–387.

Purves, L., Machab, M., and Bersohn, I. (1968). *S. Afr. J. Med.* **42**, 1138–1141.

Purves, L., Machab, M., Rolle, M., and Bersohn, I. (1969). *S. Afr. J. Med.* **44**, 1194–1196.

Purves L. R., Van der Merwe, E., and Bersohn, I. (1970a). *South Afr. J. Med.* **44**, 1264–1268.

358 G. I. ABELEV

Purves, L. R., Bersohn, I., Geddes, E., Falkson, G., and Cohen, L. (1970b). *South Afr. J. Med.* **44**, 590–594.

Purves, L. R., Bersohn, I., and Geddes, E. W. (1970c). *Cancer* **25**, 1261–1270.

Reuber, M., and Glover, E. (1970). *J. Nat. Cancer Inst.* **44**, 419–427.

Rioche, M., Quelin, S., Seck, J., Jacquesson, M., Basteris, B., and Masseyeff, R. (1970). *C. R. Acad. Sci. (Paris)* **271**, 1148–1151.

Rosentahl, M., Wishnow, R., and Sato, G. (1970). *J. Nat. Cancer Inst.* **44**, 1001.

Rowe, D. S. (1969). *Bull. W. H. O.* **40**, 613.

Rowe, D. S. (1970a). *Lancet* **1**, 1340.

Rowe, D. S. (1970b). WHO Immunoglobulins Reference Center, Lausanne. Personal communication.

Sainte-Marie, G. (1962). *J. Histochem. Cytochem.* **10**, 250–256.

Schapira, F., Dreyefus, J., and Schapira, G. (1963). *Nature (London)* **200**, 995–997.

Schapira, F., Reuber, M., and Hatzfeld, A. (1970). *Biochem. Biophys. Res. Commun.* **40**, 321–327.

Shipova, L. Ja., Abelev, G. I., Gusev, A. I., and Engelhardt, N. V. (1971). In preparation.

Smith, J. B., and Blumberg, B. S. (1969). *Lancet* **2**, 953.

Smith, J. B., and Todd, D. (1968). *Lancet* **2**, 833.

Spiro, R. (1960). *J. Biol. Chem.* **235**, 2860–2869.

Stanislawski-Birencwajg, M. (1965). *C. R. Acad. Sci.* **260**, 364–366.

Stanislawski-Birencwajg, M. (1967). *Cancer Res.* **27**, 1982–1989.

Stanislawski-Birencwajg, M., Uriel, J., and Grabar, P. (1967). *Cancer Res.* **27**, 1900–1907.

Tatarinov, Ju. S. (1964a). *Vopr. Med. Khim.* **10**, 90–91.

Tatarinov, Ju. S. (1964b). *Vopr. Med. Khim.* **10**, 218–219.

Tatarinov, Ju. S. (1964c). *Vopr. Med. Khim.* **10**, 584–588.

Tatarinov, Ju. S. (1965a). *Vopr. Med. Khim.* **11**, No. 2, 20–24.

Tatarinov, Ju. S. (1965b). *Vopr. Med. Khim.* **11**, No. 3, 98–99.

Tatarinov, Ju. S. (1967). *Vopr. Med. Khim.* **13**, 37–42.

Tatarinov, Ju. S. (1968). *Nature (London)* **217**, 964–965.

Tatarinov, Ju. S. (1970). *Vestn. Akad. Med. Nauk SSSR* **25**, No. 9, 68–72.

Tatarinov, Ju. S., and Afanassieva, A. V. (1965). *Byull. Eksp. Biol. Med.* No. 6, 65–59.

Tatarinov, Ju. S., and Nogaller, A. I. (1966). *Vopr. Onkol.* **12**, No. 12, 26–30.

Tatarinov, Ju. S., Massiukevitch, V. N., Mesnyankina, N. V., and Parfenova, L. F. (1967). *Akusherstvo i Ginecol. (USSR)* No. 8, 20–22.

Thomson, D., Krupey, J., Freedman, S., and Gold, P. (1969). *Proc. Nat. Acad. Sci.* **64**, 161–167.

Uriel, J. (1969). *Pathol. Biol.* **17**, 877–884.

Uriel, J., de Nechaud, B., Stanislawski-Birencwajg, M., Masseyeff, R., Leblanc, L., Quenum, C., Loisillier, F. and Grabar, P. (1967). *C. R. Acad. Sci.* **265**, 75–78.

Van Furth, R., and Adinolfi, M. (1969). *Nature (London)* **222**, 1296–1299.

Van Gool, J., and Ladiges, N. (1969). *J. Pathol.* **97**, 115–126.

Vasileysky, S. S. (1966). *Biokhimiya* **31**, 959–961.

Vasileysky, S. S., and Yablokova, V. (1964). *Byull. Eksp. Biol. Med.* No. 4, 52–54.

Weimer, H., and Benjamin, D. (1965). *Amer. J. Physiol.* **209**, 736–745.

Wise, R., and Oliver, J. (1966). *Biochem. J.* **100**, 330–333.

Wise, R., Ballard, F., and Ezekiel, E. (1963). *Comp. Biochem. Physiol.* **9**, 23.

Zizkovsky, V., Masopust, J., and Prokes, J. (1971). *Protides Biol. Fluids, Proc. Colloq.* **18** (in press).

LOW DOSE RADIATION CANCERS IN MAN

Alice Stewart

Department of Social Medicine, Oxford University, Oxford, England

I. Introduction

Ever since Muller (1927) discovered that the mutagenic effects of X-rays were directly proportional to the intensity of the exposures—a relationship which implies a linear dose-response relationship and no safety threshold—biologists have been uneasily aware that any increase in background radiation might add not only to the population load of unfavorable genes but also to the prevalence of malignant diseases. Since relationships between germ cell mutations and inherited diseases were on a firmer footing than relationships between somatic mutations and neoplasms, the genetic hazard was considered to be more certain than the cancer hazard (Wallace and Dobzhanski, 1960). On the other hand, pathologists have long felt that neoplastic diseases must be the result of fundamental changes in the structure and function of cell nuclei (Lockhart-Mummery, 1934), and there was no escaping the fact that radiations had carcinogenic as well as mutagenic effects (Medical Research Council, 1956).

Ten years after the atomic bomb explosions in Japan, radiobiologists felt reasonably certain that small doses of X-rays did not carry a general cancer hazard, but did carry a leukemia hazard, or, more precisely, a danger of developing the myeloid form of this disease. For instance, a committee appointed by the Medical Research Council (1956) to report on the hazards to man of nuclear and allied radiations had no hesitation in saying it would only be necessary to expose the whole population to relatively small doses of X-rays to increase the prevalence of myeloid leukemia by an observable amount. However, the committee also agreed that the equivalent of 200 rads in relatively concentrated amounts would be needed to produce a noteworthy increase in a normally small chance of developing this disease, and that no other type of cancer was likely to be caused by such small doses. Four years later the council issued a second report, having in the meantime considered the results of several enquiries into the long-term effects of low doses of X-rays which were not available in 1956. Although the second report was more factual than the first one, the conclusions were essentially the same except that "the risks of developing leukemia as a result of exposure to radiations may be somewhat less than we assumed in 1956" (Medical Research Council, 1960). Finally, a member of the advisory committee used the following words when addressing a recent symposium on radiation-induced cancers: "It appears clear on several grounds that leukemia, in the acute and in the chronic myeloid forms, is the type of malignancy which is most frequently induced by whole-body exposures of several hundred rads, and is the type in which incidence is the most greatly increased as compared with the normal incidence" (Pochin, 1969).

These views reflected world opinion and were widely interpreted as implying that there was a threshold dose below which radiations only had leukemogenic effects, and a second threshold below which they ceased to have any carcinogenic effects. They did not, however, explain how the basically "no-threshold" or mutagenic action of X-rays came to be associated with a "double-threshold" phenomenon in relation to malignant diseases. Nor did they account for the findings of several surveys which, individually and collectively, suggested that fetal tissues were so sensitive to the carcinogenic effects of radiations that even obstetric radiography should be regarded as a general cancer hazard, or as an agency capable of causing solid tumors as well as leukemias (Oxford Survey, see Stewart et al., 1958; Louisiana Survey, see Ford et al., 1959; New England Survey, see MacMahon, 1962).

The disparity between the surveys made exclusively on children and the ones concerned mainly or solely with adults would have been explicable if the delayed effects of radiation were determined by factors which were common to all tissues before birth and only became tissue selective after birth. However, the International Commission on Radiological Protection (1969) finally came to the conclusion that the sensitivity of individual organs to the tumor induction effects of radiation was no greater during childhood than during adult life and that, if anything, immature tissues other than the bone marrow were less likely to produce malignant tumors when exposed to radiation than adult tissues. So there were evidently strong influences at work which were making it difficult for radiobiologists to accept at face value the results of the childhood surveys.

It is not uncommon for laboratory workers to mistrust the findings of epidemiological enquiries. When, however, one finds even epidemiologists doubting the results of a nationwide enquiry (i.e., the Oxford Survey) after they have been confirmed in a much larger sample of cases (Stewart and Kneale, 1968) and reproduced in a follow-up of nearly a million live births (i.e., the New England Survey), one is clearly dealing with a very unusual situation. The trouble was that no one had succeeded in producing fetal tumors by deliberately exposing pregnant mammals to small doses of radiation (Sikov and Mahlum, 1969), thus making it possible for epidemiologists to disagree among themselves and to voice the opinion that "some fault in the methods, difficult or impossible to escape, may be implicating radiation spuriously" (Miller, 1969). A series of experiments had, in fact, shown that exposing pregnant mice and rats to relatively small doses of X-rays was liable to kill the embryos and to cause congenital defects. As, however, none of the animals who were normal at birth developed radiation cancers, the disturbing idea that there might be a cancer hazard associated with obstetric radiography gradually receded into the background.

Faced with various interpretations of the experimental data which were unfavorable to the childhood surveys, and knowing that several enquiries had failed to establish any connection between prenatal X-rays and childhood cancers (MacMahon and Hutchinson, 1964), radiobiologists became increasingly inclined to ignore the surveys with positive findings on the grounds that there must have been faulty interpretation of the available facts. For instance, in spite of much evidence to the contrary, they still considered that the extra X-rayed cases in the Oxford Survey might be due to the biased reporting of antenatal events by mothers of live and dead children (artefact theory), and that the extra cancer deaths in the New England Survey might be due to children whose fatal illnesses and X-ray experiences were the result of both events being independently correlated with a third variable which resided either in the mother or in the unborn child (hidden association theory).

These theories were difficult to refute and they exerted a powerful influence on committees which were naturally anxious not to exaggerate the dangers of radiations, and naturally suspicious of findings which were seemingly impossible to reconcile (a) with experimental data, (b) with data from the Atomic Bomb Casualty Commission, and (c) with data from a nationwide radiotherapy survey (Court Brown and Doll, 1957 and 1965). Unfortunately, it is easy to mistake theories for facts and to use the former rather than the latter as yardsticks for credibility. On this occasion the committees were probably allowing three basically implausible theories (the artefact theory, the hidden association theory and the double-threshold theory) to come between them and the realization that opportunities for the propagation of cancer cells might be totally different before and after birth.

Meanwhile the Oxford Survey had been converted into an ongoing survey because it was realized that the theories which loomed so large in the minds of radiobiologists were vulnerable on two points which, given time and perseverance, could be tested within the framework of an enquiry which had stumbled across the connection between obstetric X-rays and childhood cancers while looking for something else. The original purpose of the Oxford Survey was not to observe the long-term effects of pre-natal irradiation, but to discover why infants had escaped the postwar increase in leukemia mortality when slightly older children had been so severely affected (see Fig. 8, also see Hewitt, 1955).

Any hypothesis which denies the existence of low dose radiation cancers in children automatically attaches no importance to two variables which—in the event of obstetric X-ray examinations being the cause of some cases—would be expected to influence the proportions of exposed and nonexposed cases in certain age groups (Stewart and Hewitt, 1965). The two variables are (a) the number of films needed to complete each of the examinations and (b) the age of the exposed children when symptoms developed or death occurred (onset age and age at death). The effect of the first variable would depend upon how closely fetal doses approximated to numbers of exposures or films, and the effect of the second variable would depend partly on the number of radiogenic cases among the X-rayed cases, and partly on the nature of the correlations between initiation dates, onset dates, and dates of death. In other words film-number correlations would probably depend upon when the radiographs were taken and where they were taken (i.e., dates and places of birth) and onset-age correlations would probably depend upon the types of cancer caused by the radiations (i.e., cancer latent periods or tumor growth rates) and upon how many events are needed to set a cancer process in motion (Burch, 1965). Nevertheless, provided a survey of childhood cancers included a sufficiently large number of cases to allow birth dates, dates of death, and cell types to be held constant while studying other variables, it should be possible to confirm or refute all theories based on the assumption that in no circumstances can a diagnostic X-ray be the sole initiator of a malignant disease.

II. Oxford Survey

From this point of view the Oxford Survey was exceptionally well placed because the basic strategy incorporated the idea that until the body has stopped growing, small differences in age might have effects on cancer sensitivity which could only be detected if one had national or near-national coverage of all juvenile cancers. What is more, by establishing a nationwide network of data collecting centers (i.e., County and County Borough Public Health Departments), the survey had shown that this type of coverage was possible and that it was even possible to obtain information direct from mothers of dead children or cases, and mothers of live children or controls. In fact, the data collecting centers had already traced over 80% of the deaths between 1953 and 1955, and matched all the traced cases with live children picked at random from official birth registers (Stewart et al., 1958). So it was only necessary to regard the original (short-term) enquiry as the pilot phase of an ongoing retrospective survey to be partway toward achieving a 10- or 15-year "cancer surveillance" of all children born in Britain after 1952.

Because the findings in respect of obstetric radiography had taken everyone by surprise, only mothers who actually claimed these events had had their statements checked against contemporary records during the pilot enquiry. For the main survey (which is still continuing) a scheme was devised which allowed all negative and positive claims in respect of several events during the relevant pregnancies to be checked against clinic and hospital records (Stewart and Barber, 1962). With these additional records, it was eventually possible to refute the artefact theory by showing that the mothers of live and dead children were equally reliable in their reporting of at least four antenatal events, namely, abdominal X-rays, chest X-rays, toxemia and anemia (Hewitt, et al., 1966b).

For more than a decade the data collecting and data processing activities of the Oxford Survey of necessity had to take precedence over data analysis. Even so, it was possible to extract (from relatively inaccessible files of semiprocessed data) information which showed that for at least one malignant disease the age distributions of the exposed and nonexposed cases were significantly different, and that the differences implied relatively small numbers of irradiated leukemias in the youngest age groups (Wise, 1961; Stewart and Hewitt, 1965). This finding was important because, according to one variant of the hidden association theory, some or all of the extra X-rayed cases were the result of fetal conditions which had attracted the attention of obstetricians and thus been the cause of radiographic examinations which would not otherwise have been considered necessary. On this assumption, the extra X-rayed cases should be concentrated among the youngest cases, or children whose cancers are diagnosed at or shortly after birth (see below; also Stewart and Hewitt, 1965).

By 1966 an Oxford-survey based study of twins had shown that there was an abortion hazard associated with near-conception cancer initiations (Hewitt *et al.*, 1966a; Hewitt and Stewart, 1971). These early deaths were obviously masking the prevalence of exceptionally early (i.e., paraconception) cancer initiations. So it was reasonable to suppose that similar risks might be making it difficult or impossible to study the carcinogenic potentialities of prenatal irradiation in animals with short gestation periods. The facts were as follows: The overall number of twins with cancer exceeded the expected number by 20%, but the excess was entirely due to children who were X-rayed *in utero*, and was actually accompanied by a deficit of nonexposed twins. The extra X-rayed twins included the usual proportions of children from like and unlike sex pairs (which is what one would expect of cancers initiated too late to be the cause of an abortion) but the nonexposed cases were deficient in twins from like sex pairs (which is what one would expect if some of the missing twins had aborted). From here it was a short step to discovering that there was a shortage of males (who are more abortion-prone than females) (a) among twin-concordant cancers in the literature, (b) among healthy members of sibships in which there were two or more cases of juvenile neoplasms (familial cancers), and (c) among children who developed cancers within 15 months of nearly aborting (i.e., their mothers reported a threatened abortion).

These findings were important because they showed that there was no basic incompatibility between the childhood surveys and the animal experiments. Mice and rats have gestation periods which are measured in days and therefore have nothing in their life span which corresponds to the third trimester of a human pregnancy, or a period of several weeks during which a fully fashioned and sizable organism is living in a very protected environment. Consequently, the situation *vis à vis* obstetric radiography is a peculiarly difficult one to imitate in experimental animals because it is largely concerned with exposures which are too small and too late to have either lethal or teratogenic consequences. What is more, a viable human fetus belongs to a population which is unlikely to allow either stillbirths or later deaths to go unrecorded, and has these events recorded in ways which make it possible for epidemiologists to discover the circumstances in which they happened and to reconstruct the main sequence of events between conception and death before 10 years of age. Provided, therefore, a survey had taken as its starting point, not a group of irradiated fetuses (the starting point of the animal experiments), but a group of children who had recently died from malignant diseases (the starting point of the Oxford Survey), the fact that prenatal irradiation is liable to cause abortions and congenital defects would not prevent recognition of a concomitant cancer hazard, since, by definition, a group of fatal cancers would exclude any children who, for any reason, had failed to survive to the end of a cancer latent period.

Even a cursory inspection of the animal experiments which were supposed to argue against the existence of low dose radiation cancers in man shows that they never came near to mimicking the human situation. They not only allowed possible carcinogenic effects to be masked by actual lethal and teratogenic effects, they also described the results of using continuous and discrete exposures and varying both the dates of the exposures and the doses. In short, the discovery of an abortion hazard which is affecting the prevalence of recognizable cancers finally

TABLE I

OXFORD SURVEY—SOURCE OF 6347 TRACED CASES IN THE AGE
RANGE 0–9 YEARS

Year of death	England, Scotland, and Wales—cancers (0–9 yr) notifications	Pending series[a]	Traced cases or case/control pairs[b]	
			No.	%
1953[c]	634	—	526	83
1954[c]	619	—	502	81
1955[c]	647	—	558	86
1956	671	—	512	76
1957	592	—	445	75
1958	682	—	509	75
1959	644	—	519	81
1960	667	—	533	80
1961	657	54	484	74
1962	639	64	473	74
1963	704	98	508	72
1964	655	141	436	67
1965	563	145	342	61
Total	8374	502	6347	76

[a] Data collection not yet completed.

[b] Each traced case was matched for sex, date of birth, and region with a live control.

[c] Included in the 1958 report.

TABLE II

Oxford Survey—140 Sets of Case/Control Pairs, Classified by Year of Birth and Age at Death of the Cases

| | Traced cases | | | | | | | | | | | X-rayed *in utero* | |
| | Birth dates classified by age at death in years | | | | | | | | | | | Observed % | Expected % |
	0	1	2	3	4	5	6	7	8	9	Total		
1943	—	—	—	—	—	—	—	—	—	17	17		
1944	—	—	—	—	—	—	—	—	14	28	42	10.4	6.0
1945	—	—	—	—	—	—	—	13	32	21	66		
1946	—	—	—	—	—	—	21	38	35	35	129	13.2	2.3
1947	—	—	—	—	—	25	53	49	43	30	200	12.0	3.0
1948	—	—	—	—	32	61	53	46	35	31	258	13.6	8.1
1949	—	—	—	39	61	55	52	44	29	40	320	15.3	7.8
1950	—	—	26	71	56	53	42	44	48	31	371	16.2	9.2
1951	—	27	71	75	70	44	40	43	43	43	456	17.5	8.8
1952	24	43	91	63	55	47	46	42	31	37	479	17.7	11.8
1953	49	64	69	64	75	49	53	32	35	39	529	14.2	12.7
1954	46	60	55	77	61	43	48	27	40	29	486	17.3	14.4
1955	31	52	58	78	56	57	46	32	33	28	471	21.7	11.3
1956	50	43	69	71	63	45	42	46	28	14	471	21.4	14.6
1957	41	52	62	58	46	64	34	31	—	—	393	17.3	10.4
1958	47	62	88	59	63	52	34	18	—	—	423	13.9	11.1
1959	45	61	68	74	57	53	24	—	—	—	382	8.1	7.6
1960	39	53	73	62	45	17	—	—	—	—	289	12.5	9.3
1961	41	55	51	45	28	—	—	—	—	—	220	10.9	8.6
1962	42	51	53	12	—	—	—	—	—	—	158	12.0	7.0
1963	54	46	20	—	—	—	—	—	—	—	120	} 12.3	} 9.6
1964	32	22	—	—	—	—	—	—	—	—	54		
1965	13	—	—	—	—	—	—	—	—	—	13		
Totals	554	691	854	848	768	655	588	505	461	423	6347	15.5	10.2

TABLE III

OXFORD SURVEY—DIAGNOSTIC CLASSIFICATION OF 6347 TRACED
CASES AND 985 X-RAYED CASES

Diagnostic group	Traced cases	X-rayed *in utero*	
		No.	%
Leukemias	2947	458	15.5
Lymphosarcomas	500	78	15.6
Cerebral tumors	1030	154	15.0
Neuroblastomas	636	99	15.6
Wilms' tumors	572	93	16.3
Other cancers[a]	662	103	15.6
All cancers	6347	985	15.5
Controls	6347	645	10.2

[a] Including sarcomas of bone (122), reproductive organs (94), connective tissue (91), liver (78), retina (47), bladder (34), mouth and nasopharynx (33), and endocrine glands (11).

disposed of the idea that there was any difficulty in reconciling the findings of the childhood surveys and the animal experiments, and paved the way for a final refutation of the double threshold theory.

By 1968 the Oxford Survey had assembled a group of traced cases which included three-quarters of all juvenile cancer deaths in Britain between 1953 and 1965 (see Table I) and subsequently included an even larger proportion of these cases (see Table VI). For these children there were records of birth dates, dates of death, onset dates, and causes of death (see Tables II and III). As previously mentioned, all the traced cases were matched for sex, date of birth, and region with live controls, and for each case/control pair there were records of which members had or had not been exposed to radiations before birth (see Table IV). Finally, for most of the children who had been X-rayed before birth, there were also records of when the radiographs were taken, how many films were actually or probably used, and what was found.

The classifications by year of birth and age at death (see Tables II and IV) allow one to see how many of the birth cohorts were truncated (in the sense that they had not been screened for cancer deaths in all ten age groups) and which of the ten age groups were affected by the truncations, that is to say, by the fact that the cases were not ascertained until after death (note the empty cells in Table II and the asymmetrical appearance compared to the rest of the table). For children who were born before the survey began, there will never be a complete set of records, but there is no reason why children who were born later than 1965 should not eventually feature as fully screened or standard

TABLE IV

Oxford Survey—Estimated Imbalance of Prenatal X-Rays in 140 Sets of Case/Control Pairs

Cohorts	"Extra" X-rayed children classified by age at death of the cases[a]										Traced cases	
	0	1	2	3	4	5	6	7	8	9	Radiogenic	Non-radiogenic
1943	—	—	—	—	—	—	—	—	—	−2.1		
1944	—	—	—	—	—	—	—	—	+2.6	+1.6	2	123
1945	—	—	—	—	—	—	—	−2.4	−0.9	+3.1	14	115
1946	—	—	—	—	—	—	+1.0	+1.1	+5.7	+5.9	20	180
1947	—	—	—	—	—	+2.3	+8.9	+3.3	+1.6	+4.2	12	146
1948	—	—	—	—	−1.3	−1.0	−0.4	+7.4	+3.4	+3.8	27	293
1949	—	—	—	+4.0	+10.3	+0.8	+2.1	+5.0	+6.3	−1.1	31	340
1950	—	—	+7.3	+1.5	+2.9	+7.4	+0.2	+5.5	+5.0	+1.2	45	411
1951	+2.5	+7.3	+2.8	+5.4	+10.1	+3.5	+0.6	+8.9	+4.4	+2.4	33	446
1952	−0.2	+4.1	+6.5	+0.7	+6.3	−0.6	+6.3	+3.3	+3.8	−0.4	9	520[a]
1953[a]	−1.8	−0.1	+4.6	+6.8	+1.8	−1.3	−0.7	+3.4	−3.4	−2.3	16	470[a]
1954[a]	+5.8	+0.3	+1.2	+4.5	+7.1	+0.8	+1.2	+0.1	+2.7	−0.3	55	416[a]
1955[a]	+2.0	+2.4	+1.7	+9.1	+10.4	+8.5	+7.9	+6.3	−0.9	+3.8	41	430
1956	+5.4	−0.3	+6.8	+11.8	+5.6	−0.7	+5.9	+2.9	+1.3	+5.7	33	360
1957	+0.8	+0.7	+4.9	+5.5	−0.9	+2.8	+6.7	+6.4	+1.2	—	14	409
1958	−0.4	+7.5	+0.2	+2.8	+2.3	−2.3	+0.3	+2.8	—	—	1	381
1959	+1.5	−0.6	+5.4	+0.5	−0.4	−1.3	−2.2	—	—	—	14	275
1960	−2.8	+5.8	−3.2	+5.2	−1.5	+6.6	—	—	—	—	7	213
1961	+4.5	+9.4	−1.6	+0.2	+1.6	—	—	—	—	—	8	150
1962	−3.0	+1.7	+4.2	−2.2	—	—	—	—	—	—		
1963	+6.6	+1.8	−2.8	—	—	—	—	—	—	—		
1964	0.0	+4.6	—	—	—	—	—	—	—	—	7	180
1965	—	—	—	—	—	—	—	—	—	—		
Totals	+20.9	+44.6	+38.0	+55.8	+54.3	+25.5	+37.8	+54.0	+32.8	+25.5	389	5958

[a] + = the "extra" X-rayed children were cases } in each set (see Table II).
    − = the "extra" X-rayed children were controls }

cohorts. The data collection period already covers more years than are shown in Table I, which means that the groups of children with both age at death and date of birth in common (i.e., the number of occupied cells in Table II) are already more numerous than they were when this table was compiled. Nevertheless, however long the survey continues there will never be any reduction in the number of empty cells or "missing data sets."

By 1968 a new method of analyzing asymmetrical contingency tables had been developed in relation to the Oxford Survey which made it possible to replace missing data sets with estimated numbers, and thus to include partially screened as well as fully screened cohorts in various analyses necessitating standardization of year of birth and age at death (Kneale, 1971b). This method, which is applicable to all diseases with long latent periods, is based on the fact that adjacent columns in asymmetrical contingency tables necessarily have more in common than widely separated columns. For instance, in Table II the first two columns describe the two youngest age groups and have thirteen rows or years of birth or exposure years in common, whereas the first and last columns (i.e., the youngest and oldest age groups) only share five rows or exposure years. The detailed procedures which are needed to bring tables with empty cells into line with "complete" tables need not concern the reader (the equations leading to the best estimates can only be solved on an electronic computer), provided he realizes that the effect of the method is to bring ongoing retrospective surveys into line with conventional prospective surveys. For instance, the data in Table IV provided the basis for obtaining estimates of the radiation hazards of 17 birth cohorts from data describing 13 years of death (Stewart and Kneale, 1968). They also made it possible to convert a dose-response curve based on numbers of films into one based on estimated fetal doses (Stewart and Kneale, 1970a); and to produce latent period estimates for all the disease groups shown in Table III (Stewart and Kneale, 1970b).

A. Cohort Risks

In their review of the cancer hazards associated with prenatal irradiation, MacMahon and Hutchinson (1964) finally came to the conclusion that the "extra" cancer risk for children involved in obstetric X-ray examinations was equal to 40% of the normal risk of dying from a malignant disease before the age of 10 years. Since the normal risk would be expected to produce about 600 juvenile cancer deaths in cohorts which originally included 700,000 liveborn children (a figure which approximates the size of the birth cohorts in the Oxford Survey), this estimate would imply an extra 240 deaths if all children were X-rayed *in utero*,

or an extra 24 deaths if only one in ten members of a birth cohort were
exposed (Stewart and Kneale, 1968). If, however, the radiation cancer
hazard is dose-dependent, we should not expect diagnostic radiography
to be equally dangerous in different parts of the world or to remain
equally dangerous during a period of rapid improvement in machine
design (Ardran, 1956). On the contrary, we should expect the extra
cancer risk to vary both with mechanical factors, or relationships between films and fetal doses, and with clinical factors, or relationships
between numbers of radiographs and reasons for the examinations
(Clayton *et al.*, 1957). In other words, even if the number of X-ray

TABLE V

Oxford Survey—Estimates of the Radiogenic Component of the Juvenile
Cancer Load Sustained by 17 Cohorts, Cancer Risk Associated with
Obstetric Radiography, and the Risk of Being X-Rayed during
the Years 1946–62

Birth cohorts	Radiogenic component of the juvenile cancer load		Extra cancer risk if X-rayed *in utero*[a]		Risk of being X-rayed *in utero*[b]
	No.[c]	Standard error	%	Standard error	%
1946	34	10.5	322	241	2.3
1947	45	10.9	329	183	3.0
1948	21	12.4	55	42	8.1
1949	39	11.9	114	49	7.8
1950	39	11.8	94	38	9.2
1951	49	11.5	125	41	8.8
1952	33	11.6	62	27	11.8
1953	9	11.7	15	22	12.7
1954	16	12.4	24	21	14.4
1955	55	12.5	109	34	11.3
1956	41	13.2	62	24	14.6
1957	35	11.5	76	32	10.4
1958	17	12.5	34	27	11.1
1959	1	11.4	4	35	7.6
1960	24	13.9	58	39	9.3
1961	13	12.7	32	37	8.6
1962	19	13.7	62	57	7.0
Total	490				

[a] As % of normal risk of dying from cancer before age 10 (about 1 in 1200).

[b] Control data.

[c] The corresponding numbers of nonradiogenic cases would have been in the region
of 470 per cohort (total 8000). Had all cases been traced, the totals for radiogenic and
nonradiogenic cancers would have been about 645 and 10,500 (i.e., 6% and 94%) of the
cancer deaths, respectively.

examinations remained constant over a long period of time, the number of cancers induced by the radiations would not remain constant unless film doses and numbers of films also remained unchanged.

A recent analysis of cohort risks based on data from the Oxford Survey indicated a trend toward safer obstetric X-ray examinations between 1946 and 1955 (see Table V). There were, however, exceptionally large numbers of radiogenic cancer deaths affecting the 1955–56 cohorts without any corresponding increase in the proportion of X-rayed children. Since there was no certainty that multiple exposures were exceptionally common during this period, Miller (1969) could still insist that no childhood survey had produced convincing evidence of a dose-response effect. In fact, a much earlier analysis of the Oxford data had shown higher case/control ratios for four-film examinations than for one-film examinations (Stewart *et al.*, 1958), and there was also a table in the 1962 report of the New England Survey which showed that the cancer death rate for 67 children with records of several exposures was higher than the rate for 183 children whose examinations only entailed one or two films (MacMahon, 1962). As, however, it was possible that the first result was due to biased reporting of case and control histories, and the second was a chance finding, neither of these claims carried much weight. Eventually 7649 pairs of cases and controls from the Oxford Survey were included in an analysis which showed not only how the extra cancer risk was related to numbers of radiographs, but what this implied in the way of a dose-response curve (see Table VI and

TABLE VI

Obstetric X-Ray Records by Date of Birth and Numbers of Films

Group	Year of birth	X-rayed in utero		No. of films					No record	Totals
		Yes	No	1	2	3	4	>5		
Cases	1943–49	212	1610	29	34	19	8	14	108	1822
	1950–54	437	2298	92	80	45	30	33	157	2735
	1955–59	381	1772	109	71	35	19	15	132	2153
	1960–65	111	828	44	16	4	3	3	41	939
	Total	1141	6508	274	201	103	60	65	438	7649
Controls	1943–49	110	1712	19	11	5	3	1	71	1822
	1950–54	316	2419	73	74	30	15	17	107	2735
	1955–59	248	1905	79	52	18	9	10	80	2153
	1960–65	100	839	47	14	5	1	1	32	939
	Total	774	6875	218	151	58	28	29	290	7649
Cases/control ratios		*1.48*	*0.95*	*1.26*	*1.33*	*1.78*	*2.14*	*2.24*	*1.51*	*1.00*

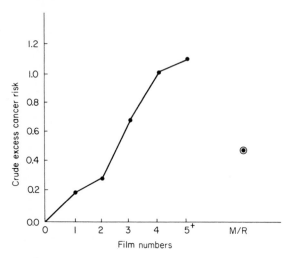

Fig. 1. Crude dose response curve for the radiogenic cancers included in the Oxford Survey.

Fig. 1). The curve relating numbers of radiographs to the extra cancer risk was described by Stewart and Kneale (1970a) as a "crude" dose-response curve because they had in the meantime discovered that dates of birth were affecting both radiographic doses and numbers of radiographs per examination. They were, however, able to show, first, that the cancer yield following prenatal irradiation was directly proportional to the dose (i.e., there appeared to be a linear dose-response relationship of the type which had been observed by Müller in relation to the mutagenic effect of radiations). Second, the extra cancer risk was the same for solid tumors as for leukemias. Third, the number of cancer deaths which would result if one million children were exposed to 1 rad of ionizing radiations shortly before birth was in the region of 600 (see Table VII and Fig. 2). Fourth, when stating the cancer risk associated with prenatal irradiation it was important to state the age of the fetus because first trimester exposures are more dangerous than later ones.

The discovery than an immature fetus is more vulnerable to the tumor induction effects of radiation than a mature fetus is difficult to reconcile with the conclusion that organ sensitivity is not age dependent (International Commission on Radiation Protection, 1969). It is, however, in line with the suggestion that it is the cell population requirements of a tissue which determine cancer sensitivity, and that it is not possible for mutant cells to hold in abeyance their newly acquired properties for any length of time (Stewart, 1970).

Lying at the root of many theories of cancer causation are two

TABLE VII

CALCULATION OF CANCER RISK INCURRED BY CHILDREN WHO ARE EXPOSED TO 1 RAD OF IONIZING RADIATIONS SHORTLY BEFORE BIRTH BASED ON OXFORD SURVEY DATA[a]

Period	Live births (Great Britain)	N.C.R. estimates[b]			E.C.R. estimates[c]			
		No. of cancer deaths (0–9 yr)	Rate per million live births	Risk per single film	S.E.	Extra cancer deaths (0–9 yr) per million children exposed to 1 film	Mean fetal dose per single film millirads
1943–49	6,014,408	3688	613.2	0.581	0.208	365.3	460
1950–54	3,863,300	3024	782.8	0.226	0.095	176.9	400
1955–59	4,065,304	3163	778.0	0.357	0.129	277.7	250
1960–65	5,642,275	3532	626.0	0.098	0.110	61.3	200

[a] Absolute radiation risk expressed as numbers of extra cancer deaths (0–9 yr) per rad per million children at risk* = 572 (S.E. 133). (From the regression of E.C.R. rates on mean fetal doses.)

[b] N.C.R. = Normal cancer risk. 1943–59 estimates based on actual deaths during the period 1943–68; 1960–65 estimates based on expected deaths during the period 1960–74.

[c] E.C.R. = Extra cancer risk for children X-rayed before birth (see text).

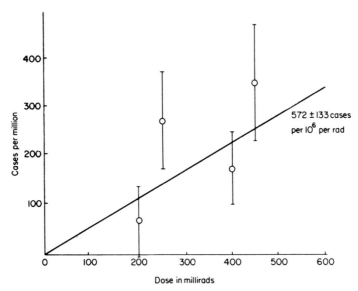

FIG. 2. Fetal dose response curve (Oxford data, see Tables VI and VII).

assumptions. First, it is not until neoplastic cells are "provoked" by environmental influences that they are at all likely to reveal their abnormal growth potential and freedom of movement. Second, the relationship between advancing age and cancer mortality is such as to rule out the possibility of cancers being caused by a single somatic mutation (one-hit hypothesis, see Burch, 1965). Hence the idea that cancers must be the result of a long-drawn-out process which in some unexplained fashion allows an obligatory event, or *cancer initiation*, to have such a profound effect on the cellular environment that normally harmless events proceed to operate as *cancer promoters* (multi-stage hypothesis, see Salaman, 1958). If, however, it is typical of healthy tissues that they give no encouragement to mutant cells, and if it is essential for mutant cells to divide in order to survive, then events which precede or accompany cancer initiation could be of much greater importance than later events.

The theory which is based on the assumption that a cancer cell has no option but to multiply or disappear is known as the gene selection theory of cancer causation (Stewart, 1970) because it postulates the need for a particular change in a controlling gene at a particular moment. In other words, initiation and promotion remain obligatory events in tumor formation, but they occur in such rapid sequence that the conditions which are needed to ensure promotion either precede or accompany the initiating event. In other words, a cancer-potent cell—or a cell in which a nonlethal mutation has "liberated" a normally restricted growth-potential and migration-potential by destroying the restricting mechanisms—is regarded as a rare consequence of relatively common events which (by means of lethal mutations) destroy cells and thus create "cancer-sensitivity," or tissues which are temporarily or permanently short of mitotically competent cells. On this basis there is no difficulty in understanding how the ageing process (which includes both growth and decay) has diametrically opposite effects before and after maturity, but it is difficult to believe that intervals between the initiating event and the onset of symptoms are more often measured in decades than in years (Medical Research Council, 1956).

B. CANCER LATENT PERIODS

The subject of cancer latent periods is a very confused one because there is no general agreement about the esssential steps in the neoplastic process and therefore no agreement either about what constitutes the start of the cancer process or about the precise action of carcinogens, including radiations. For instance, Willis considers (1960) that "neoplastic change does *not* take place suddenly, but in a gradual or cumulative manner, hyperplasia often passing insensibly into neoplasia or benign non-invasive neoplasia into malignant invasive neoplasia without any change in cell structure or behavior," and he includes in cancer latent periods both the time that it takes for invasive and metastatic tumors to draw attention to their presence, and the periods during which erstwhile healthy tissues are in danger of developing cancers because they are in a "conditioned" or premalignant stage (i.e., he forgets that an insensible change at tissue level could be due to a sudden change in one cell followed by an exponential increase in the number of changed or mutant cells).

An obvious alternative to the Willis hypothesis is to regard the numerous factors which predispose to cancers (including benign non-invasive neoplasia) not as *essential* steps in the cancer process, but as contributory factors, that is to say, changes which are comparable to the ones which predispose to infections and were deemed to be an essential part of the infective process until bacteria were discovered. On this assumption cancer latent periods should be of relatively short duration because, however long drawn out the period of heightened cancer sensitivity, the neoplastic process would not be deemed to have started until a definitive mutation had introduced a totally new factor into the situation by creating the first of many malignant cells. On the other hand, since the precise timing of such an event would be difficult to determine, and since it is reasonable to suppose that *recognizable* carcinogens not only create cancer-potent cells but also create the conditions which are necessary for the propagation of such cells (i.e., they operate both as initiators and as promoters of cancers), there could be great difficulty in discriminating between the older theories of cancer causation and the gene selection theory.

For instance, although we have learned from the atomic explosions that myeloid leukemia often takes less than 5 years to produce symptoms, the radiations caused such widespread tissue damage that the cancers which are currently causing concern (Wanebo *et al.*, 1968a,b) could well be due to mutations which happened much later than 1945 and succeeded in producing tumors because the aftermath of the explosions had rendered several tissues permanently cancer-prone by introducing an element of premature senility. Moreover, in view of how many individuals survived the immediate effects of the explosions only to succumb to radiation sickness and related infections, we might have hazarded a guess that the "extra" myeloid leukemia deaths would be equally common in all age groups (Bizzozero *et al.*, 1966). For although young adults are much less leukemia-prone than children or older adults, the earlier infection deaths should have exerted a counterbalancing effect by being *least* common in young adults (Jablon *et al.*, 1965).

A better opportunity for observing the effects of age on the tumor induction effects of radiations was provided by a follow-up of several thousand patients who were given radiotherapy for ankylosing spondylitis (Court Brown and Doll, 1957, 1965). In this series of patients there were 16 deaths from aplastic anemia, which meant that some of the treatments had caused extensive tissue damage. There were, however, many more patients who developed myeloid leukemia 3 to 5 years after their treatments, and enough of these (adult) cases to show that the extra cancer hazard increased with age. Latent periods of 3 to 5 years were also found in a group of adults who had probably developed myeloid leukemia as a result of being involved in radiographic investigations which necessitated several exposures of the bone marrow to much smaller doses of X-rays (Stewart *et al.*, 1962). But it was not until the Oxford Survey had assembled over 6000 case/control pairs that it was possible to use a group of radiation-induced cancers to measure latent periods in circumstances which ensured that the initiating events coincided with the X-ray exposures, and that the consequences included more solid tumors than leukemias.

Because the Oxford Survey was based on a nationwide sample of X-rayed and non-X-rayed cases, children who died before the age of 10 years could be used to measure the latent periods of cancers which

TABLE VIII

OXFORD SURVEY—ONSET-AGE DISTRIBUTIONS OF JUVENILE NEOPLASMS CLASSIFIED BY CELL TYPES AND X-RAY EXPERIENCES

X-ray classification	Onset age (years)	Leukemias Lymphatic %	Leukemias Stem-cell %	Leukemias Myeloid and monocytic %	Lymphomas %	Cerebral tumors %	Neuroblastomas %	Wilms' tumors %	Osteogenic sarcomas %	Mixed types Series I %	Mixed types Series II %	All cancers Series Hemopoietic %	All cancers Solid %	All types %	All types No. of cases
Spontaneous (not X-rayed) cases	0	8.3	12.8	12.7	11.9	14.8	21.1	17.1	3.1	29.6	24.5	10.1	18.2	13.8	799
	1	13.7	12.5	11.8	10.3	16.0	20.5	17.0	8.7	24.2	18.5	11.9	17.8	14.0	810
	2	17.5	19.0	13.0	11.7	11.9	15.6	19.4	5.4	15.6	13.5	15.8	14.1	15.2	881
	3	16.6	14.1	11.7	11.5	11.5	11.8	16.2	6.4	8.8	9.9	15.3	11.8	14.5	840
	4	12.8	12.9	12.9	14.5	10.3	10.6	13.7	12.1	6.0	9.4	13.1	11.2	12.7	736
	5	9.4	9.1	8.2	10.1	10.2	8.8	7.0	9.3	4.5	6.4	10.2	8.0	8.4	487
	6	7.6	7.1	11.0	10.3	10.1	4.6	4.5	18.0	5.4	4.7	7.9	7.2	7.6	440
	7	6.6	5.7	8.0	7.2	10.1	3.1	3.0	15.0	2.7	4.7	7.0	5.1	6.4	371
	8	5.2	5.4	7.4	8.2	7.0	2.9	1.8	19.6	2.9	7.9	5.9	4.8	5.3	307
	9–	2.3	1.4	3.3	3.7	0.2	1.2	0.3	2.4	0.3	0.5	2.8	1.8	2.1	122
No. of cases		*1478*	*708*	*536*	*417*	*886*	*563*	*497*	*118*	*349*	*241*	*3139*	*2654*	*5793*	*5793*
"Extra" X-rayed cases	0	0.3	1.0	1.3	0.1	30.0	20.9	6.0	0.0	28.8	28.9	0.1	27.6	9.0	38
	1	6.3	6.7	13.7	8.6	0.9	34.9	23.0	0.0	10.5	22.1	8.9	15.6	11.8	50
	2	17.2	15.6	10.0	21.0	3.1	9.2	25.9	0.0	16.5	0.0	11.7	16.0	19.3	81
	3	22.0	19.0	5.3	14.0	9.3	3.0	13.8	0.0	13.7	0.0	20.4	5.7	13.6	57
	4	21.3	17.3	5.0	6.8	9.2	2.5	6.0	7.0	5.7	0.1	17.6	4.2	10.2	43
	5	16.4	14.6	8.3	4.8	8.0	4.4	3.5	11.4	3.0	20.9	14.2	6.7	8.4	36
	6	9.3	12.3	14.3	5.9	15.6	8.4	3.6	6.2	4.6	23.7	9.5	9.2	10.8	46
	7	3.7	9.0	15.7	10.5	23.6	9.0	6.1	75.4	13.1	0.0	8.7	10.8	10.2	43
	8	1.6	4.0	11.4	16.3	0.3	4.8	9.0	0.0	4.1	0.0	3.5	2.2	3.7	16
	9	1.9	0.5	15.0	11.1	0.0	2.9	3.1	0.0	0.0	4.3	5.4	2.0	3.0	13
No. of cases		*99*	*59*	*32*	*25*	*73*	*42*	*41*	*7*	*30*	*15*	*215*	*208*	*423*	*423*

normally take less than 10 years to run their full course, and to distinguish between rival theories of cancer causation. For instance, the continuous process described by Willis (1960) and the discontinuous process implicit in other multistage theories (Burch, 1965) would lead one to expect that the X-rayed cases either had the same age distributions as the non-X-rayed cases (i.e., none of the exposures had influenced the outcome) or were younger than average (i.e., some of the exposures had hastened the onset of symptoms, but none had been the initiating event). If, however, the action of the X-rays was either to have *no* effect on the fetus or to be a *definitive* cause of a juvenile cancer, then (knowing that some of the spontaneous cancers had weathered an abortion hazard and that most of the X-rays were taken during the third trimester), one would expect the extra X-rayed cases to be older than average and to have onset ages which corresponded to cancer latent periods and were more compact than the onset ages of the spontaneous cases (see Table VIII).

Table VIII is taken from a paper by Stewart and Kneale (1970b) and illustrates several points of interest. For instance, the figures for the non-X-rayed cases show that cancer initiation risks normally de-

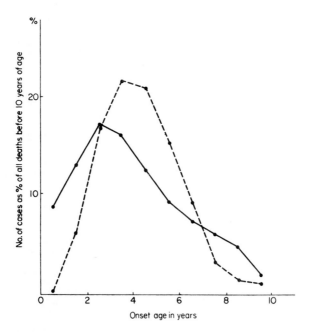

Fig. 3. Onset age distributions of two types of lymphatic leukemia: radiogenic and spontaneous (estimates see Table VII). - - - radiogenic; ——— spontaneous.

crease with age between conception and puberty, and the figures for the extra X-rayed cases show that the radiation-induced cases must have been initiated later than the first (and largest) batch of spontaneous cases, but earlier than the last (and smallest) batch. For instance, 40% of the non-X-rayed lymphatic leukemias were diagnosed within 3 years of birth and 30% after the age of 5 years. For the corresponding group of extra X-rayed leukemias, the figures were 24% and 17%, respectively (see Fig. 3). The table also shows that most of the solid tumors had shorter latent periods than the leukemias (see neuroblastomas and Wilms' tumors in Table VIII, also Figs. 4 and 5), but there were some malignant diseases which characteristically take more than 6 years to produce symptoms (see lymphomas, cerebral tumors, and bone sarcomas in Table VIII; also Fig. 6).

In view of the suggestion that the fetal condition of cancer-prone children would be likely to "attract" obstetric X-ray examinations (see

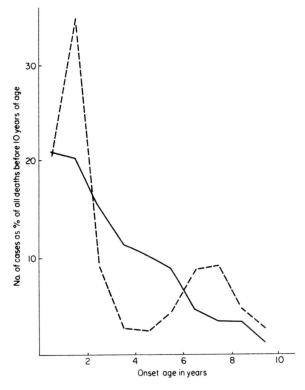

Fig. 4. Onset age distributions of two types of neuroblastomas: radiogenic and spontaneous (estimates, see Table VIII). - - - radiogenic; —— spontaneous.

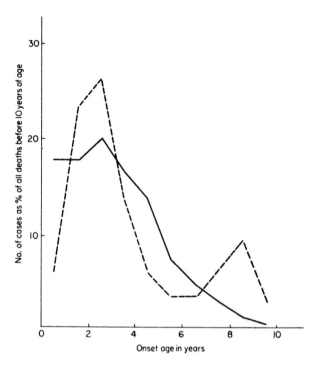

FIG. 5. Onset age distribution of two types of Wilms' tumors: radiogenic and spontaneous (estimates, see Table VIII). - - - radiogenic; —— spontaneous.

hidden association theory above), it is important to note that the cerebral tumors produced no extra X-rayed cases in the second youngest age group and about 20 such cases in the youngest age group (see Fig. 7). This apparent exception to the rule that cerebral tumors have longer latent periods than leukemias was explained when it transpired that nearly half of a small group of cases which presented with a congenital hydrocephalus had been X-rayed *in utero* because a large head was threatening to obstruct labor. In other words, about 2% of the cerebral tumors and about 0.5% of all the cancers which feature as extra X-rayed in Table VIII were not, in fact, radiation-induced.

To sum up, the Oxford Survey has been able to show that there was no difficulty in distinguishing between additional (X-rayed) cases which were not radiation-induced and the genuinely radiogenic cases; and that when they are recognizable, cancer initiation dates are separated from cancer onsets by relatively constant intervals. The survey has also shown that solid tumors of children often have shorter latent periods than hemopoietic neoplasms, and that the acute lymphatic leukemias of children take the same length of time to produce symptoms as the

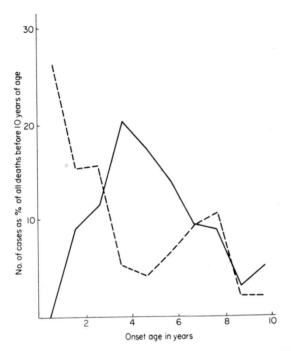

Fɪɢ. 6. Onset age distributions of two sets of radiogenic cancers: solid tumors and hemopoietic neoplasms (estimates, see Table VIII). --- solid tumors; —— hemopoietic.

acute myeloid leukemias of adults. Thus the idea that a cancer cell is forced to multiply or disappear would seem to apply to all childhood cancers and to the one type of adult cancer which it has been possible to study in circumstances which ensured recognition of the initiation dates.

III. Tissue Destructive Doses of Radiation

Although solid tumors are as easily produced by obstetric radiography as leukemia, there is no escaping the fact that in adults acute myeloid leukemia has more often followed whole or partial body exposure than other forms of cancer. According to the double threshold theory, this is because the bone marrow is the only tissue to remain sensitive to small doses of radiation. But according to the gene selection theory, the leukemia bias is due to the fact that the RES reacts more sharply to tissue destructive doses of radiation than other tissues, and thus give any mutant stem cells formed by the radiations an exceptionally good chance to multiply in the bone marrow.

The gene selection theory also assumes that Cronkite's observations

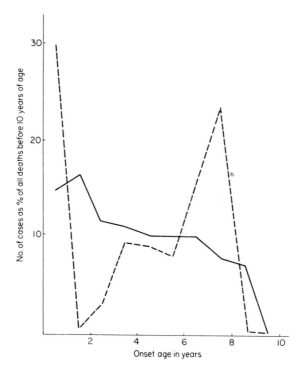

FIG. 7. Onset age distributions of three types of cerebral tumors: (a) Radiogenic, (b) spontaneous and not X-rayed, (c) Spontaneous and attracting X-ray examinations (estimates, see Table VIII). - - - "extra" X-rayed cases; ———"non" X-rayed cases.

in relation to malignant leukocytes mean that these cells divide at the same rate as their normal counterparts and remain equally sensitive to the need for extra cells (Cronkite, 1965). Consequently, doses of radiation which are too small to cause tissue damage, but happen to coincide with a period of rapid tissue expansion, are bound to have totally different effects from doses which cause tissue destruction *and* lower resistance to infections, because one of the injured tissues is the RES. In the first situation, which is typified by obstetric radiography, all the tissues are equally cancer sensitive and there is no call for extra leukocytes. In the second situation, which is typified by radiotherapy, some or all of the tissues may be forced to produce extra cells, but the leukocytosis which follows in the wake of the agranulocytosis is of a different order of magnitude from the reactions of other tissues.

It is also possible to have a situation in which the tissue destructive effects of the radiations are so variable that, at one end of the scale, there are individuals dying from septic complications of the acute or subacute effects, and at the other end of the scale, individuals who remain in perfect health until they develop leukemia. In this situation, which is typified by the atomic bomb explosions, the experiences of individuals who survive the acute and subacute effects of the radiations cannot be used to estimate the population effects of small doses; not because there is any difficulty in classifying survivors according to the doses of radiations they received, but because individuals who failed to survive the acute and subacute effects are biased to an unknown extent in favor of embryos, infants, old people, pregnant women, and sick persons of both sexes (Jablon *et al.*, 1965; Jablon and Kato, 1970).

In short, the gene selection theory provides relatively simple solutions for several problems raised by radiation cancers in man, and also allows us to assume that the rapid increase in leukemia mortality which characterized the period 1945 to 1955 was due to an equally rapid increase in the number of individuals with incipient leukemia who survived to the end of an exceptionally dangerous latent period because they had leukemia-induced infections treated with antibiotics.

IV. Infections and Leukemia

Ever since the Oxford Survey succeeded in uncovering a high incidence of pneumonic complications of childhood infections during the 2 years preceding the onset of leukemia, a hidden association between infections and hemopoietic neoplasms has been suspected (Stewart *et al.*, 1958; Stewart, 1961), but it was not until much later that a negative correlation between the trends of mortality for pneumonia and leukemia was finally established (see Fig. 8; also Stewart and Kneale, 1969; Kneale, 1971a). By this time the latent period studies had shown that for young children, the amount of the leukemia latent period which is spent in an *in utero* setting is negatively correlated with age at the onset of symptoms. If, therefore, the risk of an infection death while incubating leukemia is in any way related to the amount of the latent period which is spent in a *postnatal* setting, this should make children under 2 years of age less likely to be affected by a rising trend of leukemia mortality than slightly older children (see Fig. 9). Following this line of thought, Stewart and Kneale finally succeeded in showing that the risk of dying from pneumonia while incubating leukemia was much greater for children between 2 and 4 years of age than for younger children, and so great as to make it likely that at least half of the observed increase in leukemia mortality between 1920 and 1960 was due to deaths which were ascribed to pneumonia but should have been ascribed to pneumonic complications of leukemia.

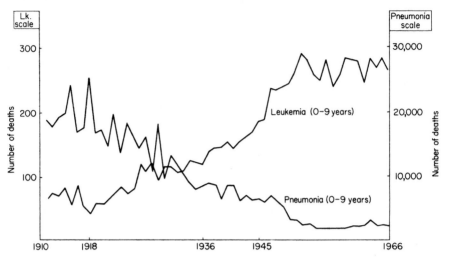

FIG. 8. Secular trends of leukemia and pneumonia deaths (0–9 years). England and Wales, 1911–1966.

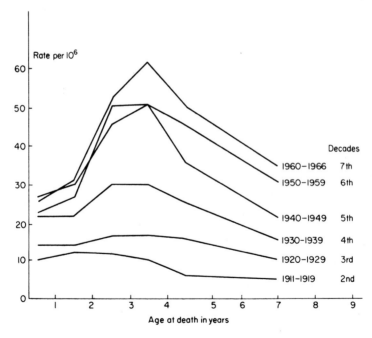

FIG. 9. Leukemia mortality (0–9 years) in six consecutive decades. England and Wales, 1911–1966.

Since these findings implied continual multiplication of leukemia cells during the latent period, they provided further support for the idea that cancer initiation is followed immediately by multiplication of the cancer cells. They also served as a warning that it may not be safe to compare leukemia death rates in different parts of the world unless one has an intimate knowledge of the prevailing infections and how they are treated. For instance, the odd geographic distribution of Burkitt's lymphoma—which follows the line of endemic malaria but tends to disappear in hyperendemic areas—is supposed to indicate a viral origin for this unusual form of lymphosarcoma (Burkitt, 1962; Woodall and Haddow, 1962; Pike et al., 1967). But according to the gene selection theory, the coexistence of a lymphatic neoplasm and chronic malaria is bound to affect the anatomical positions of metastatic deposits and might account not only for the jaw and eye tumors of Burkitt's lymphoma, but also for the fact that these oddly positioned and exceptionally large tumors react better to cytotoxic drugs than the more centrally placed tumors.

The process envisaged is one which makes it easier to produce one large tumor in an unusual position than to produce several small tumors scattered throughout the RES. When this happens chemotherapy becomes more effective because it is possible for relatively strong concentrations of a cytotoxic drug to build up inside a large encapsulated tumor. One also has the (false) impression that lymphoma is a rare disease in areas of hyperendemic malaria, because in these localities the risk of dying during the latent period is so high; and the (true) impression that African type lymphoma is drifting away from certain areas because as soon as malaria comes under control the unusual type of lymphoma reverts to the common type.

From the point of view of radiation cancers the precise reasons for the clinical and histological differences between African and European lymphomas are not important. What is important is the possibility that indigenous infections have a powerful say, both in the forms that hemopoietic neoplasms take, and in their geographical distributions. For instance, infections which are common in temperate zones might account for the fact that it is possible to classify myeloid and lymphatic leukemias as acute, subacute, or chronic, and to observe a steady increase in the proportion of chronic leukemias with advancing age (Registrar General of England and Wales, 1968). It is also possible that the negative correlation between birth order and leukemia incidence observed by MacMahon and Newill (1962) is related to the fact that infection risks for children who are too young to go to school are positively correlated with birth order (Dykes, 1951) and to the fact that it is only before the age of 5 years that leukemia is exceptionally common in first-born children (Stewart *et al.*, 1958). Finally, the clustering which has been observed in relation to childhood leukemias (Knox, 1964) is obviously too weak to be due to case-to-case transmission of the disease. But this type of space–time interaction could easily be due to epidemics of, say, measles, causing some children with incipient leukemia to have their deaths ascribed to measles, and others having their leukemia diagnosed earlier than usual because they developed measles.

V. Conclusions

For adults, the risk of dying from a malignant disease increases five or six times as fast as one would expect if each increment of age increased the risk by an equal amount (Cook *et al.*, 1969). This so called power-law relationship lies at the root of several multistage theories of cancer causation because one way of explaining an age dependence as steep as this is to assume that malignant tumors are the result of several mutations whose cumulative effects are responsible for the final or invasive stage of the disease. For instance, Fisher and Holloman (1951) showed that the rule would be met if a colony or compact group of six or seven cells was needed to initiate independent tumor growth, and other authors have suggested that somatic mutations or discrete changes may accumulate randomly in the cell line, which eventually becomes neoplastic, and that even the premalignant changes give the affected cells an advantage over neighboring cells (Armitage and Doll, 1957). But unless one is prepared to accept yet another suggestion— namely, that it is not until a controlling gene has accumulated five or six mutations that the behavior of a cell is altered (Burch, 1965), there is no multistage theory which explains why the power-law generalization operates in reverse during childhood. And even if we accept the Burch hypothesis, it is still necessary to explain why the radiogenic cases in the Oxford survey had later onsets than the nonradiogenic cases, and why the power-law relationship applies to all numerically important causes of death (see Fig. 10).

In short, there is a need for a working hypothesis which allows tissue reactions to all pathological processes (including cancer initiations) to be age dependent and also allows the delayed reactions to radiation damage to be tissue selective in some, but not all, circumstances. To satisfy these needs it is tentatively suggested that cancers are the result of somatic mutations whose effects are of little consequence unless the demand for mitotically competent cells is well above average. This is only likely to happen if (a) the event which causes the mutation also has tissue destructive effects; (b) the body has not stopped growing

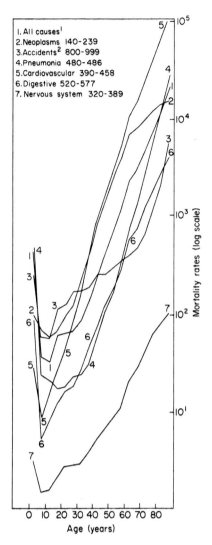

FIG. 10. Age specific mortality from various causes (Registrar General of England and Wales, 1968).
  [1] All causes of deaths on a different scale (10^6) than other causes (10^5).
  [2] Car accidents not included.

before the mutation occurs; and (c) for any reason the number of mitotically competent cells has fallen below the level which is needed to keep the tissue in a steady state.

According to this theory, even if all cancers were caused by something as randomly distributed as background radiation, we should still have cancer mortality rates which varied with age, sex, occupation, climate, social status, eating habits, drinking habits, smoking, etc.

Opposition to the idea that there is a cancer hazard associated with diagnostic radiography was voiced before it was realized how much events which follow fast on the heels of a cancer initiation affect the outcome. Today, there is less difficulty in understanding why small doses of radiation have totally different cancer yields from ones which necessitate widespread tissue repair at a time when any increase in cell production rates not only increases the risk of cancer initiations being followed by tumor formation but also increases the leukemia risk relative to the solid tumor risk.

For instance, the experiences of three groups of individuals (A-bomb survivors, patients with ankylosing spondylitis, and children) have all shown that the delayed effects of radiations are dose dependent. But on one occasion, the tissue destructive effects of the radiations masked the fact that cancer sensitivity (or the risk of a cancer mutation producing a tumor) increases with adult age. On another occasion, tissue destruction failed to mask the effects of age on cancer sensitivity, but made it difficult to detect the general cancer hazard, and on the third occasion, the fact that cell destruction was reduced to a minimum allowed one to see that between birth and conception, cancer sensitivity decreases with age. In short, we are clearly dealing with a threshold situation in relation to whole-body exposure to radiations but instead of a fall to a low level of dose marking a change from a general cancer hazard to a leukemia hazard, a rising dose will sooner or later reach the point where the demand for new cells to replace ones destroyed by the radiations may give mutant stem cells a chance to infiltrate the bone marrow and other sources of myelocytes.

Acknowledgments

The Oxford Survey of Childhood Cancers is supported by grants from the U. S. Public Health Service (Grant No. CA-05392), the Medical Research Council (Grant No. G.964/230/C), and the British Empire Cancer Campaign for Research. The data were collected by a nationwide network of Public Health Departments.

References

Ardran, G. W. (1956). *Brit. J. Radiol.* **26,** 266.
Armitage, D., and Doll, R. (1957). *Brit. J. Cancer* **11,** 161.
Bizzozero, O. J., Johnson, K. G., and Ciocco, A. (1966). *N. Engl. J. Med.* **274,** 1095.
Burch, P. (1965). *Proc. Roy. Soc. Ser. B* **162,** 223–287.
Burkitt, D. (1962). *Postgrad. Med. J.* **38,** 71.
Clayton, C. M., Farne, R. F. T., and Warrick, C. K. (1957). *Brit. J. Radiol.* **30,** 291.

Cook, P., Doll, R., and Fellingham, S. A. (1969). *Int. J. Cancer* **4**, 93.

Court Brown, W. M., and Doll, R. (1957). *Med. Res. Counc. (Gt. Brit.), Spec. Rep. Ser.* **SRS-295**.

Court Brown, W. M., and Doll, R. (1965). *Brit. Med. J.* **ii**, 1327.

Cronkite, E. P. (1965). *In* "Perspectives in Leukemia," p. 158. Grune & Stratton, New York.

Dykes, R. M. (1951). *Proc. Roy. Soc. Med.* **45**, 118.

Fisher, J. C., and Holloman, J. H. (1951). *Cancer* **4**, 916.

Ford, D., Paterson, J. C., and Trueting, W. L. (1959). *J. Nat. Cancer Inst.* **22**, 1093–1104.

Hewitt, D. (1955). *Brit. J. Soc. Med.* **9**, 81.

Hewitt, D., and Stewart, A. M. (1971). *Proc. 1st Intern. Conf. Twins, Rome, 1970 Acta Genet. Med. Gemell.* **19**, 83.

Hewitt, D., Lashof, J. C., and Stewart, A. M. (1966a). *Cancer* **19**, 157.

Hewitt, D., Sanders, B., and Stewart, A. M. (1966b). *Mon. Bull. Min. Health Pub. Health Lab. Serv.* **25**, 80.

International Commission on Radiological Protection. (1969). No. 14. Pergamon Press, Oxford.

Jablon, S., and Kato, H. (1970). *Lancet* **ii**, 1000.

Jablon, S., Ishida, M., and Yamasaki, M. (1965). *Radiat. Res.* **25**, 25.

Kneale, G. (1971a). *Brit. J. Prev. Soc. Med.* (to be published).

Kneale, G. (1971b). *Biometrics* (to be published).

Knox, E. G. (1964). *Brit. J. Prev. Soc. Med.* **18**, 17.

Lockhart-Mummery, J. P. (1934). "The Origin of Cancer."

MacMahon, B. (1962). *J. Nat. Cancer Inst.* **28**, 1173.

MacMahon, B., and Hutchinson, G. (1964). *Acta Uni. Int. Contra Cancrum* **20**, 1172–1174.

MacMahon, B., and Newill, V. A. (1962). *J. Nat. Cancer Inst.* **28**, 231–244.

Medical Research Council. (1956). Command No. 9780.

Medical Research Council. (1960). Command No. 1225.

Miller, R. W. (1969). *Science* **166**, 569.

Muller, H. J. (1927). *Science* **66**, 84.

Pike, M. C., Williams, E. H., and Wright, B. (1967). *Brit. Med. J.* **1**, 395.

Pochin, E. E. (1969). *U.I.C.C. Conf. Thyroid Cancer Ser., 1968* Vol. 12, p. 12.

Registrar General of England and Wales (1968). Statist. Rev. Table 17.

Salaman, M. H. (1958). *Brit. Med. Bull.* **14**, 116.

Sikov, M. R., and Mahlum, D. D., eds. (1969). "Radiation Biology of the Fetal and Juvenile Mammal," pp. 229–391. U. S. At. Energy Comm., Washington, D. C.

Stewart, A. M. (1961). *Brit. Med. J.* **1**, 452.

Stewart, A. M. (1970). *Lancet* **1**, 923.

Stewart, A. M., and Barber, R. (1962). *Pub. Health Rep.* **77**, 129.

Stewart, A. M., and Hewitt, D. (1965). *In* "Current Topics in Radiation Research" (M. Ebert and A. Howard, eds.). North-Holland Publ., Amsterdam.

Stewart, A. M., and Kneale, G. (1968). *Lancet* **1**, 104.

Stewart, A. M., and Kneale, G. (1969). *Nature* **223**, 741.

Stewart, A. M., and Kneale, G. (1970a). *Lancet* **1**, 1185.

Stewart, A. M., and Kneale, G. (1970b). *Lancet* **2**, 4.

Stewart, A. M., Webb, J., and Hewitt, D. (1958). *Brit. Med. J.* **1**, 1495.

Stewart, A. M., Pennybacker, W., and Barber, R. (1962). *Brit. Med. J.* **2**, 882.

Wallace, J., and Dobzhansky, T. (1960). "Radiation, Genes and Man." Methuen, London.

Wanebo, C. K., Johnson, K. G., Sato, K., and Thorslund, T. W. (1968a). *Amer. Rev. Resp. Dis.* **98,** 778.

Wanebo, C. K., Johnson, K. G., Sato, K., and Thorslund, T. W. (1968b). *N. Engl. J. Med.* **279,** 667.

Willis, R. P. (1960). "Pathology of Tumors," 3rd ed., p. 198. London.

Wise, M. (1961). *Brit. Med. J.* **2,** 48.

Woodall, J. P., and Haddow, A. J. (1962). *East Afr. Virus Res. Inst. Rep.* p. 30.

AUTHOR INDEX

Numbers in italics refer to the pages on which the complete references are listed.

H

Katz, M., 139, *159*
Katz, R., 193, *226*
Kavaklieva-Dimitrova, J., 28, *33*
Kawachi, S., 233, 235, 250, 262, 263, *290, 291*
Kawamura, A., 234, 239, 241, 263, *290*
Kawamura, A., Jr., 241, 245, *288, 291*
Kawana, T., 253, 268, *290*
Kaye, A. M., 42, 66, *69, 70*
Keeling, J., 352, *355*
Keighley, G., 186, *227*
Kelemen, E., 190, *227, 229*
Kelly, M., 324, 327, 328, 329, 331, 340, 342, *356*
Kent, R., 43, *70*
Kern, J., 107, 109, 110, *155*
Kesden, D., 5, *36*
Kessel, R. W. I., 14, *32*
Ketcham, A. S., 18, *35*
Keydar, J., 67, *70, 72, 158*
Khasanov, A. I., 297, 320, 321, 336, 343, 347, 348, 351, *354, 356*
Khramkova, N. I., 4, *31*, 296, 301, 302, 318, 324, 327, 328, 340, *354, 356*
Kidwai, J. R., 59, 60, 61, *70*, 113, 114, *158*
Kiernan, J. A., 120, *156*
Kim, C. A., 163, *178*
Kinsky, C. B., 275, *287, 288*
Kinsky, R., 163, 164, *178*
Kinsky, S. C., 275, *287, 288*
Kinugawa, H., 276, *290, 292*
Kirchmyer, R., 187, 198, *225*
Kirschbaum, A., 194, *227*
Kirschstein, R. L., 38, *68*
Kirsh, I., 301, 307, 311, *356*
Kisljak, N. S., 26, *36*
Kit, S., 66, *69, 71*, 80, 86, 107, 108, 109, 111, *155, 156*
Kitahara, T., 66, *69*, 107, 108, 109, 111, *156*
Kithier, K., 296, 299, 301, 302, 304, 314, 327, 333, 350, 351, *356, 357*
Kitzes, J., 308, 310, *356*
Kiviniemi, K., 211, *229*
Klein, E., 10, 29, 30, *33, 34, 36*, 139, *156, 162*, 163, 168, 169, 172, *175, 176, 177, 178*, 246, 247, 257, 269, *288, 290, 291*
Klein, G., 10, 18, 29, *32, 33, 34*, 38, 49, *69, 70*, 117, 139, *156, 158*, 162, 164, 167,

168, *175, 176, 177, 178*, 245, 246, 247, 257, 267, 269, 271, *285, 287, 288, 290, 291*
Klein, J. J., 189, *227*
Klein, P. A., 8, *34*
Kleinschmit, L., 349, 352, *356*
Kleist, S., 353, *356*
Kline, I., *34*
Kluchareva, T. E., 4, *32*
Kneale, G., 361, 369, 370, 372, 378, 383, *389*
Knowles, B. B., 86, 112, *156, 158*
Knox, E. G., 386, *389*
Knyszynski, A., 204, *224*
Kobayashi, H., 8, *34*
Koch, M. A., 38, 54, *67, 69*, 85, 87, *158*
Kodama, T., 8, *34*
Kodovsky, P., 163, *177*
Kohn, J., 333, *356*
Kohne, D. E., 64, *67*
Kojima, K., 263, *288*
Kolar, V., 165, *177*
Koldovsky, P., 163, 164, *175*
Koller, P. C., 189, *225*
Komeiji, T., 276, *292*
Kondi, A., 327, 329, 333, 342, *355*
Kondo, K., 15, *33*
Kooistra, J. B., 168, *178*
Koprowski, H., 38, 44, 60, *69*, 85, 86, 87, 95, 112, 115, 133, *156, 158, 159*
Korenchevsky, V., 194, *229*
Kotal, L., 296, 314, 333, 350, *357*
Koulirsky, R., 237, *288*
Koulirsky, S., 237, *288*
Kout, M., 169, *176*
Koutecky, J., 296, 333, 350, *357*
Kraemer, W. H., 165, *176*
Kraevsky, N. A., 296, 301, 331, 341, *354*
Kramer, P. I., 166, *174*
Krantz, S. B., 186, 214, *227*
Krementz, E. T., 26, *34*
Kresno, S., 335, *356*
Kritchewsky, I. L., 235, *288*
Krizsa, G., 190, *227*
Kröger, H., 167, *177*
Kronman, B. S., 3, *34*, 247, *288*
Kropackova, L., 346, *355*
Krupey, J., 172, *176, 177*, 246, *292*, 353, *358*
Krzymowska, H., 191, *227*

SUBJECT INDEX

A

Adenovirus, cells transformed by, in study of oncogenic viral genomes, 48–49

Alpha-fetoprotein (AFP), 295–358
definition and identification of, 299–302
detection of, 302–304
in hepatocellular cancer, 324–345
in blood, 326–334
factors influencing, 328–345
quantitative aspects, 334–338
site of synthesis, 324–326
immunochemical properties, 300–301
isolation of, 304–305.
in ontogenesis, 307–310
dynamics of, 310–317
site of synthesis, 307–310
physiochemical properties, 300–301, 304–305
synthesis during liver regeneration, 318–323
in teratocarcinoma, 349–352
terminology of, 300–301

Antigen-antibody complement complex, cell receptor for, 234–238

B

BCG, in nonspecific immunotherapy, 4–5
Bordetalla pertussa, in nonspecific immunotherapy, 5
Burkitt lymphoma cells, in study of oncogenic viral genomes, 49

C

Cancer
of endocrine glands, see Endocrine tumors
from low-dose radiation in man, 359–390
cancer latent periods, 375–381
cohort risks, 369–375
infections and leukemia, 383–386

Oxford Survey, 363–386
tissue destructive doses, 381–383
role of antibodies in development of, 162–163
use of active immunotherapy in, 15–18

Cell receptors
as immunological cell markers, 234–245
use in tumor cell characterization, 240–245

Cellular antigen, as immunological markers, 245–249

Chalones, in regulation of hematopoiesis, 190–191

Colony-stimulating factor (CSF)
in preleukemic period, 198–200
in regulation of hematopoiesis, 187–188
role in leukemia, 205–209

Complement and tumor immunology, 231–293
C1 fixation and transfer reaction, 265–272
cell receptors, 234–245
cellular antigen, 245–249
complement fixation test, 272–275
immune adherence, 249–265
immune cytotoxicity, 275–283

Cortisone, in leukemia therapy, 192–193

Corynebacterium parvum, in nonspecific immunotherapy, 5

D

DNA
of oncogenic viruses
coding potential of, 53–55
functions as studied with temperature-sensitive mutants, 77–79
properties of different fractions, 76–79
of SV40 and cell, homology between, 49–52

DNA viruses, transformation by, 95–97, 98–99